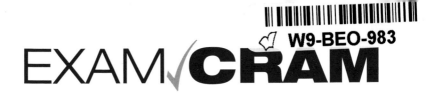

EXAM✓CRAM

The NCLEX-RN® Cram Sheet

This cram sheet contains the distilled, key facts about the licensure exam. Review this information just before you enter the testing center, paying special attention to those areas where you feel you need the most review. You can transfer any of these facts from your head onto a blank sheet provided by the testing center. Good luck.

GENERAL TEST INFORMATION

1. **Minimum 75/maximum 265**—The maximum time allotted for the test is 6 hours. Don't get frustrated if you need to take the entire number of items or take the entire allotted time. Get up and move around and take breaks if you need a time-out.

2. **Take deep breaths and imagine yourself studying in your favorite location**—Take a small item with you that you have had with you during your study time.

3. **Read the question and all answers carefully**—Don't jump to conclusions or make wild guesses.

4. **Look for keywords**—Avoid answers that include *always, never, all, every, only, must, no, except,* or *none.*

5. **Watch for specific details**—Avoid vague answers. Look for adjectives and adverbs.

6. **Eliminate answers that are clearly wrong or incorrect**— Eliminating any incorrect answer increases the probability of selecting the correct answer by 25%.

7. **Look for information given within the question and the answers**—For example, the phrase "client with *diabetic ketoacidosis*" should bring to mind the range of 7.35–7.45 or normal pH.

8. **Look for the same or similar wording in the question and the answers.**

9. **Watch for grammatical inconsistencies**—Subjects and verbs should agree, meaning singular subject, singular verb or plural subject, plural verb. If the question is an incomplete sentence, the correct answer should complete the question in a grammatically correct manner.

10. **Don't read into questions**—Reading into the question can create errors in judgment. If the question asks for an immediate response or prioritization of action, choose the answer that is critical to the life and safety of the client.

11. **Make an educated guess**—If you are unsure after carefully reading the question and all the answers, choose C or the answer with the most information.

12. **Don't hurry, you are not penalized for running out of time.** If you run out of time the computer calculates the last 60 items for consistency above or below the pass-point.

13. **Serum electrolytes**—It is important for you to remember these normal lab values because they might be included in questions throughout the test.
    ▶ Sodium: 135–145 mEq/L
    ▶ Potassium: 3.5–5.5 mEq/L
    ▶ Calcium: 8.5–10.9 mg/L
    ▶ Chloride: 95–105 mEq/L
    ▶ Magnesium: 1.5-2.5 mEq/L
    ▶ Phosphorus: 2.5–4.5 mg/dL

14. **Hematology values**
    ▶ RBC: 4.5–5.0 million/cu mm
    ▶ WBC: 5,000–10,000/cu mm
    ▶ Plt.: 200,000–400,000/cu mm
    ▶ Hgb: 12–16 gms/dL females; 14–18 gms/dL males

15. **ABG values**
    ▶ HCO_3: 24–26 mEq/L
    ▶ CO_2: 35–45 mEq/L
    ▶ PaO_2: 80%–100%
    ▶ SaO_2: > 95%

16. **Chemistry values**
    ▶ Glucose: 70–110 mg/dL
    ▶ Urine specific gravity: 1.010–1.030
    ▶ BUN: 7–22 mg/dL
    ▶ Serum creatinine: 0.6–1.35 mg/dL (< 2 in older adults)

*Information included in laboratory tests may vary slightly according to methods used
    ▶ LDH: 100–190 U/L
    ▶ CPK: 21–232 U/L
    ▶ Uric acid: 3.5–7.5 mg/dL
    ▶ Triglyceride: <150 mg/dL
    ▶ Total cholesterol: 130–200 mg/dL
    ▶ Bilirubin: < 1.0 mg/dL
    ▶ Protein: 6.2–8.1 g/dL
    ▶ Albumin: 3.4–5.0 g/dL

17. **Therapeutic drug levels**
    ▶ Digoxin: 0.5–2.0 ng/ml
    ▶ Lithium: 0.6-1.5 mEq/L
    ▶ Dilantin: 10–20 mcg/dL
    ▶ Aminophylline: 10–20 mcg/dL

18. **Vital signs (adult)**
    ▶ Heart rate: 80–100
    ▶ Respiratory rate: 12–20
    ▶ Blood pressure: 110–120 (systolic); 60–90 (diastolic)
    ▶ Temperature: 98.6° +/–1

19. **Maternity normals**
    ▶ FHR: 120–160 BPM.
    ▶ Variability: 6–10 BPM.
    ▶ Contractions: normal frequency 2–5 minutes apart; normal duration < 90 sec.; intensity < 100 mm/hg.
    ▶ Amniotic fluid: 500–1200 ml (nitrozine urine-litmus paper green/ amniotic fluid-litmus paper blue).
    ▶ Apgar scoring: A = appearance, P = pulses, G = grimace, A = activity, R = reflexes (Done at 1 and 5 minutes with a score of 0 for absent, 1 for decreased, and 2 for strongly positive.)
    ▶ AVA: The umbilical cord has two arteries and one vein. (Arteries carry deoxygenated blood. The vein carries oxygenated blood.)

20. **FAB 9**—Folic acid = B9. Hint: B stands for brain (decreases the incidence of neural tube defects); the client should begin taking B9 three months prior to becoming pregnant.

21. **Abnormalities in the laboring obstetric client**—Decelerations are abnormal findings on the fetal monitoring strip. Decelerations are classified as
    ▶ **Early decelerations**—Begin prior to the peak of the contraction and end by the end of the contraction. They are caused by head compression. There is no need for intervention if the variability is within normal range (that is, there is a rapid return to the baseline fetal heart rate) and the fetal heart rate is within normal range.
    ▶ **Variable decelerations**—Are noted as V-shaped on the monitoring strip. Variable decelerations can occur anytime during monitoring of the fetus. They are caused by cord compression. The intervention is to change the mother's position; if pitocin is infusing, stop the infusion; apply oxygen; and increase the rate of IV fluids. Contact the doctor if the problem persists.

    ▶ **Late decelerations**—Occur after the peak of the contraction and mirror the contraction in length and intensity. These are caused by uteroplacental insuffiency. The intervention is to change the mother's position; if pitocin is infusing, stop the infusion; apply oxygen;, and increase the rate of IV fluids. Contact the doctor if the problem persists.

22. **TORCHS syndrome in the neonate**—This is a combination of diseases. These include toxoplasmosis, rubella (German measles), cytomegalovirus, herpes, and syphyllis. Pregnant nurses should not be assigned to care for the client with toxoplasmosis or cytomegalovirus.

23. **STOP**—This is the treatment for maternal hypotension after an epidural anesthesia:
    1. **Stop** the infusion of pitocin
    2. **Turn** the client to the left side
    3. **Oxygen** administered by tight face mask
    4. **Push** IV fluids for hypotension/hypovolemia

24. **Anticoagulant therapy and monitoring**
    ▶ Coumadin (sodium warfarin) PT
    ▶ Antidote: The antidote for Coumadin is vitamin K.
    ▶ Heparin/Lovenox/Dalteparin PTT
    ▶ Antidote: The antidote for Heparin is protamine sulfate.
    ▶ Therapeutic level: It is important to maintain a bleeding time that is slightly prolonged so that clotting will not occur; therefore, the bleeding time with medication should be 1 1/2–2 times the control.

    *The control is the premedication bleeding time.

25. **Rule of Nines for calculating TBSA for burns**
    ▶ Head = 9%
    ▶ Arms = 18% (9% each)
    ▶ Back (posterior torso) = 18%
    ▶ Chest and abdomen (anterior torso) = 18%
    ▶ Legs = 36% (18% each)
    ▶ Genitalia = 1%

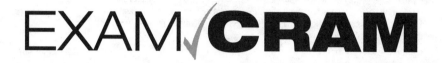

NCLEX-RN®

Practice Questions

Fifth Edition

Wilda Rinehart
Diann Sloan
Clara Hurd

800 East 96th Street, Indianapolis, Indiana 46240 USA

NCLEX-RN® Practice Questions Exam Cram, Fifth Edition

ISBN-13: 978-0-7897-5753-1

ISBN-10: 0-7897-5753-2

Library of Congress Control Number: 2016958162

Printed in the United States of America

1   16

Trademarks

All terms mentioned in this book that are known to be trademarks or service marks have been appropriately capitalized. Pearson cannot attest to the accuracy of this information. Use of a term in this book should not be regarded as affecting the validity of any trademark or service mark.

NCLEX® is a registered trademark of the National Council of State Boards of Nursing, Inc. (NCSBN), which does not sponsor or endorse this product.

Warning and Disclaimer

Every effort has been made to make this book as complete and as accurate as possible, but no warranty or fitness is implied. The information provided is on an "as is" basis. The author and the publisher shall have neither liability nor responsibility to any person or entity with respect to any loss or damages arising from the information contained in this book.

Special Sales

For information about buying this title in bulk quantities, or for special sales opportunities (which may include electronic versions; custom cover designs; and content particular to your business, training goals, marketing focus, or branding interests), please contact our corporate sales department at corpsales@pearsoned.com or (800) 382-3419.

For government sales inquiries, please contact governmentsales@pearsoned.com.

For questions about sales outside the United States, please contact intlcs@pearson.com.

Editor-in-Chief
Mark Taub

Product Line Manager
Brett Bartow

Acquisitions Editor
Michelle Newcomb

Development Editor
Christopher Cleveland

Managing Editor
Sandra Schroeder

Project Editor
Mandie Frank

Copy Editor
Bart Reed

Proofreader
The Wordsmithery LLC

Technical Editor
Steve Picray

Publishing Coordinator
Vanessa Evans

Designer
Chuti Prasertsith

Page Layout
Studio Galou

Contents at a Glance

Table of Contents

About the Authors

Wilda Rinehart Gardner received an Associate Degree in Nursing in 1973 from Northeast Mississippi Community College in Booneville, Mississippi. After working as a staff nurse and charge nurse, she became a public health nurse and served in that capacity for a number of years. In 1975, she received her certification as a family planning nurse practitioner from the midwifery program at the University of Mississippi Medical Center in Jackson, Mississippi. She completed her BSN in 1979 and MSN in 1980 from Mississippi University for Women. She retired after 26 years as nursing instructor at Northeast Mississippi Community College where she taught medical-surgical nursing and maternal newborn nursing. From 1982 to 2012, she operated Rinehart and Associates Nursing Review to assist graduate nurses to pass the National Council of Licensure Exam. She also worked as a curriculum consultant with nursing faculty in the improvement of test construction. Ms. Rinehart has served as a convention speaker in several states in the southeast and has been a reviewer of medical-surgical and obstetric texts.

Dr. Diann Sloan received an Associate Degree in Nursing from Northeast Mississippi Community College, a Bachelor of Science degree in Nursing from the University of Mississippi, and a Master of Science degree in Nursing from Mississippi University for Women. In addition to her nursing degrees, she holds a Master of Science in Counseling Psychology from Georgia State University and a Doctor of Philosophy in Counselor Education, with minors in both Psychology and Educational Psychology, from Mississippi State University. She has completed additional graduate studies in healthcare administration at Western New England College and the University of Mississippi. Dr. Sloan has taught pediatric nursing, psychiatric mental health nursing, and medical surgical nursing in both associate degree and baccalaureate nursing programs. Dr. Sloan has conducted test construction workshops for both RN and PN faculty and is coauthor of the Pearson Online Review.

Clara Hurd received an Associate Degree in Nursing from Northeast Mississippi Community College in Booneville, Mississippi (1975). Her experiences in nursing are clinically based, having served as a staff nurse in medical-surgical nursing. She has worked as an oncology, intensive care, orthopedic, neurological, and pediatric nurse. She received her Bachelor of Science degree in Nursing from the University of North Alabama in Florence, Alabama, and her Master of Science degree in Nursing from the Mississippi University for Women in Columbus, Mississippi. Ms. Hurd is a certified nurse educator. She currently serves as a nurse educator consultant and an independent contractor. Ms. Hurd has taught in both associate degree and baccalaureate degree nursing programs. She was a faculty member of Mississippi University for Women; Austin Peay State University in Clarksville, Tennessee; Tennessee State University in Nashville, Tennessee; and Northeast Mississippi Community College. Ms. Hurd joined Rinehart and Associates in 1993. She has worked with students in preparing for the National Council Licensure Exam and with faculty as a consultant in writing test items. Ms. Hurd has also been a presenter at nursing conventions on various topics, including item-writing for nursing faculty. Her primary professional goal is to prepare the student and graduate for excellence in the delivery of healthcare.

Dedication

We would like to thank our families for tolerating our late nights and long hours. Special thanks to all the graduates who have attended Rinehart and Associates Review Seminars. Thanks for allowing us to be a part of your success.

We are also delighted that Jessica Rinehart Wentz, RN, Whitney Hurd Miller, RN, and Brad Sloan, RN, chose nursing as their profession above so many other professions.

Acknowledgments

Our special thanks to our editors, support staff, and nurse reviewers for helping us to organize our thoughts and experiences into a text for students and practicing professionals. You made the task before us challenging and enjoyable.

We Want to Hear from You!

As the reader of this book, *you* are our most important critic and commentator. We value your opinion and want to know what we're doing right, what we could do better, what areas you'd like to see us publish in, and any other words of wisdom you're willing to pass our way.

We welcome your comments. You can email or write to let us know what you did or didn't like about this book—as well as what we can do to make our books better.

Please note that we cannot help you with technical problems related to the topic of this book.

When you write, please be sure to include this book's title and author as well as your name and email address. We will carefully review your comments and share them with the author and editors who worked on the book.

Email: feedback@pearsonitcertification.com

Mail: Pearson IT Certification
            ATTN: Reader Feedback
            800 East 96th Street
            Indianapolis, IN 46240 USA

Reader Services

Register your copy of *NCLEX-RN Practice Questions Exam Cram* at quepublishing.com for convenient access to downloads, updates, and corrections as they become available. To start the registration process, go to quepublishing.com/register and log in or create an account*. Enter the product ISBN, 9780789757531, and click Submit. Once the process is complete, you will find any available bonus content under Registered Products.

*Be sure to check the box that you would like to hear from us in order to receive exclusive discounts on future editions of this product.

Pearson Test Prep Practice Test Software

As noted previously, this book comes complete with the Pearson Test Prep practice test software containing four full exams (the two from the back of the book as well as two additional tests). These practice tests are available to you either online or as an offline Windows application. To access the practice exams that were developed with this book, please see the instructions in the card inserted in the sleeve in the back of the book. This card includes a unique access code that enables you to activate your exams in the Pearson Test Prep software.

Accessing the Pearson Test Prep Software Online

The online version of this software can be used on any device with a browser and connectivity to the Internet including desktop machines, tablets, and smartphones. To start using your practice exams online, simply follow these steps:

1. Go to: http://www.PearsonTestPrep.com

2. Select **Pearson IT Certification** as your product group

3. Enter your email/password for your account. If you don't have an account on PearsonITCertification.com or CiscoPress.com, you will need to establish one by going to PearsonITCertification.com/join.

4. In the **My Products** tab, click the Activate **New Product** button.

5. Enter the access code printed on the insert card in the back of your book to activate your product.

6. The product will now be listed in your My Products page. Click the **Exams** button to launch the exam settings screen and start your exam.

Accessing the Pearson Test Prep Software Offline

If you wish to study offline, you can download and install the Windows version of the Pearson Test Prep software. There is a download link for this software on the book's companion web site, or you can just enter this link in your browser: http://www.pearsonitcertification.com/content/downloads/pcpt/engine.zip

To access the book's companion web site and the software, simply follow these steps:

1. Register your book by going to: PearsonITCertification.com/register and entering the ISBN: 9780789757531

2. Respond to the challenge questions

3. Go to your account page and select the **Registered Products** tab

4. Click on the **Access Bonus Content** link under the product listing

5. Click the **Install Pearson Test Prep Desktop Version** link under the Practice Exams section of the page to download the software

6. Once the software finishes downloading, unzip all the files on your computer

7. Double click the application file to start the installation, and follow the on-screen instructions to complete the registration.

8. Once the installation is complete, launch the application and select **Activate Exam** button on the My Products tab

9. Click the **Activate a Product** button in the Activate Product Wizard

10. Enter the unique access code found on the card in the sleeve in the back of your book and click the **Activate** button

11. Click **Next** and then the **Finish** button to download the exam data to your application

12. You can now start using the practice exams by selecting the product and clicking the **Open Exam** button to open the exam settings screen

Note that the offline and online versions will synch together, so saved exams and grade results recorded on one version will be available to you on the other as well.

Customizing Your Exams

Once you are in the exam settings screen, you can choose to take exams in one of three modes:

- ▶ Study Mode
- ▶ Practice Exam Mode
- ▶ Flash Card Mode

Study Mode allows you to fully customize your exams and review answers as you are taking the exam. This is typically the mode you would use first to assess your knowledge and identify information gaps. Practice Exam Mode locks certain customization options, as it is presenting a realistic exam experience. Use this mode when you are preparing to test your exam readiness. Flash Card Mode strips out the answers and presents you with only the question stem. This mode is great for late stage preparation when you really want to challenge yourself to provide answers without the benefit of seeing multiple choice options. This mode will not provide the

detailed score reports that the other two modes will, so it should not be used if you are trying to identify knowledge gaps.

In addition to these three modes, you will be able to select the source of your questions. You can choose to take exams that cover all of the chapters or you can narrow your selection to just a single chapter or the chapters that make up specific parts in the book. All chapters are selected by default. If you want to narrow your focus to individual chapters, simply deselect all the chapters then select only those on which you wish to focus in the Objectives area.

You can also select the exam banks on which to focus. Each exam bank comes complete with a full exam of questions that cover topics in every chapter. The two exams printed in the book are available to you as well as two additional exams of unique questions. You can have the test engine serve up exams from all four banks or just from one individual bank by selecting the desired banks in the exam bank area.

There are several other customizations you can make to your exam from the exam settings screen, such as the time of the exam, the number of questions served up, whether to randomize questions and answers, whether to show the number of correct answers for multiple answer questions, or whether to serve up only specific types of questions. You can also create custom test banks by selecting only questions that you have marked or questions on which you have added notes.

Updating Your Exams

If you are using the online version of the Pearson Test Prep software, you should always have access to the latest version of the software as well as the exam data. If you are using the Windows desktop version, every time you launch the software, it will check to see if there are any updates to your exam data and automatically download any changes that were made since the last time you used the software. This requires that you are connected to the Internet at the time you launch the software.

Sometimes, due to many factors, the exam data may not fully download when you activate your exam. If you find that figures or exhibits are missing, you may need to manually update your exams.

To update a particular exam you have already activated and downloaded, simply select the **Tools** tab and select the **Update Products** button. Again, this is only an issue with the desktop Windows application.

If you wish to check for updates to the Pearson Test Prep exam engine software, Windows desktop version, simply select the **Tools** tab and select the **Update Application** button. This will ensure you are running the latest version of the software engine.

Introduction

Welcome to the NCLEX-RN® Practice Questions Exam Cram

This book helps you get ready to take and pass the Licensure Exam for Registered Nurses. This portion of the book discusses the NCLEX-RN® exam in general and how this Exam Cram can help you prepare for the test. It doesn't matter whether this is the first time you're going to take the exam or whether you have taken it previously; this book gives you the necessary information and techniques to obtain licensure.

The *NCLEX-RN® Practice Questions Exam Cram* helps you practice taking questions that are written in the NCLEX® format. Used with the *NCLEX-RN® Exam Cram*, it will help you understand and appreciate the subjects and materials you need to pass. Both books are aimed at test preparation and review. They do not teach you everything you need to know about the subject of nursing. Instead, they present you with materials that you are likely to encounter on the exam. Using a simple approach, we help you understand the "need to know" information.

To be able to pass the NCLEX®, you must understand how the exam is developed. The NCLEX-RN® consists of questions from the cognitive levels of knowledge, comprehension, application, and analysis. The majority of questions are written at the application and analysis level. Questions incorporate the five stages of the Nursing Process (assessment, diagnosis, planning, implementation, and evaluation) and the four categories of Client Needs. Client Needs are divided into subcategories that define the content within each of the four major categories. These categories and subcategories are

A. Safe effective care:
    Management of care: 17%–23%
    Safety and infection control: 7%–15%

B. Health promotion and maintenance: 6%–12%

C. Psychosocial integrity: 6%–12%

D. Physiological integrity:
    Basic care and comfort: 6%–12%
    Pharmacological and parenteral therapy: 12%–18%
    Reduction of risk: 9%–15%
    Physiological adaptation: 11%–17%

Taking the Computerized Adaptive Test

Computer-adaptive testing, commonly known as CAT, offers the candidate several advantages. The graduate can schedule the exam at a time that is convenient for him or her. It's also possible that you will not be tested on the entire 265-question range; if you answer the beginning questions correctly, the CAT might stop early in the session, with far fewer than the 265 questions you were expecting. The first questions will be difficult and should remain difficult. When the exam engine has determined your ability level and is satisfied that you are qualified to be a registered nurse, it will stop. The disadvantage of a CAT is that you cannot go back and change answers. When you choose an answer and move to the next question, that's it—no second guessing like on a paper exam.

The Pearson Vue testing group is responsible for administering the exam. You can locate a Pearson Vue center nearest you by visiting www.pearsonvue.com. Because you might not be familiar with the Pearson Vue testing centers, we recommend that you arrive at least 30 minutes early. If you are late, you will not be allowed to take the test. Bring two forms of identification with you, one of which must be a picture ID. Be sure that your form of identification matches your application. You will be photographed and fingerprinted upon entering the testing site, so don't let this increase your stress. The allotted time is six hours, and the candidate can receive results within approximately seven days (in some states, even sooner). Remember, the exam is written at approximately the tenth-grade reading level, so keep a good dictionary handy during your studies.

The Cost of the Exam

A candidate wanting to write the licensure exam must fill out two applications: one to the National Council State Boards of Nursing and one to the state board of nursing where he or she wants to be licensed. A separate fee must accompany each application. One must be paid to the National Council and one to the state where the candidate wishes to be licensed. State licensing fees vary. Licensure applications can be obtained at www.ncsbn.org. Several states are members of the multistate licensure compact. This means that if you are issued a multistate license, you pay only one fee to practice within the states in the compact. This information also can be obtained by visiting the National Council's website at https://www.ncsbn.org/contact-bon.htm.

How to Prepare for the Exam

Judicious use of this book and its sister books, the *NCLEX-RN® Exam Cram* and *NCLEX® RN Exam Prep* either alone or with a review seminar such as that provided by Rinehart and Associates, will help you achieve your goal of becoming a registered nurse. As you review for the NCLEX® exam, we suggest that you find a location where you can concentrate on the material each day. A minimum of two hours per day for at least two weeks is suggested. In the *NCLEX-RN® Exam Cram* and *NCLEX® RN Exam Prep*, we provide you with exam alerts, tips, notes, and sample questions, both multiple choice and alternative items. Using these books allows you to practice taking hundreds of questions much like those on the actual licensure exam. We have also formulated a "mock" exam with those difficult management and delegation questions that you can score to determine your readiness to test. Pay particular attention to the helpful hints and the Cram Sheet. Using these will help you gain and retain knowledge, and will help reduce your stress as you prepare to test.

What You Will Find in This Book

As seems obvious from the title, this book is all about practice questions! There are five full exams in this book, totaling 1,250 questions. Each chapter is set up with the questions and their possible answers first; the correct answers and rationales appear at the end of each chapter. In the margins next to each question, you will see a quick key to finding the location of its answer and rationales. Here's exactly what you will find in the chapters:

▶ *Practice Questions multiple choice and alternative format*—These are the numerous questions that will help you learn, drill, and review.

▶ *Quick Check Answers*—When you finish answering the questions, you can quickly grade your exam from this section. Only correct answers are given here; no rationales are offered yet. These appear in the Answers and Rationales section.

▶ *Answers and Rationales*—This section offers you the correct answers, as well as further explanation about the content posed in that question. Use this information to learn why an answer is correct and to reinforce the content in your mind for exam day.

You will also find a Cram Sheet at the beginning of this book specifically written for this exam. This is a popular element that is also found in *NCLEX_RN® Exam Cram* (ISBN 978-0-7897-5752-4). This item condenses all the necessary facts found in this exam into one easy-to-handle tearout card. The Cram Sheet is something you can carry with you to the exam location and use as a last-minute study aide. However, be aware that you cannot take it or any other resource into the room where the test is being given.

Hints for Using This Book

We suggest that you score your exam by subtracting the missed items from the total and then dividing the total answered correctly by the total number of questions. This gives you the percentage answered correctly. We also suggest that you achieve a score of at least 77% before you schedule your exam.

If you do not score at least 77%, repeat the exam. The higher the score, the better your chance to do well on the NCLEX® exam!

You should also take advantage of the Pearson Test Prep practice test software; it provides you with a computer-adaptive test, or CAT, very similar to the one you will experience during the NCLEX® exam. Every question in this book is available in the Pearson Test Prep practice test software, including the answers and rationales.

Aside from being a test-preparation book, this book is useful if you are brushing up on your nursing knowledge. It is an excellent quick reference for the licensed nurse.

Need Further Study?

If you are having a hard time correctly answering questions, be sure to see this book's sister books, the *NCLEX®RN Exam Cram* (ISBN: 978-0-7897-5752-4) and the *NCLEX® RN Exam Prep* (ISBN: 978-0-7897-5313-7). If you still need further study, you might want to take an NCLEX® review seminar or look at one of the many other books available at your local bookstore.

Contact the Authors

The authors of this text are interested in you and want you to pass on your first attempt. If, after reviewing with this text, you want to contact the authors, you may do so at Pearson at feedback@pearsonitcertification.com.

CHAPTER ONE

Practice Exam 1 and Rationales

1. A client with a renal failure is prescribed a low potassium diet. Which food choice would be best for this client?

   ○ **A.** 1 cup beef broth

   ○ **B.** 1 baked potato with the skin

   ○ **C.** 1/2 cup raisins

   ● **D.** 1 cup rice

   Quick Answer: **58**
   Detailed Answer: **61**

2. An appropriate nursing intervention for the client with borderline personality disorder is:

   ● **A.** Observing the client for signs of depression or suicidal thinking

   ○ **B.** Allowing the client to lead unit group sessions

   ○ **C.** Restricting the client's activity to the assigned unit of care throughout hospitalization

   ○ **D.** Allowing the client to select a primary caregiver

   Quick Answer: **58**
   Detailed Answer: **61**

3. Which of the following is an expected finding in the assessment of a client with bulimia nervosa?

   ○ **A.** Extreme weight loss

   ○ **B.** Presence of lanugo over body

   ● **C.** Erosion of tooth enamel

   ○ **D.** Muscle wasting

   Quick Answer: **58**
   Detailed Answer: **61**

4. Assuming that all have achieved normal cognitive and emotional development, which of the following children is at greatest risk for accidental poisoning?

   ○ **A.** One-year-old

   ● **B.** Four-year-old

   ○ **C.** Eight-year-old

   ○ **D.** Twelve-year-old

   Quick Answer: **58**
   Detailed Answer: **61**

5. Which term describes the play activity of the preschool aged child?

Quick Answer: **58**
Detailed Answer: **61**

- ○ **A.** Cooperative
- ○ **B.** Associative
- ● **C.** Parallel
- ○ **D.** Solitary

6. The nurse is ready to begin an exam on a nine-month-old infant who is sitting quietly on his mother's lap. Which should the nurse do first?

Quick Answer: **58**
Detailed Answer: **61**

- ○ **A.** Check the Babinski reflex
- ● **B.** Listen to the heart and lung sounds
- ○ **C.** Palpate the abdomen
- ○ **D.** Check tympanic membranes

7. In terms of cognitive development, a three-year-old would be expected to:

Quick Answer: **58**
Detailed Answer: **61**

- ○ **A.** Think abstractly
- ● **B.** Use magical thinking
- ○ **C.** Understand conservation of matter
- ○ **D.** See things from the perspective of others

8. Which of the following describes the language development of a two-year-old?

Quick Answer: **58**
Detailed Answer: **61**

- ○ **A.** Doesn't understand yes and no
- ○ **B.** Understands the meaning of all words
- ● **C.** Can combine three or four words
- ○ **D.** Repeatedly asks "why?"

9. A client who has been receiving Urokinase (uPA) for deep vein thrombosis is noted to have dark brown urine in the urine collection bag. Which action should the nurse take immediately?

Quick Answer: **58**
Detailed Answer: **61**

- ○ **A.** Prepare an injection of vitamin K
- ○ **B.** Irrigate the urinary catheter with 50 mL of normal saline
- ● **C.** Offer the client additional oral fluids
- ○ **D.** Withhold the medication and notify the physician

10. Which of the following can occur with the frequent use of calcium-based antacids?

  ○ **A.** Constipation

  ◉ **B.** Hyperperistalsis

  ○ **C.** Delayed gastric emptying

  ○ **D.** Diarrhea

Quick Answer: **58**
Detailed Answer: **62**

11. Which statement made by the student nurse indicates the need for further teaching regarding the administration of heparin?

  ○ **A.** "I will administer the medication 1–2 inches away from the umbilicus."

  ○ **B.** "I will not massage the injection site after administering the heparin."

  ○ **C.** "I will check the PTT before administering the heparin."

  ◉ **D.** "I will need to gently aspirate when I give the heparin."

Quick Answer: **58**
Detailed Answer: **62**

12. To correctly assess the oxygen saturation level of an adult client, the pulse oximeter should <u>not</u> be placed on the:

  ○ **A.** Finger

  ○ **B.** Earlobe

  ○ **C.** Extremity with noninvasive BP cuff

  ◉ **D.** Nose

Quick Answer: **58**
Detailed Answer: **62**

13. While caring for an elderly patient with hypertension, the nurse notes the following vital signs: BP of 140/40, pulse 120, respirations 36. The nurse's initial action should be to:

  ○ **A.** Report the findings to the physician

  ○ **B.** Recheck the vital signs in one hour

  ◉ **C.** Ask the patient if he is in pain

  ○ **D.** Compare the current vital signs with those on admission

Quick Answer: **58**
Detailed Answer: **62**

14. The nurse is preparing a client with an axillopopliteal bypass graft for discharge. The client should be taught to avoid:

  ○ **A.** Using a recliner to rest

  ○ **B.** Resting in supine position

  ○ **C.** Sitting in a straight chair

  ◉ **D.** Sleeping in right Sim's position

Quick Answer: **58**
Detailed Answer: **62**

15. The doctor has ordered antithrombotic stockings to be applied to the legs of a client with peripheral vascular disease. The nurse knows antithrombotic stockings should be applied:

Quick Answer: **58**
Detailed Answer: **62**

- ○ **A.** Before the client arises in the morning
- ○ **B.** With the client in a standing position
- ◉ **C.** After the client has bathed and applied lotion to the legs
- ○ **D.** Before the client retires in the evening

16. The nurse has just received the change of shift report and is preparing to make rounds. Which client should the nurse assess first?

Quick Answer: **58**
Detailed Answer: **62**

- ○ **A.** A client recovering from a stroke with an oxygen saturation rate of 99%
- ○ **B.** A client three days post-coronary artery bypass graft with an oral temperature of 100.2°F
- ◉ **C.** A client admitted one hour ago with rales and shortness of breath
- ○ **D.** A client being prepared for discharge following a right colectomy

17. A client with a femoral popliteal bypass graft is assigned to a semiprivate room. The most suitable roommate for this client is the client with:

Quick Answer: **58**
Detailed Answer: **62**

- ◉ **A.** Hypothyroidism
- ○ **B.** Diabetic ulcers
- ○ **C.** Gastroenteritis
- ○ **D.** Bacterial pneumonia

18. The nurse is teaching the client regarding use of sodium warfarin. Which statement made by the client would require further teaching?

Quick Answer: **58**
Detailed Answer: **62**

- ○ **A.** "I will have blood drawn every month."
- ○ **B.** "I will assess my skin for a rash."
- ◉ **C.** "I take aspirin for a headache."
- ○ **D.** "I will use an electric razor to shave."

19. The client returns to the recovery room following repair of an abdominal aneurysm. Which finding would require further investigation?

Quick Answer: **58**
Detailed Answer: **63**

- ○ **A.** Pedal pulses regular
- ○ **B.** Urinary output 20mL in the past hour
- ◉ **C.** Blood pressure 108/50
- ○ **D.** Oxygen saturation 97%

20. The nurse is doing bowel and bladder retraining for the client with paraplegia. Which of the following is not a factor for the nurse to consider?

    ○ **A.** Diet pattern

    ○ **B.** Mobility

    ○ **C.** Fluid intake

    ● **D.** Sexual function

Quick Answer: **58**
Detailed Answer: **63**

21. Which one of the following statements is correct when measuring the client for crutches?

    ● **A.** A distance of five fingerbreadths should exist between the top of the crutch and the axilla.

    ○ **B.** The nurse should measure three inches between the top of the crutch and the axilla.

    ○ **C.** The client's elbows should be flexed at a 10° angle.

    ○ **D.** The crutches should be extended 8 to 10 inches from the side of the foot.

Quick Answer: **58**
Detailed Answer: **63**

22. The nurse is caring for a client following a cerebral vascular accident. Which portion of the brain is responsible for changes in the client's vision?

    ○ **A.** Temporal lobe

    ○ **B.** Frontal lobe

    ● **C.** Occipital lobe

    ○ **D.** Parietal lobe

Quick Answer: **58**
Detailed Answer: **63**

23. A client with a hemorrhagic stroke has a temperature of 103°F. Efforts to reduce the temperature have not been effective. The most likely explanation for the elevated temperature is that damage has occurred to the:

    ○ **A.** Hypothalamus

    ○ **B.** Pituitary

    ● **C.** Carotid baroreceptors

    ○ **D.** Frontal lobe

Quick Answer: **58**
Detailed Answer: **63**

24. A client is admitted to the hospital in chronic renal failure. A low protein diet is ordered. The rationale for a low protein diet is that:

Quick Answer: **58**
Detailed Answer: **63**

- ○ **A.** A low protein diet helps reduce blood urea nitrogen and other wastes excreted by the kidneys.
- ○ **B.** A low protein diet increases the sodium and potassium levels.
- ○ **C.** A low protein diet increases albumin production.
- ○ **D.** A low protein diet increases the calcium and phosphorous levels.

25. The nurse has an order for the administration of intravenous heparin. The medication should be administered using a/an:

Quick Answer: **58**
Detailed Answer: **63**

- ○ **A.** Metered chamber
- ○ **B.** Infusion controller
- ○ **C.** Intravenous filter
- ○ **D.** Three-way stopcock

26. When assessing the client's blood pressure, the nurse should use a cuff with a width that is ____% of the circumference of the extremity. (Fill in the blank.)

Quick Answer: **58**
Detailed Answer: **63**

- ○ **A.** 40
- ○ **B.** 30
- ○ **C.** 20
- ○ **D.** 10

27. Which diet would the nurse expect to see ordered for a patient with nephrotic syndrome?

Quick Answer: **58**
Detailed Answer: **63**

- ○ **A.** Low carbohydrate potassium
- ○ **B.** Moderate protein
- ○ **C.** Low calcium
- ○ **D.** Increased potassium

28. A client with an abdominal aortic aneurysm is admitted in preparation for surgery. Which finding should be reported to the doctor?

Quick Answer: **58**
Detailed Answer: **63**

- ○ **A.** A WBC of 14,000 cu.mm
- ○ **B.** Auscultation of abdominal bruit
- ○ **C.** Complaints of lower back pain
- ○ **D.** A platelet count of 175,000 cu.mm

29. When assessing deep tendon reflexes, the nurse grades the client's patellar reflex as a 3+. This reading indicates that the assessed reflex is:

    ○ **A.** Stronger than normal

    ○ **B.** Hypoactive

    ○ **C.** Normal

    ○ **D.** Hyperactive

Quick Answer: **58**
Detailed Answer: **64**

30. The physician has ordered atropine sulfate 0.4milligrams IM before surgery. The medication is supplied in 0.8 milligrams per milliliter. How much medication should the nurse prepare to administer?

    ○ **A.** 0.25mL

    ○ **B.** 0.5mL

    ○ **C.** 1.0mL

    ○ **D.** 1.25mL

Quick Answer: **58**
Detailed Answer: **64**

31. The nurse is evaluating the client's pulmonary artery pressure (PAP). The nurse is aware that PAP evaluates:

    ○ **A.** Pressure in the left ventricle

    ○ **B.** Systolic, diastolic, and mean pressure in the pulmonary artery

    ○ **C.** Pressure in the pulmonary veins

    ○ **D.** Pressure in the right ventricle

Quick Answer: **58**
Detailed Answer: **64**

32. A client is being monitored using a central venous pressure monitor. If the CVP is 1 cm of water, the nurse should:

    ○ **A.** Notify the physician immediately

    ○ **B.** Slow the intravenous infusion

    ○ **C.** Auscultate the lungs for rales

    ○ **D.** Administer a diuretic

Quick Answer: **58**
Detailed Answer: **64**

33. The nurse identifies ventricular tachycardia on the cardiac monitor. The patient has a pulse rate of 160 with a regular rhythm. The nurse should give priority to:

    ○ **A.** Administering atropine sulfate

    ○ **B.** Requesting a stat potassium level

    ○ **C.** Administering amiodarone

    ○ **D.** Defibrillating at 360 joules

Quick Answer: **58**
Detailed Answer: **64**

34. In preparation for the removal of the client's chest tubes, the nurse should instruct the client to:

    ○ **A.** Breathe normally

    ○ **B.** Hold his breath and bear down

    ○ **C.** Take deep breaths

    ○ **D.** Take shallow breaths

Quick Answer: **58**
Detailed Answer: **64**

35. An elderly patient has been taking 80mg of furosemide (Lasix) bid. The nurse notes that the patient's most recent potassium level is 2.5mEq/L. The nurse should:

    ○ **A.** Continue the medication as ordered

    ○ **B.** Administer the morning dose only

    ○ **C.** Give the medication with orange juice

    ○ **D.** Withhold the medication and notify the physician

Quick Answer: **58**
Detailed Answer: **64**

36. Which one of the following lab tests should be done periodically if the client is being maintained on warfarin sodium (Coumadin)?

    ○ **A.** Platelet count

    ○ **B.** White blood cell count

    ○ **C.** Neutrophil count

    ○ **D.** Basophil count

Quick Answer: **58**
Detailed Answer: **64**

37. Which statement is true regarding therapy with Levemir (insulin detemir)?

    ○ **A.** The onset is 1–2 hours.

    ○ **B.** It may be mixed with regular insulin.

    ○ **C.** It peaks in 2–3 hours.

    ○ **D.** The duration is 24 hours.

Quick Answer: **58**
Detailed Answer: **64**

38. A client with AIDS tells the nurse that he has been using herbal supplements in addition to the regimen of drugs prescribed by the physician. The nurse should tell the client that:

    ○ **A.** Most herbals are well suited to use with prescription medications.

    ○ **B.** He should buy only FDA-approved herbal supplements for use.

    ○ **C.** The use of herbals may alter the effect of the medication he is taking.

    ○ **D.** The herbal supplements should be taken at the same time as his medication.

Quick Answer: **58**
Detailed Answer: **64**

39. The nurse is assessing the vital signs of a client with pancreatic cancer. In addition to routine vital signs, the nurse assesses the fifth vital sign of:

Quick Answer: **58**
Detailed Answer: **64**

- ○ **A.** Anorexia
- ○ **B.** Pain
- ○ **C.** Insomnia
- ○ **D.** Fatigue

40. The physician has prescribed Oxycontin (oxycodone) for a client following an exploratory laparotomy. Which of the following is an adverse effect associated with the medication?

Quick Answer: **58**
Detailed Answer: **65**

- ○ **A.** Pulmonary edema
- ○ **B.** Increased blood pressure
- ○ **C.** Nervousness
- ○ **D.** Rapid pulse

41. A patient with a PCA pump (patient controlled analgesia) asks the nurse if he can become overdosed with pain medication using this machine. Which statement made by the nurse is correct?

Quick Answer: **58**
Detailed Answer: **65**

- ○ **A.** "The machine will administer only the amount of medication needed to control pain without any action from you."
- ○ **B.** "The machine has a locking device that prevents over-dosing."
- ○ **C.** "The machine will administer one large dose every four hours to relieve your pain."
- ○ **D.** "The machine is set to deliver medication only if you need it."

42. Which information should be given to the client using a TENS unit?

Quick Answer: **58**
Detailed Answer: **65**

- ○ **A.** "Electrocution may occur if you use water with this unit."
- ○ **B.** "Skin irritation may occur with prolonged use of the unit."
- ○ **C.** "The unit can be placed anywhere on the body without fear of adverse reactions."
- ○ **D.** "A cream or lotion should be applied to the skin before applying the unit."

43. During an intake assessment, the nurse asks the client if he has an advanced directive. The reason for asking the client this question is:

Quick Answer: **58**
Detailed Answer: **65**

- ○ **A.** The nursing staff needs to know about funeral arrangements.
- ○ **B.** Much confusion regarding care can occur with the client's family if there is no advanced directive.
- ○ **C.** An advanced directive allows the medical personnel to make decisions for the client.
- ○ **D.** An advanced directive allows active euthanasia to be carried out.

44. Which measure helps reduce nipple soreness associated with breastfeeding?

Quick Answer: **58**
Detailed Answer: **65**

- ○ **A.** Feeding the baby during the first 48 hours after delivery
- ○ **B.** Placing a finger between the baby's mouth and the breast to break suction after feeding
- ○ **C.** Applying warm, moist soaks to the breast several times per day
- ○ **D.** Wearing a support bra during the day

45. The nurse is performing an assessment on an elderly client who had a total hip repair this morning. Which assessment finding indicates that the patient is in pain?

Quick Answer: **58**
Detailed Answer: **65**

- ○ **A.** The client's blood pressure is 130/86.
- ○ **B.** The client is unable to concentrate.
- ○ **C.** The client's pupils are dilated.
- ○ **D.** The client grimaces during care.

46. An obstetrical client decides to have epidural anesthesia to relieve pain during labor and delivery. Following administration of the epidural anesthesia, the nurse should monitor the client for:

Quick Answer: **58**
Detailed Answer: **65**

- ○ **A.** Seizures
- ○ **B.** Postural hypertension
- ○ **C.** Respiratory depression
- ○ **D.** Hematuria

47. Which of the following is a late sign associated with oral cancer?

Quick Answer: **58**
Detailed Answer: **65**

- ○ **A.** Warmth
- ○ **B.** Odor
- ○ **C.** Pain
- ○ **D.** Ulcer with flat edges

48. Which complaint is frequently expressed by a client with macular degeneration?

Quick Answer: **58**
Detailed Answer: **65**

- ○ **A.** Problems with activities requiring focused vision such as sewing
- ○ **B.** Severe eye and face pain accompanied by nausea and vomiting
- ○ **C.** Seeing halos around lights
- ○ **D.** Veil-like loss of vision

49. Continuous bladder irrigations are ordered for a patient following a TURP. The purpose of continuous bladder irrigations is to:

Quick Answer: **58**
Detailed Answer: **65**

- ○ **A.** Prevent formation of blood clots
- ○ **B.** Administer intravesical medication
- ○ **C.** Prevent postoperative pain
- ○ **D.** Maintain bladder tone

50. The nurse is caring for a patient following a thyroidectomy. Which of the following is an early symptom of hypocalcemia?

Quick Answer: **58**
Detailed Answer: **66**

- ○ **A.** Positive Chvostek's sign
- ○ **B.** 3+ deep tendon reflexes
- ○ **C.** Numbness or tingling of the toes and extremities
- ○ **D.** Prolonged ST and QT intervals

51. The patient states, "My stomach hurts about two hours after I eat." Based upon this information, the nurse suspects the patient likely has a:

Quick Answer: **58**
Detailed Answer: **66**

- ○ **A.** Gastric ulcer
- ○ **B.** Duodenal ulcer
- ○ **C.** Peptic ulcer
- ○ **D.** Curling's ulcer

52. The nurse is caring for a patient with suspected diverticulitis. The nurse would be most prudent in questioning an order for which of the following diagnostic tests?

Quick Answer: **58**
Detailed Answer: **66**

- ○ **A.** Abdominal ultrasound
- ○ **B.** Barium enema
- ○ **C.** Complete blood count
- ○ **D.** Computed tomography (CT) scan

53. The nurse is planning care for the patient with celiac disease. In teaching about the diet, the nurse should instruct the patient to avoid which of the following for breakfast?

    Quick Answer: **58**
    Detailed Answer: **66**

    - ○ **A.** Puffed wheat
    - ○ **B.** Banana
    - ○ **C.** Puffed rice
    - ○ **D.** Cornflakes

54. The nurse is teaching about irritable bowel syndrome (IBS). Which of the following would be most important?

    Quick Answer: **58**
    Detailed Answer: **66**

    - ○ **A.** Reinforcing the need for a balanced diet
    - ○ **B.** Encouraging the client to drink 16 ounces of fluid with each meal
    - ○ **C.** Telling the client to eat a diet low in fiber
    - ○ **D.** Instructing the client to limit his intake of fruits and vegetables

55. In planning care for the patient with ulcerative colitis, the nurse identifies which nursing diagnosis as a priority?

    Quick Answer: **58**
    Detailed Answer: **66**

    - ○ **A.** Anxiety
    - ○ **B.** Impaired skin integrity
    - ○ **C.** Fluid volume deficit
    - ○ **D.** Nutrition altered, less than body requirements

56. The patient is prescribed metronidazole (Flagyl) for adjunct treatment for a duodenal ulcer. When teaching about this medication, the nurse would include:

    Quick Answer: **58**
    Detailed Answer: **66**

    - ○ **A.** "This medication should be taken only until you begin to feel better."
    - ○ **B.** "This medication should be taken on an empty stomach to increase absorption."
    - ○ **C.** "While taking this medication, you do not have to be concerned about being in the sun."
    - ○ **D.** "While taking this medication, alcoholic beverages and products containing alcohol should be avoided."

57. The nurse is preparing to administer a feeding via a nasogastric tube. The nurse would perform which of the following before initiating the feeding?

Quick Answer: **58**
Detailed Answer: **66**

- ○ **A.** Assess for tube placement by aspirating stomach content.

- ○ **B.** Place the patient in a left-lying position.

- ○ **C.** Administer feeding with 50% Dextrose.

- ○ **D.** Ensure that the feeding solution has been warmed in a microwave for two minutes.

58. Which is true regarding the administration of antacids?

Quick Answer: **58**
Detailed Answer: **66**

- ○ **A.** Antacids should be administered without regard to mealtimes.

- ○ **B.** Antacids should be administered with each meal and snack of the day.

- ○ **C.** Antacids should not be administered with other medications.

- ○ **D.** Antacids should be administered with all other medications, for maximal absorption.

59. The nurse is caring for a patient with a colostomy. The patient asks, "Will I ever be able to swim again?" The nurse's best response would be:

Quick Answer: **58**
Detailed Answer: **66**

- ○ **A.** "Yes, you should be able to swim again, even with the colostomy."

- ○ **B.** "You should avoid immersing the colostomy in water."

- ○ **C.** "No, you should avoid getting the colostomy wet."

- ○ **D.** "Don't worry about that. You will be able to live just like you did before."

60. The nurse is assisting in the care of a patient who is two days post-operative from a hemorrhoidectomy. The nurse would be correct in instructing the patient to:

Quick Answer: **58**
Detailed Answer: **66**

- ○ **A.** Avoid a high-fiber diet

- ○ **B.** Continue to apply ice packs

- ○ **C.** Take a laxative daily to prevent constipation

- ○ **D.** Use a sitz bath after each bowel movement

61. The nurse is caring for a client with a recent laparoscopic hemi-colectomy. Which finding should be reported to the physician?

   ○ **A.** Sluggish bowel sounds

   ○ **B.** Pain and tenderness at the umbilicus

   ○ **C.** Passage of small amount of liquid stool

   ○ **D.** Increasing abdominal girth

Quick Answer: **58**
Detailed Answer: **67**

62. A client is newly diagnosed with diabetes. Which nursing diagnosis is a priority at this time?

   ○ **A.** Fluid volume deficit

   ○ **B.** Anxiety

   ○ **C.** Deficient knowledge

   ○ **D.** Activity intolerance

Quick Answer: **58**
Detailed Answer: **67**

63. Which action by the home health nurse indicates a knowledge of the needs of an elderly client?

   ○ **A.** Teaching regarding availability and services offered by hospice care

   ○ **B.** Speaking in a higher pitched voice tone to facilitate hearing

   ○ **C.** Encouraging fluid restriction to prevent nighttime voiding

   ○ **D.** Reinforcing teaching regarding the prevention of falls

Quick Answer: **58**
Detailed Answer: **67**

64. The nurse asks a patient about current medications. Which one of the patient's medications is most likely to cause abdominal pain?

   ○ **A.** Norco (hydrocodone/APAP)

   ○ **B.** Erythrocin (erythromycin)

   ○ **C.** Zyrtec (cetirizine)

   ○ **D.** Aldactone (spironolactone)

Quick Answer: **58**
Detailed Answer: **67**

65. The nurse is assessing the abdomen. The nurse knows the best sequence to perform the assessment is:

   ○ **A.** Inspection, auscultation, palpation

   ○ **B.** Auscultation, palpation, inspection

   ○ **C.** Palpation, inspection, auscultation

   ○ **D.** Inspection, palpation, auscultation

Quick Answer: **58**
Detailed Answer: **67**

66. The nurse is caring for the client who has been in a coma for two months. He has signed a donor card, but the wife is opposed to the idea of organ donation. How should the nurse handle the topic of organ donation with the wife?

- ○ **A.** Tell the wife that the hospital will honor her wishes regarding organ donation, but contact the organ-retrieval staff.
- ○ **B.** Tell her that because her husband signed a donor card, the hospital has the right to take the organs upon the death of her husband.
- ○ **C.** Explain that it is necessary for her to donate her husband's organs because he signed the permit.
- ○ **D.** Refrain from talking about the subject until after the death of her husband.

67. The client with cancer refuses to care for herself. Which action by the nurse would be best?

- ○ **A.** Alternate nurses caring for the client so that the staff will not get tired of caring for this client.
- ○ **B.** Talk to the client and explain the need for self-care.
- ○ **C.** Explore the reason for the lack of motivation seen in the client.
- ○ **D.** Talk to the physician about the client's lack of motivation.

68. The charge nurse is making assignments for the day. After accepting the assignment to care for a client with leukemia, the nurse tells the charge nurse that her child has chickenpox. Which initial action should the charge nurse take?

- ○ **A.** Change the nurse's assignment to another client.
- ○ **B.** Explain to the nurse that there is no risk to the client.
- ○ **C.** Ask the nurse if the chickenpox have crusted.
- ○ **D.** Ask the nurse if she has ever had the chickenpox.

69. The nurse is caring for the client with a mastectomy. Which action would be contraindicated?

- ○ **A.** Taking the blood pressure on the side of the mastectomy
- ○ **B.** Elevating the arm on the side of the mastectomy
- ○ **C.** Positioning the client on the unaffected side
- ○ **D.** Performing a fingerstick on the unaffected side

70. The client has an order for Garamycin (gentamicin) to be administered. Which lab test should be done before beginning the medication?

  ○ **A.** Hematocrit

  ○ **B.** Serum creatinine

  ○ **C.** White cell count

  ○ **D.** BUN

Quick Answer: **58**
Detailed Answer: **67**

71. Which of the following is the best indicator of the diagnosis of HIV?

  ○ **A.** WBC

  ○ **B.** ELISA

  ○ **C.** Western blot

  ○ **D.** CBC

Quick Answer: **58**
Detailed Answer: **68**

72. The client presents to the emergency room with a "bull's eye" rash, headache, and arthralgia. Which question would be most appropriate for the nurse to ask the client?

  ○ **A.** "Have you found any ticks on your body?"

  ○ **B.** "Have you had any diarrhea in the last 24 hours?"

  ○ **C.** "Have you been outside the country in the last six months?"

  ○ **D.** "Have you had any itching for the past few days?"

Quick Answer: **58**
Detailed Answer: **68**

73. Which client should be assigned to the nursing assistant?

  ○ **A.** The 18-year-old with a fracture to two cervical vertebrae

  ○ **B.** The infant with meningitis with a temperature of 101°F

  ○ **C.** The elderly client with a thyroidectomy four days ago

  ○ **D.** The client with a thoracotomy two days ago

Quick Answer: **58**
Detailed Answer: **68**

74. The client presents to the emergency room with a hyphema. Which action by the nurse would be appropriate?

  ○ **A.** Elevate the head of the bed and apply ice to the eye.

  ○ **B.** Place the client in a supine position and apply heat to the knee.

  ○ **C.** Insert a Foley catheter and measure the intake and output.

  ○ **D.** Perform a vaginal exam and check for a discharge.

Quick Answer: **58**
Detailed Answer: **68**

75. The client has an order for Feosol(ferrous sulfate). To promote absorption, the nurse should administer the medication with:

- ○ **A.** Milk
- ○ **B.** A meal
- ○ **C.** Orange juice
- ○ **D.** Undiluted

Quick Answer: **58**
Detailed Answer: **68**

76. A client with an ileostomy is being discharged. Which teaching should be included in the plan of care?

- ○ **A.** Using Karaya powder to seal the bag
- ○ **B.** Irrigating the ileostomy daily
- ○ **C.** Using Stomahesive as a skin protector
- ○ **D.** Using a stool softener as needed

Quick Answer: **58**
Detailed Answer: **68**

77. Why is Phytonadione(vitamin K) administered to a newborn shortly after birth?

- ○ **A.** To stop hemorrhage
- ○ **B.** To treat infection
- ○ **C.** To replace electrolytes
- ○ **D.** To facilitate clotting

Quick Answer: **58**
Detailed Answer: **68**

78. A client is admitted to the postpartal unit with a large amount of lochia rubra, uterine enlargement, and excessive clots. Which medication will likely be ordered for the client?

- ○ **A.** Fentanyl (sublimaze)
- ○ **B.** Stadol (butorphanol)
- ○ **C.** Prepidil (dinoprostone)
- ○ **D.** Hemabate (carboprost tromethamine)

Quick Answer: **58**
Detailed Answer: **68**

79. Before administering intravenous chemotherapy to the patient being treated, the nurse should:

- ○ **A.** Administer a bolus of IV fluid
- ○ **B.** Administer pain medication
- ○ **C.** Administer an antiemetic
- ○ **D.** Allow the patient a chance to eat

Quick Answer: **58**
Detailed Answer: **68**

80. The client is admitted to the postpartum unit with an order to continue the infusion of Pitocin (oxytocin). The nurse is aware that
Pitocin is working if the fundus is:

- ○ **A.** Deviated to the left
- ○ **B.** Firm and in the midline
- ○ **C.** Boggy
- ○ **D.** Two finger breadths below the umbilicus

81. A patient is diagnosed with secondary syphilis. The nurse can
expect the patient to have:

- ○ **A.** "Copper penny" rash on the palms of the hands and
soles of the feet
- ○ **B.** Localized tumors in the skin, bones, and liver
- ○ **C.** Chancres and lymphadenopathy
- ○ **D.** General paresis

82. A four-year-old with cystic fibrosis has a prescription for Creon
(pancrelipase). The medication is given to:

- ○ **A.** Thin respiratory secretions
- ○ **B.** Promote clotting
- ○ **C.** Assist with digestion
- ○ **D.** Shrink nasal polyps

83. The physician has prescribed Zyvox (linezolid) for a patient with
VRE. The concurrent use of which medication may result in
serotonin syndrome?

- ○ **A.** Nexium (esomeprazole)
- ○ **B.** Zoloft (sertraline)
- ○ **C.** Lipitor (atorvastatin)
- ○ **D.** Zyrtec (cetirizine)

84. A new diabetic is learning to administer his insulin. He receives
10 units of NPH insulin and 12 units of regular insulin each morning. Which of the following statements reflects understanding of
the nurse's teaching?

- ○ **A.** "When drawing up my insulin, I should draw up the
regular insulin first."
- ○ **B.** "When drawing up my insulin, I should draw up the
NPH insulin first."
- ○ **C.** "It doesn't matter which insulin I draw up first."
- ○ **D.** "I cannot mix the two insulins, so I will need two
injections."

85. A client is scheduled to have a cardiac CTA with contrast. Before the procedure, the nurse should assess the patient for:

    ○ **A.** Allergies to shellfish or iodine allergies

    ○ **B.** The ability to lie prone for 30 minutes

    ○ **C.** A history of reaction to nitrates

    ○ **D.** The presence of body tattoos

Quick Answer: **58**
Detailed Answer: **69**

86. Which medication does the nurse expect to be ordered for the postpartal patient with bleeding uncontrolled by Pitocin (oxytocin)?

    ○ **A.** Methergine (methylergonovine maleate)

    ○ **B.** Aquamephyton (phytonadione)

    ○ **C.** Amicar (aminocaproic acid)

    ○ **D.** Celestone (betamethasone)

Quick Answer: **58**
Detailed Answer: **69**

87. The client with a recent liver transplant asks the nurse how long he will have to take an immunosuppressant. Which response is correct?

    ○ **A.** One year

    ○ **B.** Five years

    ○ **C.** 10 years

    ○ **D.** Life

Quick Answer: **58**
Detailed Answer: **69**

88. A client admitted to the emergency room with multiple injuries develops Cullen's sign. The nurse is aware that the client has sustained damage to the:

    ○ **A.** Frontal lobe

    ○ **B.** Lungs

    ○ **C.** Abdominal organs

    ○ **D.** Spinal cord

Quick Answer: **58**
Detailed Answer: **69**

89. The physician prescribes regular insulin, five units subcutaneous. Regular insulin begins to exert an effect:

    ○ **A.** Within 5–10 minutes

    ○ **B.** Within 10–20 minutes

    ○ **C.** Within 30–60 minutes

    ○ **D.** Within 60–90 minutes

Quick Answer: **58**
Detailed Answer: **69**

90. A 60-year-old diabetic is taking glyburide (Diabeta) 1.25mg daily to treat Type II diabetes mellitus. Which statement indicates the need for further teaching?

Quick Answer: **58**
Detailed Answer: **69**

- ○ **A.** "I will keep candy with me just in case my blood sugar drops."
- ○ **B.** "I need to stay out of the sun as much as possible."
- ○ **C.** "I often skip dinner because I don't feel hungry."
- ○ **D.** "I always wear my medical identification."

91. A 20-year-old female has a prescription for Sumycin (tetracycline). While teaching the client how to take her medicine, the nurse learns that the client is also taking an oral contraceptive. Which instruction should be included in the teaching plan?

Quick Answer: **58**
Detailed Answer: **69**

- ○ **A.** Oral contraceptives will decrease the effectiveness of the tetracycline.
- ○ **B.** Anorexia often results from taking oral contraceptives with antibiotics.
- ○ **C.** Toxicity can result when taking these antibiotics and an oral contraceptive together.
- ○ **D.** Antibiotics can decrease the effectiveness of oral contraceptives.

92. A client is taking Deltasone(prednisone) each morning to treat his systemic lupus erythematosus. Which statement best explains the reason for taking the prednisone in the morning?

Quick Answer: **58**
Detailed Answer: **69**

- ○ **A.** There is less chance of forgetting the medication if taken in the morning.
- ○ **B.** There will be less fluid retention if taken in the morning.
- ○ **C.** The medication is absorbed best with the breakfast meal.
- ○ **D.** Morning administration mimics the body's natural secretion of corticosteroid.

93. A client is taking Rifadin(rifampin) 600mg PO daily for pulmonary tuberculosis. The nurse should tell the client to:

Quick Answer: **58**
Detailed Answer: **69**

- ○ **A.** Take the medication with juice
- ○ **B.** Expect red discoloration of the urine
- ○ **C.** Take the medication before going to bed at night
- ○ **D.** Take the medication only if night sweats occur

94. The client is diagnosed with multiple myeloma. The doctor has ordered cyclophosphamide (Cytoxan). Which instruction should be given to the client?

○ **A.** "Walk about a mile a day to prevent calcium loss."

○ **B.** "Increase the fiber in your diet."

○ **C.** "Report nausea to the doctor immediately."

○ **D.** "Drink at least eight large glasses of water a day."

95. A client with ovarian cancer is receiving fluorouracil (Adrucil) IV. What should the nurse do if she notices crystals in the IV medication?

○ **A.** Discard the solution and order a new bag.

○ **B.** Warm the solution.

○ **C.** Continue the infusion and document the finding.

○ **D.** Discontinue the medication.

96. Before administering Theo-Dur (theophylline), the nurse should check the patient's:

○ **A.** Urinary output

○ **B.** Blood pressure

○ **C.** Pulse

○ **D.** Temperature

97. Which information obtained from the mother of a child with cerebral palsy correlates to the diagnosis?

○ **A.** She was born at 40 weeks gestation.

○ **B.** She had meningitis when she was six months old.

○ **C.** She had physiologic jaundice after delivery.

○ **D.** She has frequent sore throats.

98. Which finding is expected in an 18-month-old with normal growth and development?

○ **A.** She dresses herself.

○ **B.** She pulls a toy behind her.

○ **C.** She can build a tower of eight blocks.

○ **D.** She can copy a horizontal or vertical line.

99. A five-year-old is admitted to the unit following a tonsillectomy. Which of the following would indicate a complication of the surgery?

Quick Answer: **58**
Detailed Answer: **70**

- ○ **A.** Decreased appetite
- ○ **B.** A low-grade fever
- ○ **C.** Chest congestion
- ○ **D.** Constant swallowing

100. The child with seizure disorder is being treated with phenytoin (Dilantin). Which of the following statements by the patient's mother indicates to the nurse that the patient is experiencing a side effect of Dilantin therapy?

Quick Answer: **58**
Detailed Answer: **70**

- ○ **A.** "She is very irritable lately."
- ○ **B.** "She sleeps quite a bit of the time."
- ○ **C.** "Her gums look too big for her teeth."
- ○ **D.** "She has gained about 10 pounds in the last six months."

101. The physician has prescribed tranylcypromine sulfate (Parnate) 10mg bid. The nurse should teach the client to refrain from eating foods containing tyramine because it may cause:

Quick Answer: **59**
Detailed Answer: **70**

- ○ **A.** Hypertension
- ○ **B.** Hyperthermia
- ○ **C.** Hypotension
- ○ **D.** Urinary retention

102. The client is admitted to the emergency room with shortness of breath, anxiety, and tachycardia. His ECG reveals atrial fibrillation with a ventricular response rate of 130 beats per minute. The doctor orders quinidine sulfate. While he is receiving quinidine, the nurse should monitor his ECG for:

Quick Answer: **59**
Detailed Answer: **70**

- ○ **A.** Peaked P wave
- ○ **B.** Elevated ST segment
- ○ **C.** Inverted T wave
- ○ **D.** Prolonged QT interval

103. Lidocaine is a medication frequently ordered for the client experiencing:

Quick Answer: **59**
Detailed Answer: **70**

- ○ **A.** Atrial tachycardia
- ○ **B.** Ventricular tachycardia
- ○ **C.** Heart block
- ○ **D.** Ventricular bradycardia

104. The doctor orders 2% nitroglycerin ointment in a 1-inch dose every 12 hours. Proper application of nitroglycerin ointment includes:

- ○ **A.** Rotating application sites
- ○ **B.** Limiting applications to the chest
- ○ **C.** Rubbing it into the skin
- ○ **D.** Covering it with a gauze dressing

105. The physician prescribes captopril (Capoten) 25mg PO bid for the client with hypertension. Which of the following adverse reactions can occur with administration of Capoten?

- ○ **A.** Tinnitus
- ○ **B.** Persistent cough
- ○ **C.** Muscle weakness
- ○ **D.** Diarrhea

106. The client is admitted with a BP of 210/100. Her doctor orders furosemide (Lasix) 40mg IV stat. How should the nurse administer the prescribed furosemide to this client?

- ○ **A.** By giving it over 1–2 minutes
- ○ **B.** By hanging it IV piggyback
- ○ **C.** With normal saline only
- ○ **D.** With a filter

107. The client is receiving heparin for thrombophlebitis of the left lower extremity. Which of the following drugs reverses the effects of heparin?

- ○ **A.** Cyanocobalamine
- ○ **B.** Protamine sulfate
- ○ **C.** Streptokinase
- ○ **D.** Sodium warfarin

108. The nurse is making assignments for the day. Which client should be assigned to the pregnant nurse?

- ○ **A.** The client receiving linear accelerator radiation therapy for lung cancer
- ○ **B.** The client with a radium implant for cervical cancer
- ○ **C.** The client who has just been administered soluble brachytherapy for thyroid cancer
- ○ **D.** The client who returned from placement of iridium seeds for prostate cancer

109. The nurse is planning room assignments for the day. Which client should be assigned to a private room if only one is available?

Quick Answer: **59**
Detailed Answer: **71**

- ○ **A.** The client with Cushing's disease
- ○ **B.** The client with diabetes
- ○ **C.** The client with acromegaly
- ○ **D.** The client with myxedema

110. The charge nurse witnesses the nursing assistant hitting an elderly client in the long-term care facility. The nursing assistant can be charged with:

Quick Answer: **59**
Detailed Answer: **71**

- ○ **A.** Negligence
- ○ **B.** Tort
- ○ **C.** Assault
- ○ **D.** Malpractice

111. Which assignment should not be delegated to the licensed practical nurse?

Quick Answer: **59**
Detailed Answer: **71**

- ○ **A.** Inserting a Foley catheter
- ○ **B.** Discontinuing a nasogastric tube
- ○ **C.** Obtaining a sputum specimen
- ○ **D.** Starting a blood transfusion

112. The client returns to the unit from surgery with a blood pressure of 90/50, pulse 132, respirations 30. Which action by the nurse should receive priority?

Quick Answer: **59**
Detailed Answer: **71**

- ○ **A.** Continue to monitor the vital signs
- ○ **B.** Contact the physician
- ○ **C.** Ask the client how he feels
- ○ **D.** Ask the LPN to continue the post-op care

113. The nurse is caring for a client with ß-thalassemia major. Which therapy is used to treat ß-thalassemia major?

Quick Answer: **59**
Detailed Answer: **71**

- ○ **A.** IV fluids
- ○ **B.** Frequent blood transfusions
- ○ **C.** Oxygen therapy
- ○ **D.** Iron therapy

114. Which medication is often used to treat the client with *N.gonorrhea?*

Quick Answer: **59**
Detailed Answer: **71**

- ○ **A.** Sitavig (acyclovir)
- ○ **B.** Vibramycin (doxycycline)
- ○ **C.** Retrovir (zidovudine)
- ○ **D.** Aldara (imiquimod)

115. Which of the following symptoms is associated with *Chlamydia?*

Quick Answer: **59**
Detailed Answer: **72**

- ○ **A.** Frequent urination and vaginal discharge
- ○ **B.** Generalized rash
- ○ **C.** Lesions on the perineum
- ○ **D.** Enlarged lymph nodes and pelvic pain

116. The physician has ordered an alkaline ash diet for a patient with recurrent cysteine kidney stones. Which of the following should be included in the patient's diet?

Quick Answer: **59**
Detailed Answer: **72**

- ○ **A.** Cranberries
- ○ **B.** Grapes
- ○ **C.** Plums
- ○ **D.** Rhubarb

117. The nurse is aware that a common mode of transmission of *clostridium difficile* is:

Quick Answer: **59**
Detailed Answer: **72**

- ○ **A.** Use of unsterile surgical equipment
- ○ **B.** Contamination of objects with sputum
- ○ **C.** Through urinary catheterization
- ○ **D.** Contamination of objects with stool

118. The nurse has just received the change of shift report. Which client should the nurse assess first?

Quick Answer: **59**
Detailed Answer: **72**

- ○ **A.** A client two hours post-lobectomy with 150mL of chest drainage
- ○ **B.** A client two days post-gastrectomy with scant drainage
- ○ **C.** A client with pneumonia with an oral temperature of 102°F
- ○ **D.** A client with a fractured hip in Buck's traction

119. The nurse is removing a peripherally inserted central catheter (PICC). The nurse should position the patient in which position?

Quick Answer: **59**
Detailed Answer: **72**

- ○ **A.** Fowlers
- ○ **B.** Right side lying
- ○ **C.** Left side lying
- ○ **D.** Trendelenburg

120. The nurse is providing discharge teaching for a client taking naltrexone (Revia). The nurse should instruct the client to avoid which over-the-counter medication:

Quick Answer: **59**
Detailed Answer: **72**

- ○ **A.** Acetaminophen
- ○ **B.** Ibuprofen
- ○ **C.** Cold medicine
- ○ **D.** Antihistamines

121. A 70-year-old male who is recovering from a stroke exhibits signs of unilateral neglect. Which behavior is suggestive of unilateral neglect?

Quick Answer: **59**
Detailed Answer: **72**

- ○ **A.** The client is observed shaving only one side of his face.
- ○ **B.** The client is unable to distinguish between two tactile stimuli presented simultaneously.
- ○ **C.** The client is unable to complete a range of vision without turning his head side to side.
- ○ **D.** The client is unable to carry out cognitive and motor activity at the same time.

122. An elderly client refuses to take her daily medication for hypertension. Which action should the nurse take at this time?

Quick Answer: **59**
Detailed Answer: **72**

- ○ **A.** Administer the medication by injection
- ○ **B.** Obtain help administering the medication
- ○ **C.** Skip the dose of medication and attempt to give it later
- ○ **D.** Explore the reason for the client's refusal to take the medication

123. A nurse indicates that she is licensed in her new state of residence even though reciprocity has not been granted. The nurse's action can result in a charge of:

Quick Answer: **59**
Detailed Answer: **72**

- ○ **A.** Fraud
- ○ **B.** Tort
- ○ **C.** Malpractice
- ○ **D.** Negligence

124. The nurse is assigning staff for the day. Which client should be assigned to the nursing assistant?

- ○ **A.** A five-month-old with bronchiolitis
- ○ **B.** A 10-year-old who is two-day post-appendectomy
- ○ **C.** A two-year-old with periorbital cellulitis
- ○ **D.** A one-year-old with a fractured tibia

125. During a change of shift, the oncoming nurse notes a discrepancy in the narcotic count. The nurse's first action should be to:

- ○ **A.** Notify the hospital pharmacist
- ○ **B.** Notify the nursing supervisor
- ○ **C.** Notify the board of nursing
- ○ **D.** Notify the director of nursing

126. Due to a high census, it has been necessary for a number of clients to be transferred to other units within the hospital. Which client should be transferred to the postpartum unit?

- ○ **A.** A 66-year-old female with gastroenteritis
- ○ **B.** A 40-year-old female with a hysterectomy
- ○ **C.** A 27-year-old male with severe depression
- ○ **D.** A 28-year-old male with ulcerative colitis

127. A client with glomerulonephritis is placed on a low-sodium diet. Which of the following snacks is suitable for the client with sodium restriction?

- ○ **A.** Peanut butter cookies
- ○ **B.** Grilled cheese sandwich
- ○ **C.** Cottage cheese and fruit
- ○ **D.** Fresh peach

128. A home health nurse is making preparations for morning visits. Which one of the following clients should the nurse visit first?

- ○ **A.** A client with a stroke with tube feedings
- ○ **B.** A client with a history of congestive heart failure complaining of nighttime dyspnea
- ○ **C.** A client with a thoracotomy six months ago
- ○ **D.** A client with Parkinson's disease

129. The nurse can help alleviate the discomfort the client is experiencing associated with xerostomia by:

- ○ **A.** Limiting fluid intake
- ○ **B.** Administering an analgesic
- ○ **C.** Splinting swollen joints
- ○ **D.** Providing sugarless hard candy

130. The nurse is making assignments for the day. The staff consists of an RN, an LPN, and a nursing assistant. Which client could the nursing assistant care for?

- ○ **A.** A client with Alzheimer's disease
- ○ **B.** A client with pneumonia
- ○ **C.** A client with cirrhosis
- ○ **D.** A client with thrombophlebitis

131. The nurse is caring for a client with cerebral palsy. The nurse should provide frequent rest periods because:

- ○ **A.** Grimacing and writhing movements decrease with relaxation and rest.
- ○ **B.** Hypoactive deep tendon reflexes become more active with rest.
- ○ **C.** Stretch reflexes are increased with rest.
- ○ **D.** Fine motor movements are improved by rest.

132. The physician has ordered a culture for a male patient suspected of having *N.gonorrhea*. Which information should the nurse give the patient?

- ○ **A.** "It will be necessary to obtain a sample of blood for an antibody screen."
- ○ **B.** "We will need to obtain a swab of nasopharyngeal secretions."
- ○ **C.** "A morning sample of urine will be needed."
- ○ **D.** "Emptying the bladder one hour before the test may affect results."

133. Which of the following post-operative diets is appropriate for the client who has had a hemorrhoidectomy?

- ○ **A.** High fiber
- ○ **B.** Lactose free
- ○ **C.** Bland
- ○ **D.** Clear liquid

134. The client delivered a nine-pound infant two days ago. An effective means of managing discomfort from an episiotomy is:

Quick Answer: 59
Detailed Answer: 73

  ○ **A.** Medicated suppository

  ○ **B.** Taking a warm shower

  ○ **C.** Sitz baths

  ○ **D.** Ice packs

135. The nurse is assessing a client recently returned from surgery. The best way to determine the client's need for pain medication is to:

Quick Answer: 59
Detailed Answer: 73

  ○ **A.** Watch for changes in the client's vital signs

  ○ **B.** Ask the client to rate his pain on a scale of 0–10

  ○ **C.** Observe the client's facial expression during dressing changes

  ○ **D.** Wait for the client to request medication for pain relief

136. The client is admitted with chronic obstructive pulmonary disease. Blood gases reveal pH 7.36, CO_2 45, O_2 84, bicarb 28. The nurse would assess the client to be in:

Quick Answer: 59
Detailed Answer: 73

  ○ **A.** Uncompensated acidosis

  ○ **B.** Compensated alkalosis

  ○ **C.** Compensated respiratory acidosis

  ○ **D.** Uncompensated metabolic acidosis

137. A client with schizophrenia has become disruptive and requires seclusion to help him regain control of his behavior. Which staff member can institute seclusion?

Quick Answer: 59
Detailed Answer: 74

  ○ **A.** The security guard

  ○ **B.** The registered nurse

  ○ **C.** The licensed practical nurse

  ○ **D.** The nursing assistant

138. The physician has ordered Coumadin (sodium warfarin) for a client with thrombophlebitis. The order should be entered to administer the medication at:

Quick Answer: 59
Detailed Answer: 74

  ○ **A.** 0900

  ○ **B.** 1200

  ○ **C.** 1700

  ○ **D.** 2100

139. A 25-year-old male is brought to the emergency room with a metal fragment in his eye. The first action the nurse should take is:

- ○ **A.** Use a magnet to remove the metal fragment.
- ○ **B.** Rinse the eye thoroughly with sterile saline.
- ○ **C.** Cover both eyes with a cupped object.
- ○ **D.** Place a patch over the affected eye.

Quick Answer: **59**
Detailed Answer: **74**

140. To ensure safety while administering a nitroglycerine patch, the nurse should:

- ○ **A.** Wear gloves while applying the patch.
- ○ **B.** Shave the area where the patch will be applied.
- ○ **C.** Wash the area thoroughly with soap and rinse with hot water.
- ○ **D.** Apply the patch to the buttocks.

Quick Answer: **59**
Detailed Answer: **74**

141. A client with ascites is scheduled for a paracentesis. Which instruction should be given to the client before the procedure?

- ○ **A.** "You will need to lay flat during the procedure."
- ○ **B.** "You need to empty your bladder before the procedure."
- ○ **C.** "You will be asleep during the procedure."
- ○ **D.** "The doctor will inject a medication during the procedure."

Quick Answer: **59**
Detailed Answer: **74**

142. A client with symptoms of myasthenia gravis is scheduled for a Tensilon (edrophoniun) test. Which medication should be kept available during the test?

- ○ **A.** Atropine sulfate
- ○ **B.** Lasix (furosemide)
- ○ **C.** Prostigmine (neostigmine)
- ○ **D.** Phenergan (promethazine)

Quick Answer: **59**
Detailed Answer: **74**

143. The first exercise that should be performed by the client who had a mastectomy one day earlier is:

- ○ **A.** Walking the hand up the wall
- ○ **B.** Sweeping the floor
- ○ **C.** Combing her hair
- ○ **D.** Squeezing a ball

Quick Answer: **59**
Detailed Answer: **74**

144. Which woman is not a candidate for RhoGAM?

Quick Answer: **59**
Detailed Answer: **74**

- ○ **A.** A gravida 4 para 3 that is Rh negative with an Rh-positive baby

- ○ **B.** A gravida 1 para 1 that is Rh negative with an Rh-positive baby

- ○ **C.** A gravida 2 para 0 that is Rh negative admitted after a stillbirth delivery

- ○ **D.** A gravida 4 para 2 that is Rh negative with an Rh-negative baby

145. Which laboratory test is not included in making the diagnosis of myocardial infarction?

Quick Answer: **59**
Detailed Answer: **74**

- ○ **A.** AST

- ○ **B.** Troponin

- ○ **C.** CK-MB

- ○ **D.** Myoglobin

146. The client with a myocardial infarction comes to the nurse's station stating that he is ready to go home because there is nothing wrong with him. Which defense mechanism is the client using?

Quick Answer: **59**
Detailed Answer: **74**

- ○ **A.** Rationalization

- ○ **B.** Denial

- ○ **C.** Projection

- ○ **D.** Conversion reaction

147. The client is receiving total parenteral nutrition (TPN). Which lab test should be evaluated while the client is receiving TPN?

Quick Answer: **59**
Detailed Answer: **74**

- ○ **A.** Hemoglobin

- ○ **B.** Creatinine

- ○ **C.** Blood glucose

- ○ **D.** White cell count

148. The client with diabetes is preparing for discharge. During discharge teaching, the nurse assesses the client's ability to care for himself. Which statement made by the client would indicate a need for follow-up after discharge?

Quick Answer: **59**
Detailed Answer: **75**

- ○ **A.** "I live by myself."

- ○ **B.** "I have trouble seeing."

- ○ **C.** "I have a cat in the house with me."

- ○ **D.** "I usually drive myself to the doctor."

149. A client with cirrhosis is receiving Cephulac (lactulose). The nurse is aware that Cephulac is given to lower:

- ○ **A.** Blood glucose
- ○ **B.** Uric acid
- ○ **C.** Ammonia
- ○ **D.** Creatinine

Quick Answer: **59**
Detailed Answer: **75**

150. A client is receiving peritoneal dialysis. If the dialysate returns are cloudy, the nurse should:

- ○ **A.** Tell the client that this is a normal occurrence
- ○ **B.** Ask the client about fever or abdominal pain
- ○ **C.** Tell the client that the dialysate should be shaken before use
- ○ **D.** Ask the client how she has been warming the dialysate

Quick Answer: **59**
Detailed Answer: **75**

151. The nurse employed in the emergency room is responsible for triage of four clients injured in a motor vehicle accident. Which of the following clients should receive priority in care?

- ○ **A.** A 10-year-old with lacerations of the face
- ○ **B.** A 15-year-old with sternal bruises
- ○ **C.** A 34-year-old with a fractured femur
- ○ **D.** A 50-year-old with dislocation of the elbow

Quick Answer: **59**
Detailed Answer: **75**

152. Which roommate would be most suitable for a client newly diagnosed with myasthenia gravis?

- ○ **A.** A client with diabetes
- ○ **B.** A client with exacerbation of ulcerative colitis
- ○ **C.** A client with a venous stasis ulcer
- ○ **D.** A client with bronchitis

Quick Answer: **59**
Detailed Answer: **75**

153. Which observation indicates that a student nurse needs further teaching in the proper way to assess central venous pressure?

- ○ **A.** The student places the client in a supine position to read the manometer.
- ○ **B.** The student places the zero reading of the monometer at the phlebostatic axis.
- ○ **C.** The student instructs the client to perform the Valsalva maneuver during the CVP reading.
- ○ **D.** The student records the CVP reading as the level noted at the top of the meniscus.

Quick Answer: **59**
Detailed Answer: **75**

154. The nurse is working with another nurse and a patient care assistant. Which of the following clients should be assigned to the registered nurse?

- ○ **A.** A client two days post-appendectomy
- ○ **B.** A client one week post-thyroidectomy
- ○ **C.** A client three days post-splenectomy
- ○ **D.** A client two days post-thoracotomy

155. The physician has ordered Prostin E2 (dinoprostone) gel to induce labor. After inserting the gel, which action should the nurse take?

- ○ **A.** Raise the head of the bed
- ○ **B.** Apply nasal oxygen at 2L/min
- ○ **C.** Help the client to the bathroom
- ○ **D.** Elevate the client's hips for 30 minutes

156. The nurse is preparing a client for mammography. To prepare the client for a mammogram, the nurse should tell the client:

- ○ **A.** To restrict her fat intake for one week before the test
- ○ **B.** To omit creams, powders, or deodorants before the exam
- ○ **C.** That mammography replaces the need for self-breast exams
- ○ **D.** That mammography requires a higher dose of radiation than x-rays

157. Which action by the novice nurse indicates a need for further teaching?

- ○ **A.** The nurse fails to wear gloves consistently when removing a dressing.
- ○ **B.** The nurse applies an oxygen saturation monitor to the ear lobe.
- ○ **C.** The nurse elevates the head of the bed to check the blood pressure.
- ○ **D.** The nurse places the arm in a dependent position to perform a fingerstick.

158. The physician has ordered the Schilling test for a patient with suspected pernicious anemia. What other vitamin level is often assessed at the same time as the B12 level?

Quick Answer: **59**
Detailed Answer: **76**

- ○ **A.** Folic acid
- ○ **B.** Pyridoxine
- ○ **C.** Ascorbic acid
- ○ **D.** Thiamine

159. The nurse is assigned to care for a newborn with physiologic jaundice. Which action by the nurse would facilitate elimination of the bilirubin?

Quick Answer: **59**
Detailed Answer: **76**

- ○ **A.** Offering the newborn water between formula feedings
- ○ **B.** Maintaining the newborn's temperature at 98.6°F
- ○ **C.** Minimizing tactile stimulation
- ○ **D.** Decreasing caloric intake

160. A home health nurse is planning for her daily visits. Which client should the home health nurse visit first?

Quick Answer: **59**
Detailed Answer: **76**

- ○ **A.** A client with AIDS being treated with Foscavir (foscarnet)
- ○ **B.** A client with a fractured femur in a long leg cast
- ○ **C.** A client with a recent laryngectomy for laryngeal cancer
- ○ **D.** A client with diabetic ulcers to the left foot

161. The charge nurse overhears the patient care assistant speaking harshly to the client with dementia. The charge nurse should:

Quick Answer: **59**
Detailed Answer: **76**

- ○ **A.** Change the nursing assistant's assignment
- ○ **B.** Explore the interaction with the nursing assistant
- ○ **C.** Discuss the matter with the client's family
- ○ **D.** Initiate a group session with the nursing assistant

162. The nurse discovers a patient care assistant looking through the client's belongings while the client is out of the room. Which action should be taken by the nurse?

Quick Answer: **59**
Detailed Answer: **76**

- ○ **A.** Discuss the nursing assistant's behavior with the family.
- ○ **B.** Report the incident to the charge nurse.
- ○ **C.** Monitor the situation and note whether any items are missing.
- ○ **D.** Ignore the situation until items are reported missing.

163. Which client is best assigned to a newly licensed nurse?

- ○ **A.** A client receiving chemotherapy
- ○ **B.** A clientpostcoronary artery bypass graft
- ○ **C.** A client with a transurethral prostatectomy
- ○ **D.** A client with diverticulosis

Quick Answer: **59**
Detailed Answer: **76**

164. A patient with acute lymphocytic leukemia is receiving intrathecal chemotherapy. Intrathecal chemotherapy is used to:

- ○ **A.** Increase the number circulating neutrophils
- ○ **B.** Prevent systemic effects common to most chemotherapeutic agents
- ○ **C.** Increase the number of mature white blood cells
- ○ **D.** Destroy leukemic cells hiding in the cerebrospinal fluid

Quick Answer: **59**
Detailed Answer: **76**

165. The client is admitted after an abdominal cholecystectomy. Montgomery straps are utilized with this client. The nurse is aware that Montgomery straps are utilized on this client because:

- ○ **A.** The client is at risk for evisceration.
- ○ **B.** The client will require frequent dressing changes.
- ○ **C.** The straps provide support for drains that are inserted into the incision.
- ○ **D.** No sutures or clips are used to secure the incision.

Quick Answer: **59**
Detailed Answer: **76**

166. Which order would the nurse anticipate for a client hospitalized with acute pancreatitis?

- ○ **A.** Vital signs once per shift
- ○ **B.** Insertion of a nasogastric tube
- ○ **C.** Patient controlled analgesia with Demerol (meperidine)
- ○ **D.** Low-fat diet as tolerated

Quick Answer: **59**
Detailed Answer: **76**

167. The nurse is caring for a client with a diagnosis of cirrhosis who is experiencing pruritis. Which of the following is an appropriate nursing intervention?

- ○ **A.** Suggesting that the client take warm showers twice daily
- ○ **B.** Applying a lotion containing menthol or camphor to the skin after bathing
- ○ **C.** Applying powder to the client's skin
- ○ **D.** Placing warm compresses on the affected areas

Quick Answer: **59**
Detailed Answer: **77**

168. Which of the following would be most appropriate for the nurse to wear when providing direct care to a client with influenza?

- ○ **A.** Mask
- ○ **B.** Gown
- ○ **C.** Gloves
- ○ **D.** Goggles

169. A client is brought to the mental health clinic by her sister after the death of their father. Which statement made by the client's sister suggests the client may have abnormal grieving?

- ○ **A.** "My sister still has episodes of crying, and it's been three months since Daddy died."
- ○ **B.** "My sister seems to have forgotten a lot of the bad things that Daddy did in his lifetime."
- ○ **C.** "My sister has really had a hard time after Daddy's funeral."
- ○ **D.** "My sister doesn't seem sad at all and acts like nothing has happened."

170. The nurse is obtaining a history on an 80-year-old client. Which statement made by the client might indicate a potential for fluid and electrolyte imbalance?

- ○ **A.** "My skin is always so dry, especially in the winter."
- ○ **B.** "I have to use laxatives two or three times a week."
- ○ **C.** "I drink three or four glasses of ice tea during the day."
- ○ **D.** "I sometimes have a problem with dribbling urine."

171. A client is admitted to the acute care unit. Initial laboratory values reveal serum sodium of 170 mEq/L. What behavior changes would be most common for this client?

- ○ **A.** Anger
- ○ **B.** Mania
- ○ **C.** Depression
- ○ **D.** Psychosis

172. The nurse is assessing a client with symptoms of hyperphos-phatemia. Which of the following is most likely related to the client's symptoms?

    ○ **A.** Radiation to the neck

    ○ **B.** Recent orthopedic surgery

    ○ **C.** Minimal physical activity

    ○ **D.** Adherence to a vegan diet

Quick Answer: **59**
Detailed Answer: **77**

173. The nurse is assessing the chart of a client scheduled for surgery in the morning and finds that the consent form has been signed, but the client is unclear about the surgery and possible complica-tions. Which is the most appropriate action?

    ○ **A.** Call the physician and ask him or her to clarify the information with the client.

    ○ **B.** Explain the procedure and complications to the client.

    ○ **C.** Check in the physician's progress notes to see if client understanding has been documented.

    ○ **D.** Talk with the client's family to determine if they under-stand the procedure fully.

Quick Answer: **59**
Detailed Answer: **77**

174. The nurse is preparing a client for surgery who requests to "go as he is." Which item is most important for the nurse to remove before sending the client to surgery?

    ○ **A.** Hearing aid

    ○ **B.** Contact lenses

    ○ **C.** Wedding ring

    ○ **D.** Dentures

Quick Answer: **59**
Detailed Answer: **77**

175. A client is two days post-operative bowel resection. After a cough-ing episode, the client's wound eviscerates. Which nursing action is appropriate?

    ○ **A.** Reinserting the protruding bowel and covering the site with sterile 4×4s

    ○ **B.** Covering the site with a sterile abdominal dressing

    ○ **C.** Covering the site with a sterile saline-soaked dressing

    ○ **D.** Applying an abdominal binder and manual pressure to the site

Quick Answer: **59**
Detailed Answer: **77**

176. A client with cervical cancer is staged as Tis. A staging of Tis indicates that:

    ○ **A.** The cancer stage cannot be assessed.

    ○ **B.** The cancer is localized to the primary site.

    ○ **C.** The cancer shows increasing lymph node involvement.

    ○ **D.** The cancer is accompanied by distant metastasis.

Quick Answer: **59**
Detailed Answer: **77**

177. A client with suspected renal cancer is to be scheduled for an intravenous pyelogram. Before the IVP, the nurse should:

Quick Answer: **59**
Detailed Answer: **78**

- ○ **A.** Offer additional fluids
- ○ **B.** Ask the client to empty his bladder
- ○ **C.** Withhold the client's medication for 8 hours before the IVP
- ○ **D.** Administer pain medication

178. A 25-year-old client arrives in the emergency room with a possible fracture of the right femur. The nurse should anticipate an order for:

Quick Answer: **59**
Detailed Answer: **78**

- ○ **A.** Bryant's traction
- ○ **B.** Ice to the entire extremity
- ○ **C.** Buck's traction
- ○ **D.** An abduction pillow

179. The nurse is performing an assessment on a client with possible pernicious anemia. Which finding is specific to pernicious anemia?

Quick Answer: **59**
Detailed Answer: **78**

- ○ **A.** A weight loss of 10 pounds in six months
- ○ **B.** Fatigue
- ○ **C.** Glossitis
- ○ **D.** Pallor

180. Which statement should be included in the teaching session of a client scheduled for a renal biopsy?

Quick Answer: **59**
Detailed Answer: **78**

- ○ **A.** "You will be placed in a sitting position for the biopsy."
- ○ **B.** "You may experience a feeling of pressure or discomfort during aspiration of the biopsy."
- ○ **C.** "You will be asleep during the procedure."
- ○ **D.** "You will not be able to drink fluids for 24 hours following the study."

181. The nurse is caring for a client scheduled for repair of an abdominal aortic aneurysm. Which pre-op assessment is most important?

Quick Answer: **59**
Detailed Answer: **78**

- ○ **A.** Level of anxiety
- ○ **B.** Exercise tolerance
- ○ **C.** Quality of peripheral pulses
- ○ **D.** Bowel sounds

182. The dysrhythmia most commonly seen during tracheal suctioning is:

- ○ **A.** Bradycardia
- ○ **B.** Tachycardia
- ○ **C.** Premature ventricular beats
- ○ **D.** Heart block

183. The nurse is performing discharge teaching for a client with an implanted defibrillator. What discharge instruction is essential?

- ○ **A.** "You cannot prepare food in a microwave."
- ○ **B.** "You should avoid shoulder movement on the side of the defibrillator for six weeks."
- ○ **C.** "You should use your cell phone on your right side."
- ○ **D.** "You won't be able to fly on a commercial airliner with an implanted defibrillator."

184. Six hours after birth, the newborn is found to have swelling over the right parietal area that does not cross the suture line. The nurse should chart this finding as:

- ○ **A.** Cephalohematoma
- ○ **B.** Molding
- ○ **C.** Subdural hematoma
- ○ **D.** Caput succedaneum

185. A left-lower lobectomy is performed on a client with lung cancer. The nurse should expect postoperative care to include:

- ○ **A.** A closed chest drainage system
- ○ **B.** Bed rest for 48 hours
- ○ **C.** Positioning supine or right-side lying
- ○ **D.** Chest physiotherapy

186. The nurse is caring for a client with laryngeal cancer. Which finding is not associated with laryngeal cancer?

- ○ **A.** Halitosis
- ○ **B.** Dysphagia
- ○ **C.** *H. pylori* infection
- ○ **D.** Chronic hiccups

187. A mother asks why her newborn has lost weight since his birth one week ago. The best explanation of weight loss in the newborn is:

Quick Answer: **59**
Detailed Answer: **79**

- ○ **A.** The newborn is dehydrated.
- ○ **B.** The newborn is hypoglycemic.
- ○ **C.** The newborn is not used to the formula.
- ○ **D.** The newborn loses weigh because of the passage of meconium stools and loss of fluid.

188. The nurse is performing discharge teaching on a client with diverticulitis who has been placed on a low-roughage diet. Which food would have to be eliminated from this client's diet?

Quick Answer: **59**
Detailed Answer: **79**

- ○ **A.** Roasted chicken
- ○ **B.** Noodles
- ○ **C.** Cooked broccoli
- ○ **D.** Custard

189. The physician has ordered Betoptic (betaxolol) ophthalmic suspension for a patient with open angle glaucoma. Which statement is true regarding the medication?

Quick Answer: **59**
Detailed Answer: **79**

- ○ **A.** Optic suspensions of Betoptic have no systemic side effects.
- ○ **B.** Betoptic is safe for use by patients who have a history of congestive heart failure.
- ○ **C.** Betoptic decreases the effects of insulin.
- ○ **D.** Betoptic may cause dizziness or vertigo.

190. The nurse is assisting a client with diverticulosis to select appropriate foods. Which food should be avoided?

Quick Answer: **59**
Detailed Answer: **79**

- ○ **A.** Bran flakes
- ○ **B.** Peaches
- ○ **C.** Cucumber and tomato salad
- ○ **D.** Whole wheat bread

191. An 18-month-old is admitted with symptoms of intussusception. Which information is helpful in establishing the diagnosis?

Quick Answer: **59**
Detailed Answer: **79**

- ○ **A.** When he last ate
- ○ **B.** The characteristic of vomitus
- ○ **C.** A description of his stools
- ○ **D.** The number of times voided in the last eight hours

192. The nurse is caring for a client with epilepsy who is being treated with carbamazepine (Tegretol). Which laboratory value indicates an adverse effect of the medication?

○　**A.** Uric acid of 5mg/dL

○　**B.** Hematocrit of 33%

○　**C.** WBC 2000 per cubic millimeter

○　**D.** Platelets 150,000 per cubic millimeter

193. A client is admitted with a Ewing's sarcoma. Which symptom would be expected due to this tumor's location?

○　**A.** Hemiplegia

○　**B.** Aphasia

○　**C.** Loss of balance

○　**D.** Bone pain

194. The mother asks the nurse when the "soft spot" on the top of her baby's head will close. The nurse should tell the mother that the anterior fontanel usually closes by:

○　**A.** Three months

○　**B.** Six months

○　**C.** Twelve months

○　**D.** Eighteen months

195. The nurse is making initial rounds on a client with a C5 fracture stabilized by Crutchfield tongs. Which equipment should be kept at the bedside?

○　**A.** Forceps

○　**B.** Torque wrench

○　**C.** Wire cutters

○　**D.** Screwdriver

196. A client with osteoporosis has a new prescription for alendronate (Fosamax). Which instruction should be given to the client?

○　**A.** Rest in bed after taking the medication for at least 30 minutes.

○　**B.** Avoid rapid movements after taking the medication.

○　**C.** Take the medication with water only.

○　**D.** Allow at least one hour between taking the medicine and taking other medications.

197. The nurse is working in the emergency room when a client arrives with severe burns of the face and neck. Which action should receive priority?

Quick Answer: **59**
Detailed Answer: **79**

- ○ **A.** Starting an IV of Ringer's lactate
- ○ **B.** Assessing the airway and applying oxygen
- ○ **C.** Obtaining blood gases
- ○ **D.** Administering pain medication

198. A client is scheduled for surgery in the morning. Which of the following is the primary preoperative responsibility of the nurse?

Quick Answer: **59**
Detailed Answer: **79**

- ○ **A.** Making sure the vital signs are recorded
- ○ **B.** Obtaining a signed permit for surgery
- ○ **C.** Explaining the surgical procedure
- ○ **D.** Answering questions about the surgery

199. A client's lab values reveal Hgb 12.6, WBC 6500cu.mm, K+ 1.9, uric acid 7.0, Na+ 136, and platelets 178,000cu.mm. The nurse evaluates that the client is experiencing which of the following?

Quick Answer: **59**
Detailed Answer: **80**

- ○ **A.** Hypernatremia
- ○ **B.** Hypokalemia
- ○ **C.** Myelosuppression
- ○ **D.** Leukopenia

200. Which of the following is the best indication of resolution of a paralytic ileus?

Quick Answer: **59**
Detailed Answer: **80**

- ○ **A.** Passage of stool
- ○ **B.** Eructation
- ○ **C.** Presence of bowel sounds
- ○ **D.** Decreasing abdominal girth

201. Which finding is expected in a client with a ruptured spleen?

Quick Answer: **59**
Detailed Answer: **80**

- ○ **A.** Kehr's sign
- ○ **B.** Chvostek's sign
- ○ **C.** Kernig's sign
- ○ **D.** Trendelenburg's sign

202. The nurse is caring for a client with chronic hepatitis. Which is the best method to use for determining the degree of early ascites?

Quick Answer: **59**
Detailed Answer: **80**

   ○ **A.** Inspection of the abdomen for enlargement

   ○ **B.** Bimanual palpation for hepatomegaly

   ○ **C.** Daily measurement of abdominal girth

   ○ **D.** Assessment for peritoneal fluid wave

203. The client arrives in the emergency department after a motor vehicle accident. Nursing assessment findings include BP 68/34, pulse rate 130, and respirations 18. Which is the client's most appropriate priority nursing diagnosis?

Quick Answer: **59**
Detailed Answer: **80**

   ○ **A.** Alteration in cerebral tissue perfusion

   ○ **B.** Fluid volume deficit

   ○ **C.** Ineffective airway clearance

   ○ **D.** Alteration in sensory perception

204. Which of the following assessment findings raises concern for a child with sickle cell anemia?

Quick Answer: **59**
Detailed Answer: **80**

   ○ **A.** He enjoys playing baseball with the school team.

   ○ **B.** He drinks several carbonated drinks per day.

   ○ **C.** He requires eight to ten hours sleep a night.

   ○ **D.** He occasionally uses ibuprofen to control minor pain.

205. The nurse on an oncology unit is caring for a client with neutropenia. During evening visitation, a visitor brings a potted plant to the room. What action should the nurse take?

Quick Answer: **59**
Detailed Answer: **80**

   ○ **A.** Allow the client to keep the plant.

   ○ **B.** Place the plant by the window.

   ○ **C.** Water the plant for the client.

   ○ **D.** Ask the family to take the plant home.

206. The nurse is caring for a postoperative patient when suddenly the patient becomes less responsive and pale, with a BP of 70/40. The nurse's initial action should be to:

Quick Answer: **59**
Detailed Answer: **80**

   ○ **A.** Increase the rate of IV fluids

   ○ **B.** Lower the head of the bed

   ○ **C.** Notify the physician

   ○ **D.** Obtain a crash cart

207. Which of the following newborns is at greatest risk for iron deficiency anemia?

Quick Answer: **59**
Detailed Answer: **80**

   ○ **A.** A newborn who is fed infant formula

   ○ **B.** A newborn delivered at 32 weeks gestation

   ○ **C.** A newborn who is one of a set of quadruplets

   ○ **D.** A newborn who is breastfed

208. A client being treated with Coumadin (sodium warfarin) has an INR of 8.0. Which intervention is appropriate based on the INR level?

Quick Answer: **59**
Detailed Answer: **80**

   ○ **A.** Assessing for signs of bleeding

   ○ **B.** Administering intranasal DDAVP

   ○ **C.** Administering an injection of protamine sulfate

   ○ **D.** Limiting the intake of foods rich in vitamin K

209. Which snack selection by a client with osteoporosis indicates that the client understands the dietary management of the disease?

Quick Answer: **60**
Detailed Answer: **80**

   ○ **A.** A granola bar

   ○ **B.** A bran muffin

   ○ **C.** Yogurt

   ○ **D.** Raisins

210. A client with preeclampsia is admitted with an order for intravenous magnesium sulfate. Which statement is true regarding the administration of magnesium sulfate?

Quick Answer: **60**
Detailed Answer: **81**

   ○ **A.** A 4 gram loading dose is administered over 20–30 minutes via infusion pump.

   ○ **B.** Side effects include feeling cold and tremulous.

   ○ **C.** IV infusion rate is adjusted to maintain urine output of 20 to 30 mL per hour.

   ○ **D.** The brachial reflex is checked prior to initiation of medication.

211. The nurse is caring for a 12-year-old who requires a blood transfusion for life-threatening injuries sustained in an automobile accident. The child's mother refuses to sign the blood permit based on her religious beliefs. What nursing action is appropriate?

○ **A.** Administer the blood transfusion without a signed permit.

○ **B.** Encourage the mother to reconsider her decision.

○ **C.** Explain the consequences if he does not receive a transfusion.

○ **D.** Notify the physician of the mother's refusal to sign the permit.

Quick Answer: **60**
Detailed Answer: **81**

212. A client is admitted with partial thickness burns to the neck, face, and anterior trunk. The nurse would be most concerned about the client developing which of the following?

○ **A.** Hypovolemia

○ **B.** Laryngeal edema

○ **C.** Hypernatremia

○ **D.** Oliguria

Quick Answer: **60**
Detailed Answer: **81**

213. The nurse is evaluating nutritional outcomes for an adolescent with anorexia nervosa. Which observation best indicates that the plan of care is effective?

○ **A.** The client selects a balanced diet from the menu.

○ **B.** The client is less interested in intense exercise.

○ **C.** The client reads magazine articles on food preparation.

○ **D.** The client has gained four pounds in the last week.

Quick Answer: **60**
Detailed Answer: **81**

214. A client is admitted following the repair of a fractured tibia with cast application. Which nursing assessment should be reported to the physician?

○ **A.** Pain beneath the cast

○ **B.** Warm toes

○ **C.** Pedal pulses weak and rapid

○ **D.** Paresthesia of the toes

Quick Answer: **60**
Detailed Answer: **81**

215. The client is having a cardiac catheterization. During the procedure, the client tells the nurse, "I'm feeling really hot." What is the correct explanation for the client's statement?

Quick Answer: **60**
Detailed Answer: **81**

- ○ **A.** He is having an allergic reaction to the contrast media.
- ○ **B.** A feeling of warmth is normal when the contrast media is injected.
- ○ **C.** "The feeling of warmth" indicates that the clots in the coronary vessels are dissolving.
- ○ **D.** He has increased anxiety due to the invasive procedure.

216. A school nurse is explaining the dangers of anabolic steroid use to a group of high school athletes. Which organ is adversely affected by the use of anabolic steroids?

Quick Answer: **60**
Detailed Answer: **81**

- ○ **A.** Kidney
- ○ **B.** Stomach
- ○ **C.** Pancreas
- ○ **D.** Liver

217. A client is having electroconvulsive therapy for treatment of severe depression. Which of the findings is expected during electroconvulsive therapy?

Quick Answer: **60**
Detailed Answer: **81**

- ○ **A.** Loss of consciousness
- ○ **B.** Nausea and vomiting
- ○ **C.** Bradycardia
- ○ **D.** Tonic clonic seizure

218. Which information should be given to the patient undergoing radiation therapy for breast cancer?

Quick Answer: **60**
Detailed Answer: **81**

- ○ **A.** Avoid exposing radiation areas to sunlight during treatment time and for a year after completion of therapy
- ○ **B.** Moisturize the radiation site with oil-based lotion to prevent blistering
- ○ **C.** Use bath oil when tub bathing to prevent drying and peeling
- ○ **D.** Report redness and soreness of the area to the physician

219. The physician has prescribed Vermox (mebendazole) for a child with pinworms. Which statement is true regarding the medication?

Quick Answer: **60**
Detailed Answer: **81**

- ○ **A.** Medication is administered intramuscularly.
- ○ **B.** The entire family will need to take the medication.
- ○ **C.** Medication will be repeated in two months.
- ○ **D.** Intravenous antibiotic therapy will be ordered.

220. The registered nurse on a pediatric unit is making assignments for the day. Which patient should not be assigned to the nurse who is pregnant?

Quick Answer: **60**
Detailed Answer: **82**

- ○ **A.** A child with cystic fibrosis who is receiving Nebcin (tobramycin)
- ○ **B.** An infant with respiratory syncytial virus receiving Virazole (ribavirin)
- ○ **C.** A child with Hirschsprung's disease scheduled for barium enema
- ○ **D.** A child with Meckel's diverticulum scheduled for radiographic scintigraphy

221. A patient of Greek descent has been prescribed Bactrim (sulfamethoxazole-trimethoprim) for treatment of a urinary tract infection. Before beginning the medication, the patient should be assessed for which of the following disorders?

Quick Answer: **60**
Detailed Answer: **82**

- ○ **A.** G6PD deficiency
- ○ B. ß-thalassemia
- ○ C. Sickle cell anemia
- ○ D. Von Willebrand disease

222. The nurse is caring for an obstetrical patient admitted with HELLP syndrome. The nurse anticipates an order for which medication?

Quick Answer: **60**
Detailed Answer: **82**

- ○ A. Yutopar (ritodrine)
- ○ B. Brethine (terbutaline)
- ○ C. Methergine (methylergonovine)
- ○ D. Pitocin (oxytocin)

223. Which assignment is not within the scope of practice of the registered nurse?

Quick Answer: **60**
Detailed Answer: **82**

- ○ **A.** Performing a vaginal exam on a patient in labor
- ○ **B.** Removing a PICC line
- ○ **C.** Monitoring central venous pressure
- ○ **D.** Performing wound closure with sutures and clips

224. An obstetrical client arrives at the women's hospital with abdominal cramping and gross bright red vaginal bleeding. Which action(s) should the nurse take?

   ○ **A.** Perform a vaginal exam

   ○ **B.** Check FHT and notify the physician

   ○ **C.** Request a stat hemoglobin and hematocrit

   ○ **D.** Perform Leopold's maneuver to check for fetal position

Quick Answer: **60**
Detailed Answer: **82**

225. The physician has ordered Brethine (terbutaline) for a patient with premature labor. The nurse is aware that the medication may cause:

   ○ **A.** Bradycardia

   ○ **B.** Hyperglycemia

   ○ **C.** Decreased muscle tone

   ○ **D.** Hot flashes

Quick Answer: **60**
Detailed Answer: **82**

226. Which medication is used to treat iron toxicity?

   ○ **A.** Narcan (naloxone)

   ○ **B.** Digibind (digoxin immune Fab)

   ○ **C.** Desferal (deferoxamine)

   ○ **D.** Zinecard (dexrazoxane)

Quick Answer: **60**
Detailed Answer: **82**

227. The nurse is suspected of charting medication administration that he did not give. The nurse can be charged with:

   ○ **A.** Fraud

   ○ **B.** Malpractice

   ○ **C.** Negligence

   ○ **D.** Tort

Quick Answer: **60**
Detailed Answer: **82**

228. The home health nurse is planning for the day's visits. Which client should be seen first?

   ○ **A.** The client with renal insufficiency

   ○ **B.** The client with Alzheimer's disease

   ○ **C.** The client with diabetes who has a decubitus ulcer

   ○ **D.** The client with multiple sclerosis who is being treated with IV cortisone

Quick Answer: **60**
Detailed Answer: **82**

229. Which clients can be assigned to share a room in the emergency department during a disaster?

Quick Answer: **60**
Detailed Answer: **82**

   ○ **A.** A client with schizophrenia having visual and auditory hallucinations and the client with ulcerative colitis

   ○ **B.** The client who is six months pregnant with abdominal pain and the client with facial lacerations and fractured arm

   ○ **C.** A child whose pupils are fixed and dilated and his parents, and a client with a frontal head injury

   ○ **D.** The client who arrives with a large puncture wound to the abdomen and the client with chest pain

230. Before administering eye drops, the nurse should recognize that it is essential to consider which of the following?

Quick Answer: **60**
Detailed Answer: **83**

   ○ **A.** The eye should be cleansed with warm water to remove any exudate before instilling the eye drops.

   ○ **B.** The patient will be more comfortable if allowed to instill his own eye drops.

   ○ **C.** Eye drops should be instilled with the patient looking down.

   ○ **D.** Eye drops should always be warmed before instilling in the patient's eyes.

231. To decrease the risk of urinary tract infections, a female client should be taught to:

Quick Answer: **60**
Detailed Answer: **83**

   ○ **A.** Drink citrus fruit juices

   ○ **B.** Avoid using tampons

   ○ **C.** Increase the intake of red meats

   ○ **D.** Clean the perineum from front to back

232. Which nursing intervention would you expect when working with a hospitalized toddler?

Quick Answer: **60**
Detailed Answer: **83**

   ○ **A.** Ask the parent to leave the room when assessments are being performed

   ○ **B.** Explain that items from home should not be brought into the hospital

   ○ **C.** Tell the parents that they may stay with the toddler

   ○ **D.** Ask the toddler if he is ready to have his temperature checked

233. Which instruction should be given to a client who is fitted with a behind-the-ear hearing aid?

- ○ **A.** Remove the ear mold and clean with alcohol
- ○ **B.** Avoid exposing the hearing aid to extremes in temperature
- ○ **C.** Use a cotton-tipped applicator to clean debris from the hole in the middle of the hearing aid
- ○ **D.** Continue to use cosmetics and spray cologne as before

234. Which statement is true regarding the measurement of fetal heart tones?

- ○ **A.** The normal range for FHT is 100–180 beats per minute.
- ○ **B.** A Doppler ultrasound can detect FHT at 18 to 20 weeks gestation.
- ○ **C.** FHT can be detected at eight weeks gestation using vaginal ultrasound.
- ○ **D.** A TOCO monitor is an invasive means of measuring FHT.

235. The physician ordered Zyprexa (olanzapine) for a patient with schizophrenia. Before administering the medication, the nurse should:

- ○ **A.** Ask the patient to void and measure the amount
- ○ **B.** Check the apical pulse rate
- ○ **C.** Check the temperature
- ○ **D.** Offer additional fluids

236. The nurse is caring for a child with suspected epiglottitis. Which finding is not associated with epiglottitis?

- ○ **A.** Drooling
- ○ **B.** Brassy cough
- ○ **C.** Muffled phonation
- ○ **D.** Inspiratory stridor

237. Which of the following is an ocular change that may be found in the patient with hyperthyroidism?

- ○ **A.** Ptosis
- ○ **B.** Open angle glaucoma
- ○ **C.** Exophthalmos
- ○ **D.** Presbyopia

238. The nurse is providing dietary instructions to the mother of a four-year-old diagnosed with celiac disease. Which food, if selected by the mother, would indicate her understanding of the dietary instructions?

Quick Answer: **60**
Detailed Answer: **83**

○ **A.** Wheat toast

○ **B.** Spaghetti

○ **C.** Oatmeal

○ **D.** Rice

239. Which infant is exempt from the recommendations of the American Academy of Pediatrics "Back to Sleep" campaign against SIDS?

Quick Answer: **60**
Detailed Answer: **83**

○ **A.** An infant with intussusception

○ **B.** An infant with pyloric stenosis

○ **C.** An infant with gastroesophageal reflux

○ **D.** An infant with a cleft palate

240. A gravida 2 para 0 is admitted to the labor and delivery unit. The doctor performs an amniotomy. Which observation would the nurse expect to make immediately after an amniotomy?

Quick Answer: **60**
Detailed Answer: **84**

○ **A.** Fetal heart tones of 160 beats per minute

○ **B.** A moderate amount of straw-colored clear vaginal fluid

○ **C.** A small amount of greenish vaginal fluid

○ **D.** A small segment of the umbilical cord protruding from the vagina

241. The vaginal exam of a laboring patient reveals that she is 3 cm dilated. Which of the following statements would the nurse expect the patient to make?

Quick Answer: **60**
Detailed Answer: **84**

○ **A.** "I can't decide what to name the baby."

○ **B.** "It feels good to push with each contraction."

○ **C.** "Don't touch me. I'm trying to concentrate."

○ **D.** "When can I get my epidural?"

242. The laboring client is having fetal heart rates of 100–110 beats per minute during contractions. The first action/actions the nurse should take is to:

Quick Answer: **60**
Detailed Answer: **84**

○ **A.** Apply an internal fetal monitor

○ **B.** Turn the client on her left side and apply oxygen

○ **C.** Get the client up and walk her in the hall

○ **D.** Move the client to the delivery room

243. In evaluating the effectiveness of IV Pitocin (oxytocin) for a client with secondary dystocia, the nurse should expect:

Quick Answer: **60**
Detailed Answer: **84**

- ○ **A.** A rapid delivery
- ○ **B.** Cervical effacement
- ○ **C.** Infrequent contractions
- ○ **D.** Progressive cervical dilation

244. Vaginal exam of a term gravida 2 para 1 reveals a breech presentation. The nurse should take which action at this time?

Quick Answer: **60**
Detailed Answer: **84**

- ○ **A.** Prepare the client for a Caesarean section
- ○ **B.** Apply the fetal heart monitor
- ○ **C.** Place the client in the Trendelenburg position
- ○ **D.** Perform an ultrasound exam

245. The nurse is caring for a client admitted to labor and delivery. Which finding indicates fetal distress?

Quick Answer: **60**
Detailed Answer: **84**

- ○ **A.** Contractions every three minutes
- ○ **B.** Absent variability
- ○ **C.** Fetal heart tone accelerations with movement
- ○ **D.** Fetal heart tone 120–130 beats per minute

246. The following are all nursing diagnoses appropriate for a gravida 4 para 3 in labor. Which one would be most appropriate for the client as she completes the latent phase of labor?

Quick Answer: **60**
Detailed Answer: **84**

- ○ **A.** Impaired gas exchange related to hyperventilation
- ○ **B.** Alteration in placental perfusion related to maternal position
- ○ **C.** Impaired physical mobility related to fetal-monitoring equipment
- ○ **D.** Potential fluid volume deficit related to decreased fluid intake

247. As the client reaches 8 cm dilation, the nurse notes a pattern on the fetal monitor that shows a drop in the fetal heart rate of 30 beats per minute beginning at the peak of the contraction and ending at the end of the contraction. The FHR baseline is 165–175 beats per minute with a variability of 0–2 beats per minute. What is the most likely explanation of this pattern?

- ○ **A.** The fetus is asleep.
- ○ **B.** The umbilical cord is compressed.
- ○ **C.** There is a vagal response.
- ○ **D.** There is uteroplacental insufficiency.

248. The nurse notes variable decelerations on the fetal monitor strip. The most appropriate initial action would be to:

- ○ **A.** Notify the physician
- ○ **B.** Increase the rate of IV fluid
- ○ **C.** Reposition the client
- ○ **D.** Readjust the monitor

249. Which of the following is a characteristic of a reassuring fetal heart rate pattern?

- ○ **A.** A fetal heart rate of 180 beats per minute
- ○ **B.** A baseline variability of 35 beats per minute
- ○ **C.** A fetal heart rate of 90 at the baseline
- ○ **D.** Acceleration of FHR with fetal movements

250. The nurse asks the client with an epidural anesthesia to void every hour during labor. The rationale for this intervention is:

- ○ **A.** The bladder fills more rapidly because of the medication used for the epidural.
- ○ **B.** Her level of consciousness is altered.
- ○ **C.** The sensation of the bladder filling is diminished or lost.
- ○ **D.** To allow her to rest uninterrupted after delivery.

Quick Answers

1. D	26. A	51. B	76. C
2. A	27. B	52. B	77. D
3. C	28. A	53. A	78. D
4. B	29. A	54. A	79. C
5. B	30. B	55. C	80. B
6. B	31. B	56. D	81. A
7. B	32. A	57. A	82. C
8. C	33. C	58. C	83. B
9. D	34. B	59. A	84. A
10. A	35. D	60. D	85. A
11. D	36. A	61. D	86. A
12. C	37. D	62. C	87. D
13. A	38. C	63. D	88. C
14. C	39. B	64. B	89. C
15. A	40. A	65. A	90. C
16. C	41. B	66. A	91. D
17. A	42. B	67. C	92. D
18. C	43. B	68. D	93. B
19. B	44. B	69. A	94. D
20. D	45. D	70. B	95. A
21. B	46. C	71. C	96. C
22. C	47. C	72. A	97. B
23. A	48. A	73. C	98. B
24. A	49. A	74. A	99. D
25. B	50. C	75. C	100. C

101. A	**128.** B	**155.** D	**182.** A
102. D	**129.** D	**156.** B	**183.** C
103. B	**130.** A	**157.** A	**184.** A
104. A	**131.** A	**158.** A	**185.** A
105. B	**132.** D	**159.** A	**186.** C
106. A	**133.** D	**160.** C	**187.** D
107. B	**134.** C	**161.** B	**188.** C
108. A	**135.** B	**162.** B	**189.** D
109. A	**136.** C	**163.** D	**190.** C
110. C	**137.** B	**164.** D	**191.** C
111. D	**138.** C	**165.** B	**192.** C
112. B	**139.** C	**166.** B	**193.** D
113. B	**140.** A	**167.** B	**194.** D
114. B	**141.** B	**168.** A	**195.** B
115. A	**142.** A	**169.** D	**196.** C
116. D	**143.** D	**170.** B	**197.** B
117. D	**144.** D	**171.** B	**198.** A
118. A	**145.** A	**172.** A	**199.** B
119. D	**146.** B	**173.** A	**200.** A
120. C	**147.** C	**174.** B	**201.** A
121. A	**148.** B	**175.** C	**202.** C
122. D	**149.** C	**176.** B	**203.** B
123. A	**150.** B	**177.** B	**204.** A
124. B	**151.** B	**178.** C	**205.** D
125. B	**152.** A	**179.** C	**206.** B
126. B	**153.** C	**180.** B	**207.** C
127. D	**154.** D	**181.** C	**208.** A

209. C	**220.** B	**231.** D	**242.** B
210. A	**221.** A	**232.** C	**243.** D
211. D	**222.** D	**233.** B	**244.** B
212. B	**223.** D	**234.** C	**245.** B
213. D	**224.** B	**235.** A	**246.** D
214. D	**225.** B	**236.** B	**247.** D
215. B	**226.** C	**237.** C	**248.** C
216. D	**227.** A	**238.** D	**249.** D
217. D	**228.** D	**239.** C	**250.** C
218. A	**229.** B	**240.** B	
219. B	**230.** A	**241.** D	

Answers and Rationales

1. **Answer D is correct.** One cup of rice is considered a low-potassium food. The foods in Answers A, B, and C are incorrect because they contain higher amounts of potassium.

2. **Answer A is correct.** Clients with borderline personality frequently suffer from depression and suicidal thinking and should be assessed for risk of self-injury. Answers B and D are incorrect choices because they allow the client too much control of the therapeutic environment. Answer C is incorrect because the client's activities do not have to be restricted to the unit after the level of depression has been determined.

3. **Answer C is correct.** Erosion of tooth enamel caused by frequent self-induced vomiting is an expected finding in a client with bulimia nervosa. Answers A, B, and D are expected findings in the client with anorexia nervosa; therefore, they are incorrect.

4. **Answer B is correct.** Because of their increased mobility, manual dexterity and curiosity, the four-year-old is at greater risk for accidental poisoning. Other accidental injuries in this age group include being struck by a car, falls, burns, and drowning. Answer A is incorrect because the one-year-old lacks the developmental skill to be at risk for accidental poisoning. Answers C and D are incorrect because the eight-year-old and twelve-year-old are at less risk because they are aware of the dangers of accidental poisoning.

5. **Answer B is correct.** Play of the preschool aged child is described as associative. At this stage, children are more interested in playing with other children than they are with playing with toys. The child may talk to other children and exchange toys or play games without any rules. Answer A describes the play of a school-aged child. Answer C describes the play of a toddler. Answer D describes the play of an infant.

6. **Answer B is correct.** While the infant is quiet, the nurse should begin the exam by listening to the heart and lungs. If the nurse elicits the Babinski reflex, palpates the abdomen, or checks the tympanic membranes, the infant may cry and it will be difficult to adequately listen to the heart and lungs; therefore, Answers A, C, and D are incorrect.

7. **Answer B is correct.** A three-year-old is expected to use magical thinking, such as believing that a toy bear is a real bear. Answers A, C, and D are incorrect because abstract thinking, conservation of matter, and the ability to look at things from the perspective of others are cognitive abilities of an older child.

8. **Answer C is correct.** The two-year-old can combine three to four words. Answers A and B are incorrect because the two-year-old understands yes and no, but does not understand the meaning of all words. Answer D is incorrect because seeking information and asking "why?" is typical of the three-year old.

9. **Answer D is correct.** Urokinase is a thrombolytic agent used in the treatment of deep vein thrombosis, pulmonary embolus, or myocardial infarction. The presence of dark brown or rust-colored urine suggests bleeding. The nurse should withhold the medication, call the doctor immediately, and prepare to administer Amicar. Answer A is incorrect because vitamin K is not the antidote for urokinase. Answers B and C are incorrect because they do not address the adverse problem of bleeding.

10. **Answer A is correct.** The client taking calcium-based antacids will frequently develop constipation. Answers B, C, and D are not associated with the use of calcium-based antacids; therefore, they are incorrect.

11. **Answer D is correct.** The nurse should not aspirate when giving heparin; therefore, answer D indicates a need for further teaching regarding heparin administration. Answers A, B, and C indicate the student nurse understands the correct administration of heparin and are, therefore, incorrect answers.

12. **Answer C is correct.** To obtain a correct oxygen saturation reading using pulse oximetry, the probe should not be placed on the arm with a noninvasive BP cuff or intra-arterial line. Suitable sites are the finger, earlobe, or nose; therefore, Answers A, B, and D are incorrect.

13. **Answer A is correct.** The client is exhibiting a widened pulse pressure, tachycardia, and tachypnea. The first nursing action after obtaining these vital signs is to notify the physician for additional orders. Answers B, C, and D can be done after the physician is notified; therefore, they are incorrect choices as a first action.

14. **Answer C is correct.** The client with an axillo-popliteal bypass graft should avoid activities that can occlude the femoral artery graft. Sitting in the straight chair and wearing tight clothes are prohibited for this reason. Answers A, B, and D are incorrect because resting in a supine position, resting in a recliner, and sleeping in right Sim's position are allowed.

15. **Answer A is correct.** The best time to apply antithrombotic stockings to the client is in the morning before the client arises. (If the physician orders them later in the day, the client should return to bed, wait 30 minutes, and apply the stockings.) Answers B, C, and D are incorrect because there is likely to be more peripheral edema if the client has been standing or has just taken a bath; applying before retiring in the evening is wrong because late in the evening, more peripheral edema will be present.

16. **Answer C is correct.** A client admitted one hour ago with rales and shortness of breath should be seen first because the client might require respiratory interventions. The client in answer A with an oxygen saturation of 99% is stable. Answer B is incorrect because this client will have some inflammatory process after surgery, so a temperature of 100.2°F is not unusual. The client in answer D is stable and can be seen later.

17. **Answer A is correct.** The best roommate for the client with a femoral popliteal bypass graft is the client with hypothyroidism because the client poses little risk of infection. Answers B, C, and D are incorrect because they pose a risk of infection to the post-surgical client.

18. **Answer C is correct.** The client taking sodium warfarin, an anticoagulant, should not take aspirin or NSAIDS because these will further increase bleeding times. The client should return to have a protime drawn for bleeding time, report a rash, and use an electric razor for shaving; therefore, Answers A, B, and D are incorrect choices.

19. **Answer B is correct.** Because the aorta is clamped during surgery, the blood supply to the kidneys is decreased. This can result in renal damage. A urinary output of 20mL/hr is inadequate. Answers A, C, and D are expected findings and do not warrant further investigation; therefore, they are incorrect.

20. **Answer D is correct.** When assisting the client with bowel and bladder retraining, sexual function is not a considered factor. Dietary history, mobility, and fluid intake are important factors; these must be taken into consideration because they relate to constipation, urinary output, and the ability to use a urinal or bedpan; therefore, Answers A, B, and C are incorrect.

21. **Answer B is correct.** To correctly measure the client for crutches, the nurse should measure approximately three inches between the axilla and the top of the crutch. Answer A is incorrect because the distance is too great. Answer C is incorrect because the client's elbows should be flexed at approximately a 35° angle, not a 10° angle, as stated. The crutches should be approximately 6 inches from the side of the foot, not 8 to 10 inches, as stated in answer D.

22. **Answer C is correct.** The occipital lobe is responsible for vision. The temporal lobe is responsible for taste, smell, and hearing. The frontal lobe is responsible for judgment, foresight, and behavior. The parietal lobe is responsible for ideation, sensory functions, and language; therefore, Answers A, B, and D are incorrect.

23. **Answer A is correct.** Damage to the hypothalamus can result in an elevated temperature because this portion of the brain helps to regulate body temperature. Answers B, C, and D are incorrect because they are not associated with regulation of temperature.

24. **Answer A is correct.** The rationale for a low-protein diet is that protein increases the production of nitrogenous wastes and causes an increased workload on the kidneys. Answers B, C, and D are not the rationale for institution of a low-protein diet; therefore, they are incorrect.

25. **Answer B is correct.** To safely administer intravenous heparin, the nurse should use an infusion controller. Too rapid infusion of heparin can result in hemorrhage. Answers A, C, and D are incorrect. It is not necessary to have a buretrol, an infusion filter, or a three-way stopcock.

26. **Answer A is correct. When assessing the client's blood pressure,** the width of the blood pressure cuff used should be 40% of the circumference of the extremity. Answers B, C, and D are incorrect for assessing the blood pressure.

27. **Answer B is correct.** A diet containing moderate protein, low sodium, and low saturated fat will be ordered for the client with nephrotic syndrome. Answers A, C, and D do not meet the nutritional needs of the client; therefore, they are incorrect.

28. **Answer A is correct.** A white blood cell count of 14,000 cu.mm should be reported because it indicates infection. Answers B and C are incorrect choices because auscultation of an abdominal bruit and complaints of lower back pain are expected in the client with an abdominal aortic aneurysm. Answer D is incorrect because the platelet count is within normal limits.

29. **Answer A is correct.** The assessed reading of 3+ indicates that the reflex is stronger than normal. Answers B, C, and D are incorrect because a hypoactive reading is 1+, a normal reading is 2+, and a hyperactive reading is 4+.

30. **Answer B is correct.** The nurse should administer 0.5 mL of the medication. Answers A, C, and D are incorrect amounts.

31. **Answer B is correct.** The pulmonary artery pressure (PAP) measures the systolic, diastolic, and the mean pressure in the pulmonary artery. It will not measure the pressure in the left ventricle, the pressure in the pulmonary veins, or the pressure in the right ventricle; therefore, Answers A, C, and D are incorrect.

32. **Answer A is correct.** A CVP reading of 1 cm of water indicates decreased circulating volume and should be reported to the physician immediately. Answers B, C, and D indicate CVP readings greater than 8 cm of water and are associated with increased blood volume or right-sided heart failure.

33. **Answer C is correct.** The treatment for ventricular tachycardia is administration of a medication such as amiodarone that will slow and correct the abnormal rhythm. Answer A is incorrect because atropine sulfate will further increase the heart rate. Answer B is incorrect because it is not a priority at this time. Answer D is incorrect because defibrillation is used for the client with pulseless ventricular tachycardia or ventricular fibrillation. Defibrillation should begin at 200 joules and be increased to 360 joules.

34. **Answer B is correct.** The client should be asked to hold his breath and bear down (Valsalva maneuver) while the chest tube is being removed. Answers A, C, and D are not used during removal of chest tubes; therefore, they are incorrect.

35. **Answer D is correct.** The nurse should withhold the medication and notify the physician because the potassium level is extremely low. (The normal potassium range is 3.5–5.5mEq/L.) Answers A, B, and C are incorrect because continuing the medication will cause further hypokalemia.

36. **Answer A is correct.** A platelet count should be done periodically to detect the risk of bleeding in the client maintained on Coumadin therapy. Answers B, C, and D are not associated with the risks of Coumadin therapy; therefore, they are incorrect.

37. **Answer D is correct.** The duration of Levemir is 24 hours. Answers A, B, and C are incorrect choices because they do not apply to Levemir.

38. **Answer C is correct.** The use of herbal supplements may alter the effects of prescription medications. Answers A, B, and D are not true statements; therefore, they are incorrect choices. The FDA classifies herbs as dietary supplements.

39. **Answer B is correct.** The fifth vital sign is pain. Nurses should assess and record pain just as they would routine vital signs of temperature, respirations, pulse, and blood pressure. Answers A, C, and D are included in the nurse's assessment but are not considered to be the fifth vital sign and are, therefore, incorrect.

40. **Answer A is correct.** Adverse effects of opioids such as oxycodone include pulmonary edema, hypotension, seizures, hepatitis, and ventricular tachycardia. Answers B, C, and D are side effects of the medication, not adverse effects; therefore, they are incorrect choices.

41. **Answer B is correct.** PCA pumps have a locking device that prevents overdosing by limiting the amount of medication the client can self-administer. Answers A, C, and D are incorrect statements.

42. **Answer B is correct.** Skin irritation can occur if the TENS unit is used for prolonged periods of time. To prevent skin irritations, the client should change the location of the electrodes often. Electrocution is not a risk because it uses a battery pack; thus, answer A is incorrect. Answer C is incorrect because the unit should not be used on sensitive areas of the body. Answer D is incorrect because creams and lotions are not to be used with the device.

43. **Answer B is correct.** An advanced directive allows the client to make known his wishes regarding care if he becomes unable to act on his own. Much confusion regarding care and life-saving measures can occur if the client does not have an advanced directive. Answers A, C, and D are incorrect choices because the nursing staff doesn't need to know about funeral plans, the nursing staff cannot make decisions for the client, and active euthanasia is illegal in most states in the United States.

44. **Answer B is correct.** Using a finger between the baby's mouth and breast to break the suction helps to reduce nipple soreness associated with breast feeding. Answers A, C, and D do not help prevent or reduce nipple soreness; therefore, they are incorrect.

45. **Answer D is correct.** Facial grimacing is an indication of pain. The blood pressure listed in Answer A is within normal limits. The client's inability to concentrate and dilated pupils, as stated in Answers B and C, may be related to the anesthesia or medications received during surgery.

46. **Answer C is correct.** The nurse should monitor the client for respiratory depression. Epidural anesthesia involves injecting an anesthetic into the epidural space. If the anesthesia rises above the level of the diaphragm, the client will have impaired breathing. Answers A, B and D are incorrect because they are not associated with the use of epidural anesthesia.

47. **Answer C is correct.** Pain is a late sign associated with oral cancer. Answers A, B, and D are incorrect because a feeling of warmth, odor, and a flat ulcer in the mouth are all early signs associated with oral cancer.

48. **Answer A is correct.** Common complaints of the client with macular degeneration include difficulty with activities that require focused or central vision such as sewing, needlepoint, and reading. Answer B describes the client with acute glaucoma, Answer C describes the client with cataracts, and Answer D describes the client with detached retina.

49. **Answer A is correct.** Continuous bladder irrigations are ordered for the patient following a TURP to prevent blood clots from forming and blocking the catheter. Answers B, C, and D are incorrect because they are not the reason for continuous bladder irrigations.

50. **Answer C is correct.** Early symptoms of hypocalcemia include numbness and tingling of the toes and extremities as well as around the mouth. Answers A, B, and D are later symptoms; therefore, they are incorrect.

51. **Answer B is correct.** Individuals with ulcers within the duodenum typically complain of pain occurring 2–3 hours after a meal, as well as at night. The pain is usually relieved by eating. The pain associated with gastric ulcers, answer A, occurs 30 minutes after eating. Answer C is too vague and does not distinguish the type of ulcer. Answer D is associated with a stress ulcer.

52. **Answer B is correct.** A barium enema is contraindicated in the client with diverticulitis because it can cause bowel perforation. Answers A, C, and D are appropriate diagnostic studies for the client with suspected diverticulitis.

53. **Answer A is correct.** Clients with celiac disease should refrain from eating foods containing gluten. Foods with gluten include wheat, barley, oats, and rye. The other foods are allowed.

54. **Answer A is correct.** The nurse should reinforce the need for a diet balanced in all nutrients and fiber. Foods that often cause diarrhea and bloating associated with irritable bowel syndrome include fried foods, caffeinated beverages, alcohol, and spicy foods. Therefore, answers B, C, and D are incorrect.

55. **Answer C is correct.** Fluid volume deficit can lead to metabolic acidosis and electrolyte loss. The other nursing diagnoses in answers A, B, and D might be applicable but are of lesser priority.

56. **Answer D is correct.** Alcohol will cause extreme nausea if consumed with Flagyl. Answer A is incorrect because the full course of treatment should be taken. The medication should be taken with a full 8 oz. of water, with meals, and the client should avoid direct sunlight because he will most likely be photosensitive; therefore, answers A, B, and C are incorrect.

57. **Answer A is correct.** Before beginning feedings, an x-ray is often obtained to check for placement. Aspirating stomach content and checking the pH for acidity is the best method of checking for placement. Other methods include placing the end in water and checking for bubbling, and injecting air and listening over the epigastric area. Answers B and C are not correct choices. Answer D is incorrect because warming in the microwave is contraindicated.

58. **Answer C is correct.** Antacids should not be administered with other medications. If antacids are taken with many medications, they render the other medications inactive. All other answers are incorrect.

59. **Answer A is correct.** The client with a colostomy can swim and carry on activities as before the colostomy. Answers B and C are incorrect, and answer D shows a lack of empathy.

60. **Answer D is correct.** The use of a sitz bath will help with the pain and swelling associated with a hemorrhoidectomy. The client should eat foods high in fiber, so answer A is incorrect. Ice packs, as stated in answer B, are ordered immediately after surgery only. Answer C is incorrect because taking a laxative daily can result in diarrhea.

61. **Answer D is correct.** Increasing abdominal girth indicates over distention of the bowel frequently associated with the development of an ileus. Answers A, B, and C are expected following a laparoscopic hemicolectomy.

62. **Answer C is correct.** A client newly diagnosed with diabetes has deficient knowledge. Answers A, B, and D, while applicable, do not take priority at this time.

63. **Answer D is correct.** The home health nurse caring for the elderly client should assess the environment and reinforce teaching regarding the prevention of falls. Answer A is incorrect because there is no indication in the question that hospice services are needed. Answer B is incorrect because speaking in a high-pitched tone of voice will make hearing more difficult for the client. Answer C is incorrect because fluids may be restricted before bedtime, but should not be restricted in general because elderly clients tend to drink less fluid.

64. **Answer B is correct.** Antibiotics such as erythromycin are most likely to cause abdominal pain. Answers A, C, and D are not associated with causing abdominal pain; therefore, they are incorrect choices.

65. **Answer A is correct.** The nurse should inspect first, then auscultate, and finally palpate. If the nurse palpates first, the assessment might be unreliable. Therefore, answers B, C, and D are incorrect.

66. **Answer A is correct.** The hospital will certainly honor the wishes of family members even if the patient has signed a donor card. Answer B is incorrect, answer C is not empathetic to the family and is untrue, and answer D is not good nursing etiquette and, therefore, is incorrect.

67. **Answer C is correct.** The nurse should explore the cause for the lack of motivation. The client might be anemic and lack energy, or the client might be depressed. Alternating staff, as stated in answer A, will prevent a bond from being formed with the nurse. Answer B is not enough, and answer D is not necessary.

68. **Answer D is correct.** The nurse who has had the chickenpox has immunity to the illness and will not transmit chickenpox to the client. Answer A is incorrect because there could be no need to reassign the nurse. Answer B is incorrect because the nurse should be assessed before coming to the conclusion that she cannot spread the infection to the client. Answer C is incorrect because there is still a risk, even though chickenpox has formed scabs.

69. **Answer A is correct.** Taking the blood pressure on the side of the mastectomy is contraindicated. The nurse should not take the blood pressure, perform venipunctures, or fingersticks on the affected side. Answers B, C, and D are acceptable when caring for the client following a mastectomy.

70. **Answer B is correct.** Gentamicin is an aminoglycoside. Aminoglycosides are both nephrotoxic and ototoxic. Answers A, C, and D are not considerations when administering gentamicin; therefore, they are incorrect choices.

71. **Answer C is correct.** The best indicator of HIV is the Western blot. Answers A, B, and D are not the best indicators for HIV; therefore, they are incorrect.

72. **Answer A is correct.** A "bull's eye" rash, headache, and arthralgia are signs/symptoms associated with Lyme disease, a disease spread by ticks. Answers B, C, and D are important to the general history, but are not specific to Lyme disease, so they are incorrect.

73. **Answer C is correct.** The client that needs the least-skilled nursing care is the client with the thyroidectomy four days ago. Answers A, B, and D are incorrect because the other clients are less stable and require a registered nurse.

74. **Answer A is correct.** Hyphema is blood in the anterior chamber of the eye and around the eye. The client should have the head of the bed elevated and ice applied. Answers B, C, and D are incorrect and do not treat the problem.

75. **Answer C is correct.** Ferrous sulfate should be given with orange juice or other sources of ascorbic acid (vitamin C) to help absorption. It should not be given with meals or milk or given undiluted because these do not help with absorption; therefore, Answers A, B, and D are incorrect.

76. **Answer C is correct.** The nurse should teach the client with an ileostomy regarding the use of Stomahesive as a skin protector. Answer A is not correct because the bag will not seal if the client uses Karaya powder. Answer B is incorrect because there is no need to irrigate an ileostomy. Answer D is incorrect because the stools are liquid.

77. **Answer D is correct.** Phytonadione (vitamin K) is given to the newborn to facilitate clotting. Answers A, B, and C are incorrect because the medication does not stop hemorrhage, prevent infection, or replace electrolytes.

78. **Answer D is correct.** Hemabate is a prostaglandin F 2∂ used to treat postpartal hemorrhage. Answers A, B, and C are not used in the treatment of postpartal hemorrhage, so they are incorrect choices.

79. **Answer C is correct.** An antiemetic should be administered prior to chemotherapy because chemotherapeutic agents used to treat cancer cause nausea and vomiting. It is not necessary to give a bolus of IV fluids, medicate for pain, or allow the client to eat; therefore, Answers A, B, and D are incorrect.

80. **Answer B is correct.** Pitocin (oxytocin) is used to induce uterine contractions to decrease bleeding. A uterus deviated to the left, as stated in Answer A, indicates a full bladder. It is not desirable to have a boggy uterus, making Answer C incorrect. This lack of muscle tone will increase bleeding. Answer D is incorrect because Pitocin does not affect the position of the uterus.

81. **Answer A is correct.** A client with secondary syphilis will exhibit a "copper penny" rash on the palms of the hands and soles of the feet and flu-like symptoms. Answers B and D are incorrect choices because they are exhibited by the client with tertiary syphilis. Answer C is incorrect because it is exhibited by the client with primary syphilis.

82. **Answer C is correct.** Creon (pancrelipase) is given to assist digestion. Answers A, B, and D are incorrect because they are not uses for the medication.

83. **Answer B is correct.** Concurrent use of Zyvox and SSRIs as well as MAOIs may result in serotonin syndrome. Answers A, C, and D are incorrect because concurrent use with Zyvox does not cause serotonin syndrome.

84. **Answer A is correct.** Regular insulin should be withdrawn before the NPH insulin. They can be given together, so there is no need for two injections, making Answer D incorrect. Answer B is an incorrect choice because regular insulin is withdrawn first. Answer C is incorrect because it does matter which insulin is drawn up first.

85. **Answer A is correct.** Clients having cardiac CTA with contrast should be assessed for allergies to shellfish or iodine. Answers B, C, and D have no effect on the client having a cardiac CTA with contrast; therefore, they are incorrect choices.

86. **Answer A is correct.** Methergine (methylergonovine) produces uterine contractions and is used for postpartal bleeding that is not controlled by Pitocin (oxytocin). Answers B, C, and D are incorrect because they are not used to control postpartal bleeding.

87. **Answer D is correct.** Clients receiving a transplanted organ will be required to take immunosuppressant medication for life to prevent transplant rejection. Answers A, B, and C are incorrect because the client must take the medication for life.

88. **Answer C is correct.** Cullen's sign, a bluish discoloration around the umbilicus, is an indication of damage to the abdominal organs leading to hemorrhage. Answers A, B, and D are incorrect because the frontal lobe, the lungs, and the spinal cord are not involved in Cullen's sign.

89. **Answer C is correct.** The time of onset for regular insulin is within 30–60 minutes. Answers A, B, and D are incorrect because they are not the correct timeframes for onset.

90. **Answer C is correct.** The client should be taught to eat his meals even if he is not hungry, to prevent a hypoglycemic reaction. Answers A, B, and D are incorrect because they indicate knowledge of the nurse's teaching.

91. **Answer D is correct.** Taking antibiotics and oral contraceptives together decreases the effectiveness of the oral contraceptives. Answers A, B, and C are not necessarily true.

92. **Answer D is correct.** Taking prednisone in the morning mimics the body's natural release of corticosteroids. Answer A is not correct because it is not necessarily a true statement. Answers B and C are untrue statements, so they are incorrect.

93. **Answer B is correct.** Rifampin can change the color of the urine and body fluid. Answer A is not necessary, answer C is not true, and answer D is not true because this medication should be taken regularly during the course of the treatment.

94. **Answer D is correct.** Cytoxan (cyclophosphamide) can cause hemorrhagic cystitis, so the client should drink at least eight glasses of water a day. Answers A and B are not necessary and, so, are incorrect. Nausea often occurs with chemotherapy, so answer C is incorrect.

95. **Answer A is correct.** Crystals in the solution are not normal and should not be administered to the client. Discard the solution immediately. Answer B is incorrect because warming the solution will not help. Answer C is incorrect, and answer D requires a doctor's order.

96. **Answer C is correct.** Theo-Dur (theophylline) is a bronchodilator, and a side effect of bronchodilators is tachycardia, so checking the pulse is important. Extreme tachycardia should be reported to the doctor. Answers A, B, and D are not necessary.

97. **Answer B is correct.** The diagnosis of meningitis at age six months correlates to a diagnosis of cerebral palsy. Cerebral palsy, a neurological disorder, is often associated with birth trauma or infections of the brain or spinal column. Answers A, C, and D are not related to the question.

98. **Answer B is correct.** Children at 18 months of age like push-pull toys. Children at approximately three years of age begin to dress themselves and build a tower of eight blocks. At age four, children can copy a horizontal or vertical line. Therefore, Answers A, C, and D are incorrect.

99. **Answer D is correct.** A complication of a tonsillectomy is bleeding, and constant swallowing may indicate bleeding. Decreased appetite is expected after a tonsillectomy, as is a low-grade temperature; thus, Answers A and B are incorrect. In Answer C, chest congestion is not normal but is not associated with the tonsillectomy.

100. **Answer C is correct.** Hyperplasia of the gums is associated with Dilantin therapy. Answer A is not related to the therapy; Answer B is a side effect; and Answer D is not related to the question.

101. **Answer A is correct.** If the client eats foods high in tyramine, he might experience malignant hypertension. Tyramine is found in cheese, sour cream, Chianti wine, sherry, beer, pickled herring, liver, canned figs, raisins, bananas, avocados, chocolate, soy sauce, fava beans, and yeast. These episodes are treated with Regitine, an alpha-adrenergic blocking agent. Answers B, C, and D are not related to the question.

102. **Answer D is correct.** Quinidine can cause widened Q-T intervals and heart block. Other signs of myocardial toxicity are notched P waves and widened QRS complexes. The most common side effects are diarrhea, nausea, and vomiting. The client might experience tinnitus, vertigo, headache, visual disturbances, and confusion. Answers A, B, and C are not related to the use of quinidine.

103. **Answer B is correct.** Lidocaine is used to treat ventricular tachycardia. This medication slowly exerts an antiarrhythmic effect by increasing the electric stimulation threshold of the ventricles without depressing the force of ventricular contractions. It is not used for the treatment of atrial arrhythmias; thus, Answer A is incorrect. Answers C and D are incorrect choices because lidocaine slows the heart rate, so it is not used for the treatment of heart block or bradycardia.

104. **Answer A is correct.** Sites for the application of nitroglycerin should be rotated to prevent skin irritation. It can be applied to the back and upper arms, not to the lower extremities, making Answer B incorrect. Answer C is incorrect because nitroglycerine

should not be rubbed into the skin, and Answer D is incorrect because the medication should be covered with a prepared dressing made of a thin paper substance, not gauze.

105. **Answer B is correct.** A persistent cough might be related to an adverse reaction to Capoten. Answers A and D are incorrect because tinnitus and diarrhea are not associated with the medication. Muscle weakness might occur when beginning the treatment but is not an adverse effect; thus, Answer C is incorrect.

106. **Answer A is correct.** Lasix should be given over 1 to 2 minutes to prevent hypotension. Answers B, C, and D are incorrect because it is not necessary to be given in an IV piggyback, with saline, or through a filter.

107. **Answer B is correct.** The antidote for heparin is protamine sulfate. Cyanocobalamine is B12. Streptokinase is a thrombolytic, and sodium warfarin is an anticoagulant; therefore, Answers A, C, and D are incorrect.

108. **Answer A is correct.** The client receiving linear accelerator therapy for cancer does not pose a radiation risk to the nurse who is pregnant. Answers B, C, and D pose a risk because of the type of radiation being used; therefore, they are incorrect choices.

109. **Answer A is correct.** The client with Cushing's disease should receive placement in a private room since his condition makes him more susceptible to infection. The clients in Answers B, C, and D do not require a private room.

110. **Answer C is correct.** Assault is defined as striking or touching the client inappropriately, so a nurse assistant striking a client could be charged with assault. Answer A, negligence, is failing to perform care for the client. Answer B, a tort, is a wrongful act committed on the client or their belongings. Answer D, malpractice, is failure to perform an act that the nursing assistant knows should be done, or the act of doing something wrong that results in harm to the client.

111. **Answer D is correct.** The licensed practical nurse should not be delegated to start a blood transfusion, but can assist the registered nurse with identifying the client and taking vital signs. Answers A, B, and C are duties that the licensed practical nurse can perform.

112. **Answer B is correct.** The vital signs are abnormal and should be reported to the doctor immediately. Answer A, continuing to monitor the vital signs, can result in deterioration of the client's condition. Answer C, asking the client how he feels, would supply only subjective data. Involving the LPN, in answer D, is not the best solution to help this client because he is unstable.

113. **Answer B is correct.** ß-thalassemia is an inherited disorder that causes the red blood cells to have a shorter life span. Frequent blood transfusions are necessary to treat the anemia and provide oxygen to the tissues. Answer A is incorrect because fluid therapy will not help; Answer C is incorrect because oxygen therapy will also not help; and Answer D is incorrect because iron should not be given to the patient with ß-thalassemia.

114. **Answer B is correct.** *N. gonorrhea* is treated with antibiotics such as penicillin and doxycycline. Answers A, C, and D are not used in the treatment of *N.gonorrhea;* therefore, they are incorrect.

115. **Answer A is correct.** Clinical symptoms associated with *Chlamydia* include frequent urination and a vaginal discharge. Answers B, C, and D are not symptoms of *Chlamydia*; therefore, they are incorrect.

116. **Answer D is correct.** The client prescribed an alkaline ash diet should consume rhubarb, legumes, milk and milk products, and green vegetables. Answers A, B, and C are found on an acid ash diet and should be limited.

117. **Answer D is correct.** *Clostridium difficile* is transmitted by objects contaminated with stool containing *clostridium difficile*. Poor hand hygiene is a major source of transmission in the hospital. Answers A, B, and C are incorrect because the mode of transmission is not by sputum, through urinary catheterization, or by unsterile surgical equipment.

118. **Answer A is correct.** The first client to be seen is the one who recently returned from surgery. The other clients in answers B, C, and D are more stable and can be seen later.

119. **Answer D is correct.** The patient should be placed in Trendelenburg position for the removal of a PICC line in order to prevent an air embolus. Answers A, B, and C are incorrect positions for the removal of a PICC line.

120. **Answer C is correct.** The patient taking Revia (naltrexone) should be told to avoid cold medications because many contain alcohol. The patient may take acetaminophen, ibuprofen, and antihistamines, so Answers A, B, and D are incorrect.

121. **Answer A is correct.** The client with unilateral neglect will neglect one side of the body. Answers B, C, and D are not associated with unilateral neglect.

122. **Answer D is correct.** The nurse should explore the reasons for the client's refusal to take the medication. Answers A, B, and C are not appropriate for the situation; therefore, they are incorrect.

123. **Answer A is correct.** Identifying oneself as a licensed nurse without a current license to practice within the state or territory defrauds the public, and the individual doing so can be prosecuted. A tort is a wrongful act; malpractice is failing to act appropriately as a nurse or acting in a way that harm comes to the client; and negligence is failing to perform care. Therefore, Answers B, C, and D are incorrect.

124. **Answer B is correct.** The client with the appendectomy is the most stable of these clients and can be assigned to a nursing assistant. Answers A, C, and D are incorrect because they require skilled nursing care.

125. **Answer B is correct.** The first action the nurse should take is to report the discrepancy to the nursing supervisor. Answers A, C, and D are incorrect because none of these is the first action the nurse should take.

126. **Answer B is correct.** The best client to transfer to the postpartum unit is the 40-year-old female with a hysterectomy. The clients in answers A and D pose a possible risk of infection and will be best cared for in a medical unit. The client with depression in answer C should be transferred to a unit where suicide precautions can be instituted.

127. **Answer D is correct.** The fresh peach is the lowest in sodium of these choices. Answers A, B, and C have much higher amounts of sodium.

128. **Answer B is correct.** The client with congestive heart failure who is complaining of nighttime dyspnea should be seen first because nighttime dyspnea may indicate worsening of his condition. Answers A, C, and D are incorrect because the clients are more stable and can be seen later.

129. **Answer D is correct.** The nurse can help alleviate the client's discomfort caused by xerostomia dry mouth by providing sugarless hard candy. Answers A, B, and C do not relieve xerostomia (dry mouth); therefore, they are incorrect.

130. **Answer A is correct.** The client with Alzheimer's disease can be assigned to the nursing assistant, who can perform duties such as feeding and assisting the client with activities of daily living. The clients in Answers B, C, and D have less stable conditions and should be cared for by a nurse.

131. **Answer A is correct.** Frequent rest periods for the client with cerebral palsy help relax tense muscles, resulting in a decrease in grimacing and writhing movement. Answers B, C, and D are incorrect because they are untrue statements.

132. **Answer D is correct.** Male patients should not void within one hour of culture collection because voiding washes secretions out of the urethra. Answer A and C are incorrect because blood and urine are not used to detect *N. gonorrhea.* Answer B is incorrect because oropharyngeal secretions, not nasopharyngeal secretions, are used for culture.

133. **Answer D is correct.** After surgery, the client will be placed on a clear-liquid diet and progressed to a regular diet. Stool softeners will be included in the plan of care to avoid constipation. Later, a high-fiber diet, in Answer A, is encouraged, but this is not the first diet after surgery. Answers B and C are not diets for this type of surgery.

134. **Answer C is correct.** A sitz bath will help with swelling and improve healing for the client with an episiotomy. Answers A, B, and D are not effective ways of managing episiotomy discomfort in the client who is two days post delivery.

135. **Answer B is correct.** The best way to determine the client's need for pain medication is to ask the client to rate his pain on a pain scale from 0–10. Subjective descriptions of pain intensity and experience are more reliable and accurate than observable qualities of pain; therefore, Answers A, C, and D are incorrect.

136. **Answer C is correct.** The client is experiencing compensated metabolic acidosis. The pH is within the normal range but is lower than 7.40, so it is on the acidic side. The CO_2 level is elevated, the oxygen level is below normal, and the bicarbonate level is slightly elevated. In respiratory disorders, the pH will be the inverse of the CO_2 and bicarbonate levels. This means that if the pH is low, the CO_2 and bicarbonate levels will be elevated. Answers A, B, and D are incorrect because they do not fall into the range of symptoms.

137. **Answer B is correct.** The registered nurse and physician are the only staff members who can order a client be placed in seclusion; therefore, Answers A, C, and D are incorrect.

138. **Answer C is correct.** Sodium warfarin is administered in the late afternoon, at approximately 1700 hours. This allows for accurate bleeding times to be drawn in the morning. Therefore, Answers A, B, and D are incorrect.

139. **Answer C is correct.** The nurse should cover both of the client's eyes to prevent consensual eye movement that may increase the damage caused by the metal fragment. Answers A, B, and D are incorrect because the nurse should only cover both eyes with a cupped object and wait for the physician to examine the eye.

140. **Answer A is correct.** To protect herself from absorbing the medication, the nurse should wear gloves when applying a nitroglycerine patch or nitroglycerine cream. Answer B is incorrect because shaving the skin might abrade the area. Answer C is incorrect because washing with hot water will cause vasodilation and increase the absorption of the medication. The patches should be applied to areas above the waist, making Answer D incorrect.

141. **Answer B is correct.** The client scheduled for a paracentesis should be told to empty the bladder, to prevent the risk of the bladder being punctured when the needle is inserted. A paracentesis is done to remove fluid from the peritoneal cavity. The client will be positioned sitting up or leaning over a table, making Answer A incorrect. The client is usually awake during the procedure, and medications are not commonly instilled during the procedure; therefore, Answers C and D are incorrect.

142. **Answer A is correct.** Atropine sulfate is the antidote for Tensilon and is given to treat cholinergic crises that can occur during testing for myasthenia gravis. Answers B, C, and D are not used during the testing for myasthenia gravis; therefore, they are incorrect choices.

143. **Answer D is correct.** The first exercise that should be done by the client following a mastectomy is squeezing the ball. Answers A, B, and C are incorrect because they are performed later.

144. **Answer D is correct.** The mother who is Rh negative with a newborn who is Rh negative is not a candidate for RhoGAM. The mothers in Answers A, B, and C all require RhoGAM; therefore, these answers are incorrect.

145. **Answer A is correct.** The AST is indicated in diagnosing the client with liver disorders, not cardiac disorders such as myocardial infarction. Answers B, C, and D are used in making the diagnosis of myocardial infarction; therefore, they are incorrect choices for the question.

146. **Answer B is correct.** The client is using the defense mechanism of denial. Answers A, C, and D do not relate to the client's statement; therefore, they are incorrect choices.

147. **Answer C is correct.** When the client is receiving TPN, the blood glucose level should be evaluated. TPN is a solution that contains large amounts of glucose that may alter

the client's blood glucose level. Answers A, B, and D are not directly related to the question and are therefore incorrect.

148. **Answer B is correct.** A client with diabetes who has trouble seeing would require follow-up after discharge. The lack of visual acuity for the client preparing and injecting insulin might require help. Answers A, C, and D will not prevent the client from being able to care for himself and, thus, are incorrect.

149. **Answer C is correct.** Cephulac (lactulose) is administered to the client with cirrhosis to lower ammonia levels. Answers A, B, and D are incorrect because the medication does not have an effect on the other lab values.

150. **Answer B is correct.** Having cloudy dialysate returns usually indicates infection. Asking the client about abdominal pain and fever helps to establish a diagnosis of infection, which requires antibiotic therapy. Answer A is incorrect because cloudy dialysate return is not expected. Answers C and D are not related to the occurrence of cloudy dialysate return, so they are incorrect.

151. **Answer B is correct.** The 15-year-old with sternal bruising should be seen first because injury to his chest might have resulted in fractures to the ribs and damage to underlying structures that can affect oxygenation. The clients in Answers A, C, and D should be seen after the client with possible interference to breathing and oxygenation; therefore, they are incorrect.

152. **Answer A is correct.** The client newly diagnosed with myasthenia gravis will be treated with intravenous steroids; therefore, he or she should be placed with a client who poses little risk of infection. The client with diabetes would be the most suitable roommate for the client. The clients described in Answers B, C, and D are less suitable than the client with diabetes because they pose an increased risk of infection.

153. **Answer C is correct.** The client should not be instructed to perform the Valsalva maneuver during central venous pressure reading. Such a request indicates that the student needs further teaching. Answers A, B, and D are incorrect because they indicate that the student understands the teaching on how to correctly check the CVP.

154. **Answer D is correct.** The most critical client should be assigned to the registered nurse; in this case, that is the client two days post-thoracotomy. The clients in Answers A, B, and C may be assigned to the LPN or CNA according to their care needs.

155. **Answer D is correct.** After inserting the Prostin E2 gel, the nurse should elevate the client's hips for 30 minutes to prevent loss of the gel. Answers A, B, and C do not prevent loss of the gel, so they are incorrect choices.

156. **Answer B is correct.** The client having a mammogram should be instructed to omit deodorants or powders beforehand because these may show up as calcification and may cause a false positive reading. Answer A is incorrect because there is no need to restrict fat. Answer C is incorrect because doing a mammogram does not replace the need for self-breast exams. Answer D is incorrect because a mammogram does not require a higher dose of radiation than an x-ray.

157. **Answer A is correct.** The nurse who fails to wear gloves consistently when removing dressings needs further teaching. Answers B, C, and D are incorrect choices because they indicate correct teaching and learning by the nurse.

158. **Answer A is correct.** The folic acid level is often assessed at the same time a Schilling test is done. Patients with pernicious anemia often have elevated levels of folic acid. Answers B, C, and D are not often assessed at the same time as a Schilling test, so they are incorrect choices.

159. **Answer A is correct.** Bilirubin is excreted through the kidneys, thus the need for increased fluids. Maintaining the body temperature is important but will not assist in eliminating bilirubin; therefore, Answer B is incorrect. Answers C and D are incorrect choices because they do not relate to the question.

160. **Answer C is correct.** The client with a recent laryngectomy should be seen first because of potential airway and nutritional complications caused by the surgery. The types of nursing care required by the clients in Answers A, B, and D do not take priority over the client with a recent laryngectomy; therefore, they are incorrect choices.

161. **Answer B is correct.** The best action for the nurse to take is to explore the interaction with the nursing assistant. This will allow for clarification of the situation. Changing the assignment in Answer A might need to be done, but talking to the nursing assistant is the first step. Answer C is incorrect because discussing the incident with the family is not necessary at this time. Answer D is not a first step, even though initiating a group session might be a plan for the future.

162. **Answer B is correct.** The nurse should report the incident to the charge nurse. Further action might be needed, but it will be done by the charge nurse. Answers A, C, and D are incorrect because discussing the nursing assistant's behavior with family is not needed at this time, and monitoring and ignoring the situation are inadequate responses.

163. **Answer D is correct.** The best client to assign to a newly licensed nurse is the client whose condition is most stable; in this case, it is the client with diverticulosis. The client receiving chemotherapy, the client with post–coronary artery bypass graft, and the client with a transurethral prostatectomy need a nurse experienced in caring for clients with these diagnoses, so Answers A, B, and C are incorrect.

164. **Answer D is correct.** Intrathecal medications are administered to destroy leukemic cells hiding in the CSF. Answers A, B, and C are incorrect statements regarding the use of intrathecal medications, so they are incorrect.

165. **Answer B is correct.** Montgomery straps are used to secure abdominal dressings that require frequent dressing changes, such as the client with an abdominal cholecystectomy. This client is not at higher risk of evisceration than other clients, so Answer A is incorrect. Montgomery straps are not used to secure the drains, so Answer C is incorrect. Sutures or clips are used to secure the wound of the client with an abdominal cholecystectomy, so Answer D is incorrect.

166. **Answer B is correct.** The nurse should anticipate an order for insertion of a nasogastric tube because the client with acute pancreatitis frequently has nausea and vomiting. Gastric decompression using a nasogastric tube prevents gastric juices from flowing into the duodenum. Answer A is incorrect because the vital signs, especially respirations, should be checked every four to eight hours or more often, as needed. Answer

C is incorrect because morphine or hydromorphone, not meperidine, is used to control pain. Answer D is incorrect because the client with acute pancreatitis is NPO.

167. **Answer B is correct.** Applying antipruritic lotions containing menthol, camphor, or mint oil to the skin will make the client with pruritis more comfortable. Answer A is incorrect because two warm showers daily will increase dryness and itching. Answer C is incorrect because powder is drying and may increase itching. Answer D is incorrect because placing warm compresses on the affected areas will increase the itching.

168. **Answer A is correct.** If the nurse is providing direct care to a client with influenza, the best item to wear is a mask because the virus is spread through the respiratory tract. Answers B, C, and D are incorrect because they do not provide sufficient protection for infections spread through the respiratory tract.

169. **Answer D is correct.** Abnormal grieving may be exhibited by a lack of feeling sad when the circumstances would normally create such feelings. Answers A, B, and C are all normal expressions of grief.

170. **Answer B is correct.** Frequent use of laxatives can lead to diarrhea and electrolyte loss. Answers A and D are incorrect because they are associated with aging and are not causes for fluid and electrolyte loss. Answer C would improve the client's fluid status, so it is incorrect.

171. **Answer B is correct.** The client with serum sodium of 170mEq/L has hypernatremia and might exhibit manic behavior. Answers A, C, and D are not associated with hypernatremia and are, therefore, incorrect.

172. **Answer A is correct.** The most likely reason for the client's symptoms is radiation to the neck because it might have damaged the parathyroid glands that regulate calcium and phosphorus. Answers B, C, and D are not reasons for hyperphosphatemia; therefore, they are incorrect.

173. **Answer A is correct.** The nurse should notify the physician because it is the responsibility of the physician to explain and clarify the procedure to the client. Answers B, C, and D are incorrect because they are not within the nurse's responsibility.

174. **Answer B is correct.** The most important item to remove are contact lenses because leaving them in can lead to corneal drying, particularly with contact lenses that are not extended-wear lenses. At the client's request, the other items may go with the client to surgery and be removed in the holding area. The nursing staff in those areas should be notified so the items can be properly cared for and returned with the client after surgery. Therefore, Answers A, C, and D are incorrect.

175. **Answer C is correct.** If the client eviscerates, the site should be covered with a sterile saline-soaked dressing. Answers A, B and D are incorrect choices because they are not appropriate nursing interventions for the client who eviscerates.

176. **Answer B is correct.** A staging of Tis or cancer in situ means that the cancer is still localized to the primary site. *T* stands for "tumor," and the *is* stands for "in situ." Cancer is staged in terms of tumor, node involvement, and metastasis. Answers A, C, and D are incorrect because Answer A refers to a tumor staging of Tx; Answer C refers to a tumor staging of N1, N2, or N3; and Answer D refers to a tumor staging of M1.

177. **Answer B is correct.** The nurse should ask the client to empty his bladder because a full bladder or full bowel can obscure the visualization of the kidney and ureters. Answer A is incorrect because fluids are increased after the test. Answer C is incorrect because there is no need to withhold medication for 8 hours before the test. Answer D is incorrect because the client will not require pain medication.

178. **Answer C is correct.** The adult client with a fractured femur will be placed in Buck's traction to realign the leg and to decrease spasms and pain. Bryant's traction is used for children weighing less than 30 pounds with leg fractures, so answer A is incorrect. Ice might be ordered to the site after repair of the fracture, but not for the entire extremity, so Answer B is incorrect. An abduction pillow is ordered after a total hip replacement, not for a fractured femur; therefore, Answer D is incorrect.

179. **Answer C is correct.** Glossitis (red, beefy tongue) is a specific characteristic of the client with pernicious anemia. Answers A, B, and D are not specific to pernicious anemia because they may occur with other conditions; therefore, they are incorrect choices.

180. **Answer B is correct.** The client may experience a feeling of pressure or discomfort as the biopsy is aspirated. Pain medication is usually given to make the client more comfortable during the procedure. Answer A is incorrect because the client will be positioned prone, not placed in a sitting position, for the biopsy. Answer C incorrect because the client is awake. Answer D is incorrect because the client can eat and drink following the biopsy.

181. **Answer C is correct.** Assessment of the quality of peripheral pulses is most important because the aorta is clamped during AAA repair. This decreases blood flow to the kidneys and lower extremities. Answers A, B, and D are not as important pre-op assessments for the client having a AAA repair, so they are incorrect.

182. **Answer A is correct.** Suctioning can cause a vagal response, lowering the heart rate and causing bradycardia. Answers B, C, and D are less likely to occur; therefore, they are incorrect.

183. **Answer C is correct.** The client with an implanted defibrillator should use a cell phone or any battery-operated device on the right side or the side opposite the implanted device. The client should also check the pulse rate and report dizziness or fainting. Answers A, B, and D are incorrect because the client can prepare food in the microwave, move the shoulder on the affected side, and travel in an airplane.

184. **Answer A is correct.** Swelling over the right parietal area of a newborn that does not cross the suture line describes a cephalohematoma, an area of bleeding outside the cranium. Answer B, molding, is overlapping of the bones of the cranium and is, therefore, incorrect. Answer C, a subdural hematoma, can be seen only on a CAT scan or x-ray. A caput succedaneum, in Answer D, refers to edema that crosses the suture line.

185. **Answer A is correct.** Postoperative care of the client with a lobectomy will include a closed chest drainage system. Answer B is incorrect because he will not be on bed rest for 48 hours. Answer C is incorrect because he will be positioned supine or in modified left-side lying position. Answer D is incorrect because he will not have chest physiotherapy as part of his postoperative care.

186. **Answer C is correct.** *H. pylori* infection is a finding associated with gastric cancer, not laryngeal cancer. Answers A, B, and D are incorrect because they are findings associated with laryngeal cancer.

187. **Answer D is correct.** A newborn normally loses weight in the first week of life. A loss of 10% is normal due to the passage of meconium stools and fluid loss. There is no evidence to indicate dehydration, hypoglycemia, or problems with formula are the result of the weight loss; therefore, Answers A, B, and C are incorrect.

188. **Answer C is correct.** The client with diverticulitis should avoid eating foods that are gas forming and that increase abdominal discomfort, such as cooked broccoli. Foods such as those listed in Answers A, B, and D are allowed.

189. **Answer D is correct.** Betoptic (betaxolol) can cause dizziness and vertigo. Answers A, B, and C are untrue statements; therefore, they are incorrect.

190. **Answer C is correct.** The client with diverticulosis should avoid foods with seeds. The foods in Answers A, B, and D will help prevent constipation that increases the likelihood of diverticulitis.

191. **Answer C is correct.** The most helpful information is the description of his stools. The stools associated with intussusception contain blood and mucus. Answers A, B, and D are not useful in establishing a diagnosis of intussusception.

192. **Answer C is correct.** An adverse effect of Tegretol (carbamazepine) is a decrease in white blood cell count. The values in Answers A and D are within normal limits, and Answer B is a lower limit of normal; therefore, Answers A, B, and D are incorrect.

193. **Answer D is correct.** Ewing's sarcoma is a bone cancer that usually affects the flat bones such as the ribs, so bone pain would be expected. Answers A, B, and C are not associated with this type of cancer and are incorrect.

194. **Answer D is correct.** The anterior fontanel usually closes by 18 months of age. Answers A, B, and C are incorrect times for closure of the anterior fontanel.

195. **Answer B is correct.** A torque wrench is kept at the bedside of the client immobilized with Crutchfield tongs. The device is used to make sure the right amount of pressure is placed on the screws during adjustment. Forceps, wire cutters, and a screwdriver, in Answers A, C, and D, would not be used and, therefore, are incorrect.

196. **Answer C is correct.** Fosamax (alendronate) should be taken with water only. The client should remain upright for at least 30 minutes after taking the medication. Answers A, B, and D are not applicable to taking Fosamax and, thus, are incorrect.

197. **Answer B is correct.** The client with burns to the face and neck needs airway assessment and supplemental oxygen, so applying oxygen is the priority. The next action should be to start an IV and medicate for pain, making answers A and C incorrect. Answer D, obtaining blood gases, at this point is of less priority.

198. **Answer A is correct.** The primary preoperative responsibility of the nurse is making sure the vital signs are recorded. Answers B, C, and D are preoperative responsibilities of the physician and, therefore, are incorrect for this question.

199. **Answer B is correct.** A potassium level of 1.9 indicates hypokalemia. The remaining lab values are within normal range, making Answers A, C, and D incorrect.

200. **Answer A is correct.** The best indication of resolution of paralytic ileus is the passage of stool or flatus. Answers B, C, and D are not specific indicators of resolution; therefore, they are incorrect.

201. **Answer A is correct.** The client with a ruptured spleen can be expected to exhibit Kehr's sign (increased abdominal pain exaggerated by deep breathing with pain being referred to the right shoulder). Answers B, C, and D are not specific to a ruptured spleen.

202. **Answer C is correct.** Daily measurement of the abdominal girth is the best method of determining the degree of early ascites. Measuring with a paper tape measure and marking the measured area is the most objective method of estimating ascites. Answers A and B are incorrect because abdominal enlargement and hepatomegaly may occur without ascites. Answer D is incorrect because peritoneal fluid wave is associated with advanced ascites.

203. **Answer B is correct.** The vital signs indicate hypovolemic shock or fluid volume deficit. Answers A, C, and D (cerebral tissue perfusion, airway clearance, and sensory perception alterations) are not indicated by the assessment findings; therefore, they are incorrect.

204. **Answer A is correct.** Finding out that the child with sickle cell anemia is playing baseball should raise concern because extreme activity, especially in warm weather, can lead to dehydration and increased sickling. Answers B, C, and D are not reasons for concern for a child with sickle cell anemia.

205. **Answer D is correct.** The client with neutropenia should not have potted plants or cut flowers in the room because they pose a risk of infection. Answers A, B, and C will not help to prevent infections and, therefore, are incorrect.

206. **Answer B is correct.** The nurse's initial action should be to lower the head of the bed because the client is obviously hypotensive. Answers A, C, and D are measures that may be needed later; therefore, they are incorrect.

207. **Answer C is correct.** Multiple-birth babies have reduced fetal iron stores, making them at greater risk for iron deficiency anemia. The newborns mentioned in Answers A, B, and D are less likely to have iron deficiency anemia.

208. **Answer A is correct.** The nurse should assess for signs of abnormal bleeding. An INR of 8 is too high. The normal INR is 2.0–3.0. Answer B is incorrect because DDAVP is used to treat mild forms of hemophilia. Answer C is incorrect because protamine sulfate is the antidote for heparin. Answer D is incorrect because the client does not need to limit the intake of foods rich in vitamin K at this time.

209. **Answer C is correct.** The food indicating the client's understanding of dietary management of osteoporosis is the yogurt, with approximately 400 mg of calcium per cup. The other foods are good choices, but not as good as the yogurt; therefore, Answers A, B, and D are incorrect.

210. Answer A is correct. The loading dose of magnesium sulfate is usually 4 grams administered over 20–30 minutes via infusion pump. Answer B is incorrect because side effects include feeling warm and flushed. Answer C is incorrect because the IV rate is set to maintain a urine output of 30–50 mL/hr. Answer D is incorrect because the patellar reflex is assessed before dosing.

211. Answer D is correct. The nurse should notify the physician of the mother's refusal to sign the permit based on her religious beliefs. If the transfusion is deemed to be life-saving, then the courts might have to intervene because the child is a minor. Answer A is incorrect because blood cannot be administered without a signed permit. Answers B and C are incorrect choices because the nurse should not encourage or coerce the mother to consent to the transfusion. The physician should explain the need for the transfusion and the consequences of withholding treatment.

212. Answer B is correct. The nurse should be most concerned with the client developing laryngeal edema because of the burns to the face and neck. Answer A, C, and D do not take priority over airway; therefore, they are incorrect.

213. Answer D is correct. The best indication that the plan of care is effective is a weight gain of 4 pounds in the last week. Answers A, B, and C indicate an awareness of the care needed, but they are not the best indicators that the plan of care has been effective; therefore, they are incorrect.

214. Answer D is correct. Paresthesia of the toes is not normal and can indicate compartment syndrome. At this time, pain beneath the cast is normal and, therefore, would not be reported as a concern. The client's toes should be warm to the touch, and pulses should be present. Answers A, B, and C, then, are incorrect.

215. Answer B is correct. During cardiac catheterization, a warm sensation is expected when the contrast media is injected. Answers A, C, and D are incorrect explanations for the client's statement.

216. Answer D is correct. Anabolic steroids are toxic to the liver, especially if used with other drugs that are also hepatotoxic. Answers A, B, and C are not organs affected the most by the use of anabolic steroids; therefore, they are incorrect.

217. Answer D is correct. A tonic clonic seizure is expected during electroconvulsive therapy. Answers A, B, and C are incorrect because they are not expected with electroconvulsive therapy.

218. Answer A is correct. The patient receiving radiation therapy should avoid sunlight during the treatment period and for a year after radiation therapy is completed. Answers B and C are incorrect because they will remove the markings needed for radiation therapy. Answer D is incorrect because redness and sore skin are expected with radiation therapy.

219. Answer B is correct. The entire family will need to take the medication. Answers A, C, and D are untrue statements; therefore, they are incorrect choices.

220. Answer B is correct. The nurse who is pregnant should not be assigned to care for the infant with RSV treated with Virazole (aerosolized ribavirin) because the medication can harm the fetus. Answers A, C, and D are incorrect because she may be assigned to care for the child with cystic fibrosis receiving tobramycin, the child with Hirschsprung's disease scheduled for barium enema, and the child with Meckel's diverticulum going for radiographic scintigraphy.

221. Answer A is correct. The client should be assessed for G6PD deficiency. Cells with reduced levels of G6PD break more easily when exposed to some drugs such as sulfonamides, aspirin, quinine derivatives, high doses of vitamin C, and thiazide diuretics. Answers B, C, and D do not relate to the question; therefore, they are incorrect.

222. Answer D is correct. The nurse should anticipate an order for Pitocin to begin contractions. The treatment of the patient with HELLP syndrome is delivery of the fetus. Answers A, B, and C are incorrect because ritodrine and terbutaline are used to treat premature labor, and methylergonovine is used to treat postpartal hemorrhage.

223. Answer D is correct. The registered nurse should not perform wound closure using sutures or clips because these duties are out of her scope of practice. Answers A, B, and C are incorrect because performing a vaginal exam on a patient in labor, removing a PICC line, and monitoring central venous pressure are within the scope of practice of the registered nurse.

224. Answer B is correct. The nurse should assess FHT and notify the physician immediately because painful and gross vaginal bleeding are symptoms of abruptio placenta. Answers A, C, and D do not take priority for the situation; therefore, they are incorrect.

225. Answer B is correct. Hyperglycemia is one of the side effects of Brethine (terbutaline). Answers A, C, and D are not associated with Brethine, so they are incorrect choices.

226. Answer C is correct. Desferal (deferoxamine) is used to treat iron toxicity. Answers A, B, and D are incorrect because they are antidotes for other drugs: Narcan is used to treat opiate toxicity, Digibind is used to treat digitalis toxicity, and Zinecard is used to treat doxorubicin toxicity.

227. Answer A is correct. If the nurse charts information that he did not perform, he can be charged with fraud. Answer B is incorrect because malpractice is harm that results to the client due to an erroneous action taken by the nurse. Answer C is incorrect because negligence is failure to perform a duty that the nurse knows should be performed. Answer D is incorrect because a tort is a wrongful act to the client or his belongings.

228. Answer D is correct. The client who should receive priority is the client with multiple sclerosis and who is being treated with IV cortisone. This client is at highest risk for complications. Answers A, B, and C are incorrect because these clients are more stable and can be seen later.

229. Answer B is correct. Out of all of these clients, it is best to place the pregnant client and the client with a broken arm and facial lacerations in the same room. These two clients probably do not need immediate attention and are least likely to disturb each other. The clients in Answers A, C, and D need to be placed in separate rooms because their conditions are more serious, they might need immediate attention, and they are more likely to disturb other patients.

230. **Answer A is correct.** Before instilling eye drops, the nurse should cleanse the area with warm water to remove any exudates. Answers B, C, and D are not true statements, so they are incorrect.

231. **Answer D is correct.** To decrease the risk of urinary tract infections, the female should clean the perineum from front to back. Answer A is incorrect because drinking citrus juices will not decrease the risk of UTIs. Answers B and C are incorrect choices because they do not decrease the risk of UTIs.

232. **Answer C is correct.** The nurse should encourage the parents to stay, to promote parent-child attachment and make the toddler feel more secure. Answers A, B, and D are not appropriate interventions for the hospitalized toddler.

233. **Answer B is correct.** The client should be instructed to avoid exposing the hearing aid to extremes in temperature. Answer A is incorrect because the ear mold is cleaned with soap and water, not alcohol. Answer C is incorrect because a toothpick is used to clean debris from the hole in the middle of the part that goes in the ear. Answer D is incorrect because hair spray, cosmetics, oils, and spray colognes should not be used near the hearing aid.

234. **Answer C is correct.** FHT can be detected at 8 weeks gestation using vaginal ultrasound. Answers A, B, and D are untrue statements.

235. **Answer A is correct.** Before giving the medication, the nurse should ask the patient to void and measure the amount because the medication may cause urinary retention. Answers B, C, and D are not specific to the medication; therefore, they are incorrect.

236. **Answer B is correct.** Brassy cough is associated with laryngotracheobronchitis, not epiglottitis. Answers A, C, and D are associated with epiglottitis; therefore, they are incorrect choices.

237. **Answer C is correct.** Exophthalmos, protrusion of eyeballs, is an ocular change that may be found in the client with hyperthyroidism. Answers A, B, and D are not associated with hyperthyroidism.

238. **Answer D is correct.** Selection of a food that contains little or no gluten indicates that the mother understands the dietary instruction. The child with celiac disease should be on a gluten-free diet. Gluten is primarily contained in grains such as wheat, oats, barley, and rye. The grains are replaced with rice, corn, and millet. Answers A, B, and C contain gluten, so they are incorrect choices.

239. **Answer C is correct.** The infant with gastroesophageal reflux (GER) is exempted from the recommendations of the American Academy of Pediatrics "Back to Sleep" campaign against SIDS. Answers A, B, and D are incorrect because the infants should be placed on their backs for sleep.

240. Answer B is correct. Immediately after an amniotomy, the nurse should expect to see a moderate amount of straw-colored clear fluid. Answers A, C, and D are not expected after an amniotomy; therefore, they are incorrect answers.

241. Answer D is correct. The client is usually given epidural anesthesia at approximately three centimeters dilation during the latent phase. Answer A is vague, Answer B indicates the end of the first stage of labor, and Answer C indicates the transition phase, not the latent phase of labor.

242. Answer B is correct. The first actions the nurse should take is to turn the client on her left side and apply oxygen. The normal fetal heart rate is 120–160 beats per minute. Answers A, C, and D are incorrect because they are not the first actions the nurse should take.

243. Answer D is correct. The expected effect of Pitocin (oxytocin) is progressive cervical dilation. Answers A, B, and C are not associated with the use of Pitocin.

244. Answer B is correct. Applying a fetal heart monitor is the appropriate action at this time. Answers A, C, and D are not indicated at this time; therefore, they are incorrect choices.

245. Answer B is correct. Absent variability is an abnormal finding and suggests fetal distress. Answers A, C, and D are normal findings; therefore, they are incorrect choices.

246. Answer D is correct. Clients admitted in labor are not to eat or drink. Ice chips might be allowed, but the amount of fluid might not be sufficient to prevent fluid volume deficit. Answers A, B, and C are not the most appropriate for the client completing the latent phase of labor, so they are incorrect.

247. Answer D is correct. The most likely explanation for the pattern is late deceleration. This type of deceleration is caused by uteroplacental insufficiency, or lack of oxygen. Answer A is incorrect because there is no data to support the conclusion that the fetus is asleep, Answer B is incorrect because cord compression results in a variable deceleration, and Answer C is incorrect because it is indicative of an early deceleration.

248. Answer C is correct. The most appropriate initial action by the nurse observing a variable deceleration would be to reposition the client on her left side. Administering oxygen is also indicated. Answer A is incorrect because it is not called for at this time. Answer B is incorrect because it is not needed, and answer D is incorrect because there is no data to indicate that the monitor has been applied incorrectly.

249. Answer D is correct. Accelerations of FHR with fetal movements are characteristics of a reassuring pattern. Answers A, B, and C indicate ominous findings on the fetal heart monitor and are, therefore, incorrect choices.

250. Answer C is correct. Epidural anesthesia decreases bladder sensation and the need to void. A full bladder decreases the progression of labor. Answers A, B, and D are incorrect because they contain untrue statements.

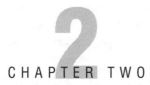

CHAPTER TWO

Practice Exam 2 and Rationales

1. The nurse is caring for a client with systemic lupus erythematosus (SLE). The major complication associated with systemic lupus erythematosus is:

   ○ **A.** Nephritis

   ○ **B.** Cardiomegaly

   ○ **C.** Desquamation

   ○ **D.** Meningitis

Quick Answer: **139**
Detailed Answer: **141**

2. A client with benign prostatic hypertrophy has been started on Proscar (finasteride). The nurse's discharge teaching should include:

   ○ **A.** Telling the client's wife not to touch the tablets

   ○ **B.** Explaining that the medication should be taken with meals

   ○ **C.** Telling the client that symptoms will improve in 1–2 weeks

   ○ **D.** Instructing the client to take the medication at bedtime, to prevent nocturia

Quick Answer: **139**
Detailed Answer: **141**

3. A five-year-old child is hospitalized for correction of congenital hip dysplasia. During the assessment of the child, the nurse can expect to find the presence of:

   ○ **A.** Scarf sign

   ○ **B.** Harlequin sign

   ○ **C.** Cullen's sign

   ○ **D.** Trendelenburg sign

Quick Answer: **139**
Detailed Answer: **141**

4. Which diet is associated with an increased risk of colorectal cancer?

Quick Answer: **139**
Detailed Answer: **141**

   ○ **A.** Low protein, complex carbohydrates

   ○ **B.** High protein, simple carbohydrates

   ○ **C.** High fat, refined carbohydrates

   ○ **D.** Low carbohydrates, complex proteins

5. The nurse is caring for an infant following a cleft lip repair. While comforting the infant, the nurse should avoid:

Quick Answer: **139**
Detailed Answer: **141**

   ○ **A.** Holding the infant

   ○ **B.** Offering a pacifier

   ○ **C.** Providing a mobile

   ○ **D.** Offering sterile water

6. The physician has diagnosed a client with cirrhosis characterized by asterixis. If the nurse assesses the client with asterixis, he can expect to find:

Quick Answer: **139**
Detailed Answer: **141**

   ○ **A.** Irregular movement of the wrist

   ○ **B.** Enlargement of the breasts

   ○ **C.** Dilated veins around the umbilicus

   ○ **D.** Redness of the palmar surfaces

7. The physician has ordered Amoxil (amoxicillin) 500mg capsules for a client with esophageal varices. The nurse can best care for the client's needs by:

Quick Answer: **139**
Detailed Answer: **141**

   ○ **A.** Giving the medication as ordered

   ○ **B.** Providing extra water with the medication

   ○ **C.** Giving the medication with an antacid

   ○ **D.** Requesting an alternate form of the medication

8. A client with an inguinal hernia asks the nurse why he should have surgery when he has had a hernia for years. The nurse understands that surgery is recommended to:

Quick Answer: **139**
Detailed Answer: **141**

   ○ **A.** Prevent strangulation of the bowel

   ○ **B.** Prevent malabsorptive disorders

   ○ **C.** Decrease secretion of bile salts

   ○ **D.** Increase intestinal motility

9. The nurse is providing dietary instructions for a client with iron-deficiency anemia. Which food is a poor source of iron?

   ○ **A.** Tomatoes

   ○ **B.** Legumes

   ○ **C.** Dried fruits

   ○ **D.** Nuts

Quick Answer: **139**
Detailed Answer: **142**

10. A client is admitted with suspected acute pancreatitis. Which lab finding confirms the diagnosis?

    ○ **A.** Blood glucose of 260mg/dL

    ○ **B.** White cell count of 21,000cu/mm

    ○ **C.** Platelet count of 250,000cu/mm

    ○ **D.** Serum amylase level of 600 units/dL

Quick Answer: **139**
Detailed Answer: **142**

11. The nurse is teaching a client with Parkinson's disease ways to prevent curvatures of the spine associated with the disease. To prevent spinal flexion, the nurse should tell the client to:

    ○ **A.** Periodically lie prone without a neck pillow.

    ○ **B.** Sleep only in dorsal recumbent position.

    ○ **C.** Rest in supine position with his head elevated.

    ○ **D.** Sleep on either side, but keep his back straight.

Quick Answer: **139**
Detailed Answer: **142**

12. The physician has ordered Dilantin (phenytoin) 100mg intravenously for a client with generalized tonic clonic seizures. The nurse should administer the medication:

    ○ **A.** Rapidly with an IV push

    ○ **B.** With IV dextrose

    ○ **C.** Slowly over 2–3 minutes

    ○ **D.** Through a small vein

Quick Answer: **139**
Detailed Answer: **142**

13. The nurse is planning dietary changes for a client following an episode of acute pancreatitis. Which diet is suitable for the client?

    ○ **A.** Low calorie, low carbohydrate

    ○ **B.** High calorie, low fat

    ○ **C.** High protein, high fat

    ○ **D.** Low protein, high carbohydrate

Quick Answer: **139**
Detailed Answer: **142**

14. A client is admitted with a diagnosis of polycythemia vera. The nurse should closely monitor the client for:

Quick Answer: **139**
Detailed Answer: **142**

- ○ **A.** Increased blood pressure
- ○ **B.** Decreased respirations
- ○ **C.** Increased urinary output
- ○ **D.** Decreased oxygen saturation

15. A client with hypothyroidism frequently complains of feeling cold. The nurse should tell the client that she will be more comfortable if she:

Quick Answer: **139**
Detailed Answer: **142**

- ○ **A.** Uses an electric blanket at night
- ○ **B.** Dresses in extra layers of clothing
- ○ **C.** Applies a heating pad to her feet
- ○ **D.** Takes a hot bath morning and evening

16. The nurse caring for a client with a closed head injury obtains an intracranial pressure (ICP) reading of 17mmHg. The nurse recognizes that:

Quick Answer: **139**
Detailed Answer: **142**

- ○ **A.** The ICP is elevated and the doctor should be notified.
- ○ **B.** The ICP is normal; therefore, no further action is needed.
- ○ **C.** The ICP is low and the client needs additional IV fluids.
- ○ **D.** The ICP reading is not as reliable as the Glascow coma scale.

17. A client has been hospitalized with a diagnosis of laryngeal cancer. Which factor is most significant in the development of laryngeal cancer?

Quick Answer: **139**
Detailed Answer: **142**

- ○ **A.** A family history of laryngeal cancer
- ○ **B.** Chronic inhalation of noxious fumes
- ○ **C.** Frequent straining of the vocal cords
- ○ **D.** A history of frequent alcohol and tobacco use

18. The nurse is completing an assessment history of a client with pernicious anemia. Which complaint differentiates pernicious anemia from other types of anemia?

Quick Answer: **139**
Detailed Answer: **142**

- ○ **A.** Difficulty in breathing after exertion
- ○ **B.** Numbness and tingling in the extremities
- ○ **C.** A faster than usual heart rate
- ○ **D.** Feelings of lightheadedness

19. A client with rheumatoid arthritis is beginning to develop flexion contractures of the knees. The nurse should tell the client to:

Quick Answer: 139
Detailed Answer: 143

   ○ **A.** Lie prone and let her feet hang over the mattress edge

   ○ **B.** Lie supine, with her feet rotated inward

   ○ **C.** Lie on her right side and point her toes downward

   ○ **D.** Lie on her left side and allow her feet to remain in a neutral position

20. The chart of a client with schizophrenia states that the client has echolalia. The nurse can expect the client to:

Quick Answer: 139
Detailed Answer: 143

   ○ **A.** Speak using words that rhyme

   ○ **B.** Repeat words or phrases used by others

   ○ **C.** Include irrelevant details in conversation

   ○ **D.** Make up new words with new meanings

21. The mother of a one-year-old with sickle cell anemia wants to know why the condition didn't show up in the nursery. The nurse's response is based on the knowledge that:

Quick Answer: 139
Detailed Answer: 143

   ○ **A.** There is no test to measure abnormal hemoglobin in newborns.

   ○ **B.** Infants do not have insensible fluid loss before a year of age.

   ○ **C.** Infants rarely have infections that would cause them to have a sickling crises.

   ○ **D.** The presence of fetal hemoglobin protects the infant.

22. Which early morning activity helps to reduce the symptoms associated with rheumatoid arthritis?

Quick Answer: 139
Detailed Answer: 143

   ○ **A.** Brushing the teeth

   ○ **B.** Drinking a glass of juice

   ○ **C.** Holding a cup of coffee

   ○ **D.** Brushing the hair

23. A client with B negative blood requires a blood transfusion during surgery. If no B negative blood is available, the client should be transfused with:

Quick Answer: 139
Detailed Answer: 143

   ○ **A.** A positive blood

   ○ **B.** B positive blood

   ○ **C.** O negative blood

   ○ **D.** AB negative blood

24. The nurse notes that a post-operative client's respirations have dropped from 14 to 6 breaths per minute. The nurse administers Narcan (naloxone) per standing order. Following administration of the medication, the nurse should assess the client for:

   ○ **A.** Pupillary changes

   ○ **B.** Projectile vomiting

   ○ **C.** Wheezing respirations

   ○ **D.** Sudden, intense pain

Quick Answer: **139**
Detailed Answer: **143**

25. A newborn weighed seven pounds at birth. At six months of age, the infant could be expected to weigh:

   ○ **A.** 14 pounds

   ○ **B.** 18 pounds

   ○ **C.** 25 pounds

   ○ **D.** 30 pounds

Quick Answer: **139**
Detailed Answer: **143**

26. A client with nontropical sprue has an exacerbation of symptoms. Which meal selection is responsible for the recurrence of the client's symptoms?

   ○ **A.** Tossed salad with oil and vinegar dressing

   ○ **B.** Baked potato with sour cream and chives

   ○ **C.** Cream of tomato soup and crackers

   ○ **D.** Mixed fruit and yogurt

Quick Answer: **139**
Detailed Answer: **143**

27. A client with congestive heart failure has been receiving digoxin (Laxoxin). Which finding indicates that the medication is having a desired effect?

   ○ **A.** Increased urinary output

   ○ **B.** Stabilized weight

   ○ **C.** Improved appetite

   ○ **D.** Increased pedal edema

Quick Answer: **139**
Detailed Answer: **143**

28. Which play activity is best suited to the gross motor skills of a toddler?

   ○ **A.** Coloring book and crayons

   ○ **B.** Ball

   ○ **C.** Building cubes

   ○ **D.** Swing set

Quick Answer: **139**
Detailed Answer: **143**

29. A client in labor admits to using alcohol throughout the pregnancy. The most recent use was the day before. Based on the client's history, the nurse should give priority to assessing the newborn for:

   ○ **A.** Respiratory depression
   ○ **B.** Wide-set eyes
   ○ **C.** Jitteriness
   ○ **D.** Low-set ears

Quick Answer: **139**
Detailed Answer: **143**

30. The physician has ordered Basaljel (aluminum carbonate gel) for a client with recurrent indigestion. The nurse should teach the client common side effects of the medication, which include:

   ○ **A.** Constipation
   ○ **B.** Urinary retention
   ○ **C.** Diarrhea
   ○ **D.** Confusion

Quick Answer: **139**
Detailed Answer: **144**

31. A client is admitted with suspected abdominal aortic aneurysm (AAA). A common complaint of the client with an abdominal aortic aneurysm is:

   ○ **A.** Loss of sensation in the lower extremities
   ○ **B.** Back pain that lessens when standing
   ○ **C.** Decreased urinary output
   ○ **D.** Pulsations in the periumbilical area

Quick Answer: **139**
Detailed Answer: **144**

32. The nurse is caring for a client hospitalized with nephrotic syndrome. Based on the client's treatment, the nurse should:

   ○ **A.** Limit the number of visitors.
   ○ **B.** Provide a low-protein diet.
   ○ **C.** Discuss the possibility of dialysis.
   ○ **D.** Offer the client additional fluids.

Quick Answer: **139**
Detailed Answer: **144**

33. A client is admitted with acute adrenal crisis. During the intake assessment, the nurse can expect to find that the client has:

   ○ **A.** Low blood pressure
   ○ **B.** A slow, regular pulse
   ○ **C.** Warm, flushed skin
   ○ **D.** Increased urination

Quick Answer: **139**
Detailed Answer: **144**

34. A five-month-old infant is admitted to the ER with a temperature of 103.6°F and irritability. The mother states that the child has been listless for the past several hours and that he had a seizure on the way to the hospital. A lumbar puncture confirms a diagnosis of bacterial meningitis. The nurse should assess the infant for:

- ○ **A.** Periorbital edema
- ○ **B.** Tenseness of the anterior fontanel
- ○ **C.** Positive Babinski reflex
- ○ **D.** Negative scarf sign

Quick Answer: **139**
Detailed Answer: **144**

35. A client with pneumocystis jiroveci pneumonia is receiving intravenous Pentam (pentamidine). While administering the medication, the nurse should give priority to checking the client's:

- ○ **A.** Deep tendon reflexes
- ○ **B.** Blood pressure
- ○ **C.** Urine output
- ○ **D.** Tissue turgor

Quick Answer: **139**
Detailed Answer: **144**

36. The doctor has ordered Ampicillin 100mg every six hours IV push for an infant weighing 7kg. The suggested dose for infants is 25–50mg/kg/day in equally divided doses. The nurse should:

- ○ **A.** Give the medication as ordered.
- ○ **B.** Give half the amount ordered.
- ○ **C.** Give the ordered amount q 12 hrs.
- ○ **D.** Check the order with the doctor.

Quick Answer: **139**
Detailed Answer: **144**

37. An elderly client is hospitalized for a transurethral prostatectomy. Which finding should be reported to the doctor immediately?

- ○ **A.** Hourly urinary output of 40–50mL
- ○ **B.** Bright red urine with many clots
- ○ **C.** Dark red urine with few clots
- ○ **D.** Requests for pain med every four hours

Quick Answer: **139**
Detailed Answer: **144**

38. Which statement by the parent of a child with sickle cell anemia indicates an understanding of the disease?

- ○ **A.** "The pain he has is due to the presence of too many red blood cells."
- ○ **B.** "He will be able to go snow skiing with his friends as long as he stays warm."
- ○ **C.** "He will need extra fluids in summer to prevent dehydration."
- ○ **D.** "There is very little chance that his brother will have sickle cell."

39. A toddler with otitis media has just completed antibiotic therapy. A recheck appointment should be made to:

- ○ **A.** Determine whether the ear infection has affected her hearing.
- ○ **B.** Make sure that she has taken all the antibiotic.
- ○ **C.** Document that the infection has completely cleared.
- ○ **D.** Obtain a new prescription, in case the infection recurs.

40. A nine-year-old is admitted with suspected rheumatic fever. Which finding is suggestive of Sydenham's chorea?

- ○ **A.** Irregular movements of the extremities and facial grimacing
- ○ **B.** Painless swellings over the extensor surfaces of the joints
- ○ **C.** Faint areas of red demarcation over the back and abdomen
- ○ **D.** Swelling, inflammation, and effusion of the joints

41. A child with croup is placed in a cool, high-humidity tent connected to room air. The primary purpose of the high-humidity tent is to:

- ○ **A.** Prevent insensible water loss
- ○ **B.** Provide a moist environment with oxygen at 30%
- ○ **C.** Prevent dehydration and reduce fever
- ○ **D.** Liquefy secretions and relieve laryngeal spasm

42. The nurse is suctioning the tracheostomy of an adult client. The recommended pressure setting for performing tracheostomy suctioning on the adult client is:

- ○ **A.** 40–60mmHg
- ○ **B.** 60–80mmHg
- ○ **C.** 80–120mmHg
- ○ **D.** 120–140mmHg

Quick Answer: **139**
Detailed Answer: **145**

43. A client is admitted with a diagnosis of myxedema. An initial assessment of the client would reveal the symptoms of:

- ○ **A.** Slow pulse rate, weight loss, diarrhea, and cardiac failure
- ○ **B.** Weight gain, lethargy, slowed speech, and decreased respiratory rate
- ○ **C.** Rapid pulse, constipation, and bulging eyes
- ○ **D.** Decreased body temperature, weight loss, and increased respirations

Quick Answer: **139**
Detailed Answer: **145**

44. Which statement describes the contagious stage of varicella?

- ○ **A.** The contagious stage is one day before the onset of the rash until the appearance of vesicles.
- ○ **B.** The contagious stage lasts during the vesicular and crusting stages of the lesions.
- ○ **C.** The contagious stage is from the onset of the rash until the rash disappears.
- ○ **D.** The contagious stage is one day before the onset of the rash until all the lesions are crusted.

Quick Answer: **139**
Detailed Answer: **145**

45. The nurse is reviewing the results of a sweat test taken from a child with cystic fibrosis. Which finding supports the client's diagnosis?

- ○ **A.** A sweat potassium concentration less than 40mEq/L
- ○ **B.** A sweat chloride concentration greater than 60mEq/L
- ○ **C.** A sweat potassium concentration greater than 40mEq/L
- ○ **D.** A sweat chloride concentration less than 40mEq/L

Quick Answer: **139**
Detailed Answer: **145**

46. A client in labor has an order for Demerol (meperidine) 75mg. IM to be administered 10 minutes before delivery. The nurse should:

Quick Answer: **139**
Detailed Answer: **145**

- ○ **A.** Wait until the client is placed on the delivery table and administer the medication.
- ○ **B.** Question the order because the medication might cause respiratory depression in the newborn.
- ○ **C.** Give the medication IM during the delivery to prevent pain from the episiotomy.
- ○ **D.** Give the medication as ordered.

47. Which of the following statements describes Piaget's stage of concrete operations?

Quick Answer: **139**
Detailed Answer: **145**

- ○ **A.** Reflex activity proceeds to imitative behavior.
- ○ **B.** The ability to see another's point of view increases.
- ○ **C.** Thought processes become more logical and coherent.
- ○ **D.** The ability to think abstractly leads to logical conclusion.

48. A client admitted to the psychiatric unit claims to be the Pope and insists that he will not be kept away from his followers. The most likely explanation for the client's delusion is:

Quick Answer: **139**
Detailed Answer: **145**

- ○ **A.** A reaction formation
- ○ **B.** A stressful event
- ○ **C.** Low self-esteem
- ○ **D.** Overwhelming anxiety

49. Which of the following statements reflects Kohlberg's theory of the moral development of the preschool-age child?

Quick Answer: **139**
Detailed Answer: **145**

- ○ **A.** Obeying adults is seen as correct behavior.
- ○ **B.** Showing respect for parents is seen as important.
- ○ **C.** Pleasing others is viewed as good behavior.
- ○ **D.** Behavior is determined by consequences.

50. The nurse is caring for an eight-year-old following a routine tonsillectomy. Which finding should be reported immediately?

Quick Answer: **139**
Detailed Answer: **146**

- ○ **A.** Reluctance to swallow
- ○ **B.** Drooling of blood-tinged saliva
- ○ **C.** An axillary temperature of 99°F
- ○ **D.** Respiratory stridor

51. The nurse is admitting a client with a suspected duodenal ulcer. The client will most likely report that his abdominal discomfort decreases when he:

Quick Answer: **139**
Detailed Answer: **146**

- ○ **A.** Avoids eating
- ○ **B.** Rests in a recumbent position
- ○ **C.** Eats a meal or snack
- ○ **D.** Sits upright after eating

52. The nurse is assessing a newborn in the well-baby nursery. Which finding should alert the nurse to the possibility of a cardiac anomaly?

Quick Answer: **139**
Detailed Answer: **146**

- ○ **A.** Diminished femoral pulses
- ○ **B.** Harlequin's sign
- ○ **C.** Circumoral pallor
- ○ **D.** Acrocyanosis

53. A two-year-old is hospitalized with a diagnosis of Kawasaki's disease. A severe complication of Kawasaki's disease is:

Quick Answer: **139**
Detailed Answer: **146**

- ○ **A.** The development of Brushfield spots
- ○ **B.** The eruption of Hutchinson's teeth
- ○ **C.** The development of coxa plana
- ○ **D.** The creation of a giant aneurysm

54. The charge nurse is formulating a discharge teaching plan for a client with mild preeclampsia. The nurse should give priority to:

Quick Answer: **139**
Detailed Answer: **146**

- ○ **A.** Teaching the client to report a nosebleed
- ○ **B.** Instructing the client to maintain strict bed rest
- ○ **C.** Telling the client to notify the doctor of pedal edema
- ○ **D.** Advising the client to avoid sodium sources in the diet

55. The nurse is preparing to discharge a client who is taking an MAOI. The nurse should instruct the client to:

Quick Answer: **139**
Detailed Answer: **146**

- ○ **A.** Wear protective clothing and sunglasses when outside.
- ○ **B.** Avoid over-the-counter cold and hay fever preparations.
- ○ **C.** Drink at least eight glasses of water a day.
- ○ **D.** Increase his intake of high-quality protein.

56. Which of the following meal selections is appropriate for the client with celiac disease?

Quick Answer: **139**
Detailed Answer: **146**

- ○ **A.** Toast, jam, and apple juice
- ○ **B.** Peanut butter cookies and milk
- ○ **C.** Rice Krispies bar and milk
- ○ **D.** Cheese pizza and Kool-Aid

57. A client with hyperthyroidism is taking Eskalith (lithium carbonate) to inhibit thyroid hormone release. Which complaint by the client should alert the nurse to a problem with the client's medication?

Quick Answer: **139**
Detailed Answer: **146**

- ○ **A.** The client complains of blurred vision.
- ○ **B.** The client complains of increased thirst and increased urination.
- ○ **C.** The client complains of increased weight gain over the past year.
- ○ **D.** The client complains of rhinorrhea.

58. The physician has ordered intravenous fluid with potassium for a client admitted with gastroenteritis and dehydration. Before adding potassium to the intravenous fluid, the nurse should:

Quick Answer: **139**
Detailed Answer: **146**

- ○ **A.** Assess the urinary output.
- ○ **B.** Obtain arterial blood gases.
- ○ **C.** Perform a dextrostick.
- ○ **D.** Obtain a stool culture.

59. A two-month-old infant has just received her first Tetramune injection. The nurse should tell the mother that the immunization:

Quick Answer: **139**
Detailed Answer: **146**

- ○ **A.** Will need to be repeated when the child is four years of age
- ○ **B.** Is given to determine whether the child is susceptible to pertussis
- ○ **C.** Is one of a series of injections that protects against diphtheria, pertussis, tetanus, and H.influenzae b
- ○ **D.** Is a one-time injection that protects against measles, mumps, rubella, and varicella

60. A client with Addison's disease has been receiving glucocorticoid therapy. Which finding indicates a need for dosage adjustment?

Quick Answer: **139**
Detailed Answer: **146**

- ○ **A.** Dryness of the skin and mucus membranes
- ○ **B.** Dizziness when rising to a standing position
- ○ **C.** A weight gain of six pounds in the past week
- ○ **D.** Difficulty in remaining asleep

61. The nurse is caring for an obstetrical client in early labor. After the rupture of membranes, the nurse should give priority to:

Quick Answer: **139**
Detailed Answer: **147**

- ○ **A.** Applying an internal monitor
- ○ **B.** Assessing fetal heart tones
- ○ **C.** Assisting with epidural anesthesia
- ○ **D.** Inserting a Foley catheter

62. The physician has prescribed Synthroid (levothyroxine) for a client with myxedema. Which statement indicates that the client understands the nurse's teaching regarding the medication?

Quick Answer: **139**
Detailed Answer: **147**

- ○ **A.** "I will take the medication each morning after breakfast."
- ○ **B.** "I will check my heart rate before taking the medication."
- ○ **C.** "I will report visual disturbances to my doctor."
- ○ **D.** "I will stop the medication if I develop gastric upset."

63. The nurse is caring for a client with a radium implant for the treatment of cervical cancer. While caring for the client with a radioactive implant, the nurse should:

Quick Answer: **139**
Detailed Answer: **147**

- ○ **A.** Provide emotional support by spending additional time with the client.
- ○ **B.** Stand at the foot of the bed when talking to the client.
- ○ **C.** Avoid handling items used by the client.
- ○ **D.** Wear a badge to monitor the amount of time spent in the client's room.

64. The nurse is caring for a client hospitalized with bipolar disorder, manic phase. Which of the following snacks would be best for the client?

Quick Answer: **139**
Detailed Answer: **147**

- ○ **A.** Potato chips
- ○ **B.** Diet cola
- ○ **C.** Apple
- ○ **D.** Milkshake

65. The physician has prescribed imipramine (Tofranil) for a client with depression. The nurse should continue to monitor the client's affect because the maximal effects of tricyclic antidepressant medication do not occur for:

- ○ **A.** 48–72 hours
- ○ **B.** 5–7 days
- ○ **C.** 2–4 weeks
- ○ **D.** 3–6 months

66. An elderly client with glaucoma has been prescribed Timoptic (timolol) eyedrops. Timoptic should be used with caution in clients with a history of:

- ○ **A.** Diabetes
- ○ **B.** Gastric ulcers
- ○ **C.** Emphysema
- ○ **D.** Pancreatitis

67. A two-year-old is hospitalized with suspected intussusception. Which finding is associated with intussusception?

- ○ **A.** "Currant jelly" stools
- ○ **B.** Projectile vomiting
- ○ **C.** "Ribbonlike" stools
- ○ **D.** Palpable mass over the flank

68. Which of the following findings would be expected in the infant with biliary atresia?

- ○ **A.** Rapid weight gain and hepatomegaly
- ○ **B.** Dark stools and poor weight gain
- ○ **C.** Abdominal distention and poor weight gain
- ○ **D.** Abdominal distention and rapid weight gain

69. A client is being treated for cancer with linear acceleration radiation. The physician has marked the radiation site with a blue marking pen. The nurse should:

- ○ **A.** Remove the unsightly markings with acetone or alcohol.
- ○ **B.** Cover the radiation site with loose gauze dressing.
- ○ **C.** Sprinkle baby powder over the radiated area.
- ○ **D.** Refrain from using soap or lotion on the marked area.

70. The blood alcohol concentration of a client admitted following a motor vehicle accident is 460mg/dL. The nurse should give priority to monitoring the client for:

- ○ **A.** Loss of coordination
- ○ **B.** Respiratory depression
- ○ **C.** Visual hallucinations
- ○ **D.** Tachycardia

Quick Answer: **139**
Detailed Answer: **147**

71. The nurse is caring for a client with acromegaly. Following a transphenoidal hypophysectomy, the nurse should:

- ○ **A.** Monitor the client's blood sugar.
- ○ **B.** Suction the mouth and pharynx every hour.
- ○ **C.** Place the client in low Trendelenburg position.
- ○ **D.** Encourage the client to cough.

Quick Answer: **139**
Detailed Answer: **148**

72. A client newly diagnosed with diabetes is started on Precose (acarbose). The nurse should tell the client that the medication should be taken:

- ○ **A.** one hour before meals
- ○ **B.** 30 minutes after meals
- ○ **C.** With the first bite of a meal
- ○ **D.** Daily at bedtime

Quick Answer: **139**
Detailed Answer: **148**

73. A client with a deep decubitus ulcer is receiving therapy in the hyperbaric oxygen chamber. Before therapy, the nurse should:

- ○ **A.** Apply a lanolin-based lotion to the skin.
- ○ **B.** Wash the skin with water and pat dry.
- ○ **C.** Cover the area with a petroleum gauze.
- ○ **D.** Apply an occlusive dressing to the site.

Quick Answer: **139**
Detailed Answer: **148**

74. The physician has ordered DDAVP (desmopressin acetate) for a client with diabetes insipidus. Which finding indicates that the medication is having its intended effect?

- ○ **A.** The client's appetite has improved.
- ○ **B.** The client's morning blood sugar was 120mg/dL.
- ○ **C.** The client's urinary output has decreased.
- ○ **D.** The client's activity level has increased.

Quick Answer: **139**
Detailed Answer: **148**

75. A client with pregnancy-induced hypertension is scheduled for a C-section. Before surgery, the nurse should keep the client:

    ○ **A.** On her right side

    ○ **B.** Supine with a small pillow

    ○ **C.** On her left side

    ○ **D.** In knee chest position

Quick Answer: **139**
Detailed Answer: **148**

76. The physician has prescribed Coumadin (sodium warfarin) for a client having transient ischemic attacks. Which laboratory test measures the therapeutic level of Coumadin?

    ○ **A.** Prothrombin time

    ○ **B.** Clot retraction time

    ○ **C.** Partial thromboplastin time

    ○ **D.** Bleeding time

Quick Answer: **139**
Detailed Answer: **148**

77. An adolescent client with cystic acne has a prescription for Accutane (isotretinoin). Which lab work is needed before beginning the medication?

    ○ **A.** Complete blood count

    ○ **B.** Clean-catch urinalysis

    ○ **C.** Liver profile

    ○ **D.** Thyroid function test

Quick Answer: **139**
Detailed Answer: **148**

78. Twenty-four hours after an uncomplicated labor and delivery, a client's WBC is 12,000cu/mm. The elevation in the client's WBC is most likely an indication of:

    ○ **A.** A normal response to the birth process

    ○ **B.** An acute bacterial infection

    ○ **C.** A sexually transmitted virus

    ○ **D.** Dehydration from being NPO during labor

Quick Answer: **139**
Detailed Answer: **148**

79. The home health nurse is visiting a client who plans to deliver her baby at home. Which statement by the client indicates an understanding regarding screening for phenylketonuria (PKU)?

    ○ **A.** "I will need to take the baby to the clinic within 24 hours of delivery to have blood drawn."

    ○ **B.** "I will need to schedule a home visit for PKU screening when the baby is three-days-old."

    ○ **C.** "I will remind the midwife to save a specimen of cord blood for the PKU test."

    ○ **D.** "I will have the PKU test done when I take her for her first immunizations."

Quick Answer: **139**
Detailed Answer: **148**

80. The physician has ordered intubation and mechanical ventilation for a client with periods of apnea following a closed head injury. Arterial blood gases reveal a pH of 7.47, PCO_2 of 28, and HCO_3 of 23. These findings indicate that the client has:

Quick Answer: **139**
Detailed Answer: **148**

- ○ **A.** Respiratory acidosis
- ○ **B.** Respiratory alkalosis
- ○ **C.** Metabolic acidosis
- ○ **D.** Metabolic alkalosis

81. A client is diagnosed with emphysema and cor pulmonale. Which findings are characteristic of cor pulmonale?

Quick Answer: **139**
Detailed Answer: **149**

- ○ **A.** Hypoxia, shortness of breath, and exertional fatigue
- ○ **B.** Weight loss, increased RBC, and fever
- ○ **C.** Rales, edema, and enlarged spleen
- ○ **D.** Edema of the lower extremities and distended neck veins

82. A client with a laryngectomy returns from surgery with a nasogastric tube in place. The primary reason for placement of the nasogastric tube is to:

Quick Answer: **139**
Detailed Answer: **149**

- ○ **A.** Prevent swelling and dysphagia
- ○ **B.** Decompress the stomach
- ○ **C.** Prevent contamination of the suture line
- ○ **D.** Promote healing of the oral mucosa

83. The physician orders the removal of an in-dwelling catheter the second post-operative day for a client with a prostatectomy. The client complains of pain and dribbling of urine the first time he voids. The nurse should tell the client that:

Quick Answer: **139**
Detailed Answer: **149**

- ○ **A.** Using warm compresses over the bladder will lessen the discomfort.
- ○ **B.** Perineal exercises will be started in a few days to help relieve his symptoms.
- ○ **C.** If the symptoms don't improve, the catheter will have to be reinserted.
- ○ **D.** His complaints are common and will improve over the next few days.

84. A client with a right lobectomy is being transported from the intensive care unit to a medical unit. The nurse understands that the client's chest drainage system:

Quick Answer: **139**
Detailed Answer: **149**

- ○ **A.** Can be disconnected from suction if the chest tube is clamped
- ○ **B.** Can be disconnected from suction, but the chest tube should remain unclamped
- ○ **C.** Must remain connected by means of a portable suction
- ○ **D.** Must be kept even with the client's shoulders during the transport

85. A nurse is caring for a client with a myocardial infarction. The nurse recognizes that the most common complication in the client following a myocardial infarction is:

Quick Answer: **139**
Detailed Answer: **149**

- ○ **A.** Right ventricular hypertrophy
- ○ **B.** Cardiac dysrhythmia
- ○ **C.** Left ventricular hypertrophy
- ○ **D.** Hyperkalemia

86. A client develops a temperature of 102°F following coronary artery bypass surgery. The nurse should notify the physician immediately because elevations in temperature:

Quick Answer: **139**
Detailed Answer: **149**

- ○ **A.** Increase cardiac output
- ○ **B.** Indicate cardiac tamponade
- ○ **C.** Decrease cardiac output
- ○ **D.** Indicate graft rejection

87. The chart indicates that a client has expressive aphasia following a stroke. The nurse understands that the client will have difficulty with:

Quick Answer: **139**
Detailed Answer: **149**

- ○ **A.** Speaking and writing
- ○ **B.** Comprehending spoken words
- ○ **C.** Carrying out purposeful motor activity
- ○ **D.** Recognizing and using an object correctly

88. A client receiving Parnate (tranylcypromine) is admitted in a hypertensive crisis. Which food is most likely to produce a hypertensive crisis when taken with the medication?

Quick Answer: **139**
Detailed Answer: **149**

   ○ **A.** Processed cheese
   ○ **B.** Cottage cheese
   ○ **C.** Cream cheese
   ○ **D.** Cheddar cheese

89. To prevent deformities of the knee joints in a client with an exacerbation of rheumatoid arthritis, the nurse should:

Quick Answer: **139**
Detailed Answer: **149**

   ○ **A.** Tell the client to remain on bed rest until swelling subsides.
   ○ **B.** Discourage passive range of motion because it will cause further swelling.
   ○ **C.** Encourage motion of the joint within the limits of pain.
   ○ **D.** Tell the client she will need joint immobilization for 2–3 weeks.

90. The nurse is assessing a trauma client in the emergency room when she notes a penetrating abdominal wound with exposed viscera. The nurse should:

Quick Answer: **139**
Detailed Answer: **150**

   ○ **A.** Apply a clean dressing to protect the wound.
   ○ **B.** Cover the exposed viscera with a sterile saline gauze.
   ○ **C.** Gently replace the abdominal contents.
   ○ **D.** Cover the area with a petroleum gauze.

91. A client is admitted to the emergency room with multiple injuries. What is the proper sequence for managing the client?

Quick Answer: **139**
Detailed Answer: **150**

   ○ **A.** Assess for head injuries, control hemorrhage, establish an airway, prevent hypovolemic shock
   ○ **B.** Control hemorrhage, prevent hypovolemic shock, establish an airway, assess for head injuries
   ○ **C.** Establish an airway, control hemorrhage, prevent hypovolemic shock, assess for head injuries
   ○ **D.** Prevent hypovolemic shock, assess for head injuries, establish an airway, control hemorrhage

92. The nurse is teaching the mother of a child with attention deficit disorder regarding the use of Ritalin (methylphenidate). The nurse recognizes that the mother understands her teaching when she states the importance of:

- ○ **A.** Offering high-calorie snacks
- ○ **B.** Watching for signs of infection
- ○ **C.** Observing for signs of oversedation
- ○ **D.** Using a sunscreen with an SPF of 30

93. A home health nurse has several elderly clients in her case load. Which of the following clients is most likely to be a victim of elder abuse?

- ○ **A.** A 76-year-old female with Alzheimer's dementia
- ○ **B.** A 70-year-old male with diabetes mellitus
- ○ **C.** A 64-year-old female with a hip replacement
- ○ **D.** A 72-year-old male with Parkinson's disease

94. A camp nurse is applying sunscreen to a group of children enrolled in swim classes. Chemical sunscreens are most effective when applied:

- ○ **A.** Just before sun exposure
- ○ **B.** Five minutes before sun exposure
- ○ **C.** 15 minutes before sun exposure
- ○ **D.** 30 minutes before sun exposure

95. The physician has made a diagnosis of "shaken child" syndrome for a 13-month-old who was brought to the emergency room after a reported fall from his highchair. Which finding supports the diagnosis of "shaken child" syndrome?

- ○ **A.** Fracture of the clavicle
- ○ **B.** Periorbital bruising
- ○ **C.** Retinal hemorrhages
- ○ **D.** Fracture of the humerus

96. A post-operative client has an order for Demerol (meperidine) 75mg and Phenergan (promethazine) 25mg IM every 3–4 hours as needed for pain. The combination of the two medications produces a/an:

- ○ **A.** Agonist effect
- ○ **B.** Synergistic effect
- ○ **C.** Antagonist effect
- ○ **D.** Excitatory effect

97. Which obstetrical client is most likely to have an infant with respiratory distress syndrome?

   Quick Answer: **139**
   Detailed Answer: **150**

   ○ **A.** A 28-year-old with a history of alcohol use during the pregnancy

   ○ **B.** A 24-year-old with a history of diabetes mellitus

   ○ **C.** A 30-year-old with a history of smoking during the pregnancy

   ○ **D.** A 32-year-old with a history of pregnancy-induced hypertension

98. A client with a C4 spinal cord injury has been placed in traction with cervical tongs. Nursing care should include:

   Quick Answer: **139**
   Detailed Answer: **150**

   ○ **A.** Releasing the traction for five minutes each shift

   ○ **B.** Loosening the pins if the client complains of headache

   ○ **C.** Elevating the head of the bed 90°

   ○ **D.** Performing sterile pin care as ordered

99. The nurse is assessing a client following a coronary artery bypass graft (CABG). The nurse should give priority to reporting:

   Quick Answer: **139**
   Detailed Answer: **151**

   ○ **A.** Chest drainage of 150mL in the past hour

   ○ **B.** Confusion and restlessness

   ○ **C.** Pallor and coolness of skin

   ○ **D.** Urinary output of 40mL per hour

100. Before administering a client's morning dose of Lanoxin (digoxin), the nurse checks the apical pulse rate and finds a rate of 54. The appropriate nursing intervention is to:

   Quick Answer: **139**
   Detailed Answer: **151**

   ○ **A.** Record the pulse rate and administer the medication

   ○ **B.** Administer the medication and monitor the heart rate

   ○ **C.** Withhold the medication and notify the doctor

   ○ **D.** Withhold the medication until the heart rate increases

101. What information should the nurse give a new mother regarding the introduction of solid foods for her infant?

   Quick Answer: **139**
   Detailed Answer: **151**

   ○ **A.** Solid foods should not be given until the extrusion reflex disappears at 8–10 months of age.

   ○ **B.** Solid foods should be introduced one at a time, with 4- to 7-day intervals.

   ○ **C.** Solid foods can be mixed in a bottle or infant feeder, to make feeding easier.

   ○ **D.** Solid foods should begin with fruits and vegetables.

102. When performing Leopold maneuvers on a client at 32 weeks gestation, the nurse would expect to find:

Quick Answer: **139**
Detailed Answer: **151**

- ○ **A.** No fetal movement
- ○ **B.** Minimal fetal movement
- ○ **C.** Moderate fetal movement
- ○ **D.** Active fetal movement

103. A client with a history of phenylketonuria (PKU) is seen in the local family planning clinic. While completing the intake history, the nurse provides information for a healthy pregnancy. Which statement indicates that the client needs further teaching?

Quick Answer: **139**
Detailed Answer: **151**

- ○ **A.** "I can use artificial sweeteners to keep me from gaining too much weight when I get pregnant."
- ○ **B.** "I need to go back on a low-phenylalanine diet before I get pregnant."
- ○ **C.** "Fresh fruits and raw vegetables will make good between-meal snacks for me."
- ○ **D.** "My baby could be mentally retarded if I don't stick to a diet eliminating phenylalanine."

104. The nurse is teaching the mother of an infant with galactosemia. Which information should be included in the nurse's teaching?

Quick Answer: **139**
Detailed Answer: **151**

- ○ **A.** Check food and drug labels for the presence of lactose.
- ○ **B.** Foods containing galactose can be gradually added.
- ○ **C.** Future children will not be affected.
- ○ **D.** Sources of galactose are essential for growth.

105. Which finding is associated with Tay Sachs disease?

Quick Answer: **139**
Detailed Answer: **151**

- ○ **A.** Pallor of the conjunctiva
- ○ **B.** Cherry-red spots on the macula
- ○ **C.** Blue-tinged sclera
- ○ **D.** White flecks in the iris

106. A client with schizophrenia is started on Zyprexa (olanzapine). Three weeks later, the client develops severe muscle rigidity and elevated temperature. The nurse should give priority to:

Quick Answer: **139**
Detailed Answer: **151**

- ○ **A.** Withholding all morning medications
- ○ **B.** Ordering a CBC and CPK
- ○ **C.** Administering prescribed anti-Parkinsonian medication
- ○ **D.** Transferring the client to a medical unit

107. A client with human immunodeficiency syndrome has gastrointestinal symptoms, including diarrhea. The nurse should teach the
client to avoid:

- ○ **A.** Calcium-rich foods
- ○ **B.** Canned or frozen vegetables
- ○ **C.** Processed meat
- ○ **D.** Raw fruits and vegetables

Quick Answer: **139**
Detailed Answer: **151**

108. A four-year-old is admitted with acute leukemia. It will be most
important to monitor the child for:

- ○ **A.** Abdominal pain and anorexia
- ○ **B.** Fatigue and bruising
- ○ **C.** Bleeding and pallor
- ○ **D.** Petechiae and mucosal ulcers

Quick Answer: **139**
Detailed Answer: **151**

109. A five-month-old is diagnosed with atopic dermatitis. Nursing
interventions will focus on:

- ○ **A.** Preventing infection
- ○ **B.** Administering antipyretics
- ○ **C.** Keeping the skin free of moisture
- ○ **D.** Limiting oral fluid intake

Quick Answer: **139**
Detailed Answer: **151**

110. A client on a mechanical ventilator begins to fight the ventilator.
Which medication will be ordered for the client?

- ○ **A.** Sublimaze (fentanyl)
- ○ **B.** Pavulon (pancuronium bromide)
- ○ **C.** Versed (midazolam)
- ○ **D.** Atarax (hydroxyzine)

Quick Answer: **139**
Detailed Answer: **152**

111. A client with a history of diverticulitis complains of abdominal
pain, fever, and diarrhea. Which food is most likely responsible for
the client's symptoms?

- ○ **A.** Mashed potatoes
- ○ **B.** Steamed carrots
- ○ **C.** Baked fish
- ○ **D.** Whole-grain cereal

Quick Answer: **139**
Detailed Answer: **152**

112. The home health nurse is visiting a client with Paget's disease. An important part of preventive care for the client with Paget's disease is:

- ○ **A.** Keeping the environment free of clutter
- ○ **B.** Advising the client to see the dentist regularly
- ○ **C.** Encouraging the client to take the influenza vaccine
- ○ **D.** Telling the client to take a daily multivitamin

113. The physician has scheduled a Whipple procedure for a client with pancreatic cancer. The nurse recognizes that the client's cancer is located in:

- ○ **A.** The tail of the pancreas
- ○ **B.** The head of the pancreas
- ○ **C.** The body of the pancreas
- ○ **D.** The entire pancreas

114. A child with cystic fibrosis is being treated with inhalation therapy with Pulmozyme (dornase alfa). A side effect of the medication is:

- ○ **A.** Weight gain
- ○ **B.** Hair loss
- ○ **C.** Sore throat
- ○ **D.** Brittle nails

115. Four days after delivery, a client develops complications of postpartal hemorrhage. The most common cause of late postpartal hemorrhage is:

- ○ **A.** Uterine atony
- ○ **B.** Retained placental fragments
- ○ **C.** Cervical laceration
- ○ **D.** Perineal tears

116. On a home visit, the nurse finds four young children alone. The youngest of the children has bruises on the face and back and circular burns on the inner aspect of the right forearm. The nurse should:

- ○ **A.** Contact child welfare services
- ○ **B.** Transport the child to the emergency room
- ○ **C.** Take the children to an abuse shelter
- ○ **D.** Stay with the children until an adult arrives

117. A client is diagnosed with post-traumatic stress disorder following a rape by an unknown assailant. The nurse should give priority to:

Quick Answer: **139**
Detailed Answer: **152**

- ○ **A.** Providing a supportive environment
- ○ **B.** Controlling the client's feelings of anger
- ○ **C.** Discussing the details of the attack
- ○ **D.** Administering a hypnotic for sleep

118. The doctor has ordered Percocet (oxycodone) for a client following abdominal surgery. The primary objective of nursing care for the client receiving an opiate analgesic is:

Quick Answer: **139**
Detailed Answer: **152**

- ○ **A.** Preventing addiction
- ○ **B.** Alleviating pain
- ○ **C.** Facilitating mobility
- ○ **D.** Preventing nausea

119. Which aminophylline level is associated with signs of toxicity?

Quick Answer: **139**
Detailed Answer: **152**

- ○ **A.** 5 micrograms/mL
- ○ **B.** 10 micrograms/mL
- ○ **C.** 20 micrograms/mL
- ○ **D.** 25 micrograms/mL

120. Which finding is the best indication that a client with ineffective airway clearance needs suctioning?

Quick Answer: **139**
Detailed Answer: **152**

- ○ **A.** Oxygen saturation
- ○ **B.** Respiratory rate
- ○ **C.** Breath sounds
- ○ **D.** Arterial blood gases

121. A client with tuberculosis has a prescription for Myambutol (ethambutol HCl). The nurse should tell the client to notify the doctor immediately if he notices:

Quick Answer: **140**
Detailed Answer: **153**

- ○ **A.** Gastric distress
- ○ **B.** Changes in hearing
- ○ **C.** Red discoloration of body fluids
- ○ **D.** Changes in color vision

122. The primary cause of anemia in a client with chronic renal failure is:

Quick Answer: **140**
Detailed Answer: **153**

- ○ **A.** Poor iron absorption
- ○ **B.** Destruction of red blood cells
- ○ **C.** Lack of intrinsic factor
- ○ **D.** Insufficient erythropoietin

123. Which of the following nursing interventions has the highest priority for the client scheduled for an intravenous pyelogram?

Quick Answer: **140**
Detailed Answer: **153**

- ○ **A.** Providing the client with a favorite meal for dinner
- ○ **B.** Asking if the client has allergies to shellfish
- ○ **C.** Encouraging fluids the evening before the test
- ○ **D.** Telling the client what to expect during the test

124. A client has ataxia following a cerebral vascular accident. The nurse should:

Quick Answer: **140**
Detailed Answer: **153**

- ○ **A.** Supervise the client's ambulation.
- ○ **B.** Measure the client's intake and output.
- ○ **C.** Request a consult for speech therapy.
- ○ **D.** Provide the client with a magic slate.

125. The doctor has prescribed aspirin 325mg daily for a client with transient ischemic attacks. The nurse explains that aspirin was prescribed to:

Quick Answer: **140**
Detailed Answer: **153**

- ○ **A.** Prevent headaches
- ○ **B.** Boost coagulation
- ○ **C.** Prevent cerebral anoxia
- ○ **D.** Decrease platelet aggregation

126. The nurse is preparing to administer regular insulin by continuous IV infusion to a client with diabetic ketoacidosis. The nurse should:

Quick Answer: **140**
Detailed Answer: **153**

- ○ **A.** Mix the insulin with Dextrose 5% in water.
- ○ **B.** Flush the IV tubing with the insulin solution and discard the first 50mL.
- ○ **C.** Avoid using a pump or controller with the infusion.
- ○ **D.** Mix the insulin with Ringer's lactate.

127. While reviewing the chart of a client with a history of hepatitis B, the nurse finds a serologic marker of HB8 AG. The nurse recognizes that the client:

Quick Answer: **140**
Detailed Answer: **153**

   ○ **A.** Has chronic hepatitis B

   ○ **B.** Has recovered from hepatitis B infection

   ○ **C.** Has immunity to infection with hepatitis C

   ○ **D.** Has no chance of spreading the infection to others

128. A client with tuberculosis who has been on combined therapy with Rifadin (rifampin) and INH (isoniazid) asks the nurse how long he will have to take medication. The nurse should tell the client that:

Quick Answer: **140**
Detailed Answer: **153**

   ○ **A.** Medication is rarely needed after two weeks.

   ○ **B.** He will need to take medication the rest of his life.

   ○ **C.** The course of combined therapy is usually six months.

   ○ **D.** He will be re-evaluated in one month to see if further medication is needed.

129. Which developmental milestone puts the four-month-old infant at greatest risk for injury?

Quick Answer: **140**
Detailed Answer: **153**

   ○ **A.** Switching objects from one hand to another

   ○ **B.** Crawling

   ○ **C.** Standing

   ○ **D.** Rolling over

130. A newborn is diagnosed with congenital syphilis. Classic signs of congenital syphilis are:

Quick Answer: **140**
Detailed Answer: **153**

   ○ **A.** Red papular rash, desquamation, white strawberry tongue

   ○ **B.** Rhinitis, maculopapular rash, hepatosplenomegaly

   ○ **C.** Red edematous cheeks, maculopapular rash on the trunk and extremities

   ○ **D.** Epicanthal folds, low-set ears, protruding tongue

131. Infants should be restrained in a car seat in a semi-reclined position facing the rear of the car until they weigh:

Quick Answer: **140**
Detailed Answer: **153**

   ○ **A.** 10 pounds

   ○ **B.** 15 pounds

   ○ **C.** 20 pounds

   ○ **D.** 25 pounds

132. The nurse is caring for a client with irritable bowel syndrome. Irritable bowel syndrome is characterized by:

   ○ **A.** Development of pouches in the wall of the intestine

   ○ **B.** Alternating bouts of constipation and diarrhea

   ○ **C.** Swelling, thickening, and abscess formation

   ○ **D.** Hypocalcemia and iron-deficiency anemia

133. A client taking Dilantin (phenytoin) for tonic-clonic seizures is preparing for discharge. Which information should be included in the client's discharge care plan?

   ○ **A.** The medication can cause dental staining.

   ○ **B.** The client will need to avoid a high-carbohydrate diet.

   ○ **C.** The client will need a regularly scheduled blood work.

   ○ **D.** The medication can cause problems with drowsiness.

134. Assessment of a newborn male reveals that the infant has hypospadias. The nurse knows that:

   ○ **A.** The infant should not be circumcised.

   ○ **B.** Surgical correction will be done by six months of age.

   ○ **C.** Surgical correction is delayed until six years of age.

   ○ **D.** The infant should be circumcised to facilitate voiding.

135. The nurse is providing dietary teaching for a client with elevated cholesterol levels. Which cooking oil is *not* suggested for the client on a low-cholesterol diet?

   ○ **A.** Safflower oil

   ○ **B.** Sunflower oil

   ○ **C.** Coconut oil

   ○ **D.** Canola oil

136. A client is hospitalized with signs of transplant rejection following a recent renal transplant. Assessment of the client would be expected to reveal:

   ○ **A.** A weight loss of two pounds in one day

   ○ **B.** A serum creatinine 1.25mg/dL

   ○ **C.** Urinary output of 50mL/hr

   ○ **D.** Rising blood pressure

137. A client is admitted with a blood alcohol level of 180mg/dL. The nurse recognizes that the alcohol in the client's system should be fully metabolized within:

    ⭘ **A.** Three hours

    ⭘ **B.** Five hours

    ⭘ **C.** Seven hours

    ⭘ **D.** Nine hours

Quick Answer: **140**
Detailed Answer: **154**

138. The nurse is caring for a client with stage III Alzheimer's disease. A characteristic of this stage is:

    ⭘ **A.** Memory loss

    ⭘ **B.** Failing to recognize familiar objects

    ⭘ **C.** Wandering at night

    ⭘ **D.** Failing to communicate

Quick Answer: **140**
Detailed Answer: **154**

139. The doctor has prescribed Cortone (cortisone) for a client with systemic lupus erythematosis. Which instruction should be given to the client?

    ⭘ **A.** Take the medication 30 minutes before eating.

    ⭘ **B.** Report changes in appetite and weight.

    ⭘ **C.** Wear sunglasses to prevent cataracts.

    ⭘ **D.** Schedule a time to take the influenza vaccine.

Quick Answer: **140**
Detailed Answer: **154**

140. The nurse is caring for a client with an above-the-knee amputation (AKA). To prevent hip flexion contractures, the nurse should:

    ⭘ **A.** Place the client in a prone position 15–30 minutes twice a day.

    ⭘ **B.** Keep the foot of the bed elevated on shock blocks.

    ⭘ **C.** Place trochanter rolls on either side of the affected leg.

    ⭘ **D.** Keep the client's leg elevated on two pillows.

Quick Answer: **140**
Detailed Answer: **154**

141. The mother of a six-month-old asks when her child will have all his baby teeth. The nurse knows that most children have all their primary teeth by age:

    ⭘ **A.** 12 months

    ⭘ **B.** 18 months

    ⭘ **C.** 24 months

    ⭘ **D.** 30 months

Quick Answer: **140**
Detailed Answer: **154**

142. A client with an esophageal tamponade develops symptoms of respiratory distress, including inspiratory stridor. The nurse should give priority to:

○ **A.** Applying oxygen at 4L via nasal cannula

○ **B.** Removing the tube after deflating the balloons

○ **C.** Elevating the head of the bed to 45°

○ **D.** Increasing the pressure in the esophageal balloon

Quick Answer: **140**
Detailed Answer: **155**

143. The nurse is assessing the heart sounds of a client with mitral stenosis following a history of rheumatic fever. To hear a mitral murmur, the nurse should place the stethoscope at:

○ **A.** The third intercostal space right of the sternum

○ **B.** The third intercostal space left of the sternum

○ **C.** The fourth intercostal space beneath the sternum

○ **D.** The fourth intercostal space mid-clavicular line

Quick Answer: **140**
Detailed Answer: **155**

144. While caring for a client with cervical cancer, the nurse notes that the radioactive implant is lying in the bed. The nurse should:

○ **A.** Place the implant in a biohazard bag and return it to the lab.

○ **B.** Give the client a pair of gloves and ask her to reinsert the implant.

○ **C.** Use tongs to pick up the implant and return it to a lead-lined container.

○ **D.** Discard the implant in the commode and double-flush.

Quick Answer: **140**
Detailed Answer: **155**

145. The nurse is preparing to discharge a client following a laparoscopic cholecystectomy. The nurse should:

○ **A.** Tell the client to avoid a tub bath for 48 hours.

○ **B.** Tell the client to expect clay-colored stools.

○ **C.** Tell the client that she can expect lower abdominal pain for the next week.

○ **D.** Tell the client to report pain in the back or shoulders.

Quick Answer: **140**
Detailed Answer: **155**

146. A high school student returns to school following a three-week absence due to mononucleosis. The school nurse knows it will be important for the client:

○ **A.** To drink additional fluids throughout the day

○ **B.** To avoid contact sports for 1–2 months

○ **C.** To have a snack twice a day to prevent hypoglycemia

○ **D.** To continue antibiotic therapy for six months

Quick Answer: **140**
Detailed Answer: **155**

147. An adolescent with cystic fibrosis has an order for pancreatic enzyme replacement. The nurse knows that the medication should be given:

Quick Answer: **140**
Detailed Answer: **155**

- ○ **A.** At bedtime
- ○ **B.** With meals and snacks
- ○ **C.** Twice daily
- ○ **D.** Daily in the morning

148. The doctor has prescribed a diet high in vitamin B12 for a client with pernicious anemia. Which foods are the best sources of B12?

Quick Answer: **140**
Detailed Answer: **155**

- ○ **A.** Meat, eggs, dairy products
- ○ **B.** Peanut butter, raisins, molasses
- ○ **C.** Broccoli, cauliflower, cabbage
- ○ **D.** Shrimp, legumes, bran cereals

149. A client with hypertension has begun an aerobic exercise program. The nurse should tell the client that the recommended exercise regimen should begin slowly and build up to:

Quick Answer: **140**
Detailed Answer: **155**

- ○ **A.** 20–30 minutes three times a week
- ○ **B.** 45 minutes two times a week
- ○ **C.** One hour four times a week
- ○ **D.** One hour two times a week

150. A home health nurse is visiting a client who is receiving diuretic therapy for congestive heart failure. Which medication places the client at risk for the development of hypokalemia?

Quick Answer: **140**
Detailed Answer: **155**

- ○ **A.** Aldactone (spironolactone)
- ○ **B.** Demadex (torsemide)
- ○ **C.** Dyrenium (triamterene)
- ○ **D.** Midamor (amiloride hydrochloride)

151. A client with breast cancer is returned to the room following a right total mastectomy. The nurse should:

Quick Answer: **140**
Detailed Answer: **155**

- ○ **A.** Elevate the client's right arm on pillows.
- ○ **B.** Place the client's right arm in a dependent sling.
- ○ **C.** Keep the client's right arm on the bed beside her.
- ○ **D.** Place the client's right arm across her body.

152. The physician has ordered Nitrostat (nitroglycerin SL) tablets for a client with stable angina. The medication:

    ○ **A.** Slows contractions of the heart

    ○ **B.** Dilates coronary blood vessels

    ○ **C.** Increases the ventricular fill time

    ○ **D.** Strengthens contractions of the heart

Quick Answer: **140**
Detailed Answer: **156**

153. A trauma client is admitted to the emergency room following a motor vehicle accident. Examination reveals that the left side of the chest moves inward when the client inhales. The finding is suggestive of:

    ○ **A.** Pneumothorax

    ○ **B.** Mediastinal shift

    ○ **C.** Pulmonary contusion

    ○ **D.** Flail chest

Quick Answer: **140**
Detailed Answer: **156**

154. A neurological consult has been ordered for a pediatric client with suspected absence seizures. The client with absence seizures can be expected to have:

    ○ **A.** Short, abrupt muscle contractions

    ○ **B.** Quick, severe bilateral jerking movements

    ○ **C.** Abrupt loss of muscle tone

    ○ **D.** Brief lapse in consciousness

Quick Answer: **140**
Detailed Answer: **156**

155. To decrease the likelihood of seizures and visual hallucinations in a client with alcohol withdrawal, the nurse should:

    ○ **A.** Keep the room darkened by pulling the curtains.

    ○ **B.** Keep the light over the bed on at all times.

    ○ **C.** Keep the room quiet and dim the lights.

    ○ **D.** Keep the television or radio turned on.

Quick Answer: **140**
Detailed Answer: **156**

156. A client with schizoaffective disorder is exhibiting Parkinsonian symptoms. Which medication is responsible for the development of Parkinsonian symptoms?

    ○ **A.** Zyprexa (olanzapine)

    ○ **B.** Cogentin (benzatropine mesylate)

    ○ **C.** Benadryl (diphenhydramine)

    ○ **D.** Depakote (divalproex sodium)

Quick Answer: **140**
Detailed Answer: **156**

157. Which activity is best suited to the 12-year-old with juvenile rheumatoid arthritis?

Quick Answer: **140**
Detailed Answer: **156**

- ○ **A.** Playing video games
- ○ **B.** Swimming
- ○ **C.** Working crossword puzzles
- ○ **D.** Playing slow-pitch softball

158. The home health nurse is scheduled to visit four clients. Which client should she visit first?

Quick Answer: **140**
Detailed Answer: **156**

- ○ **A.** A client with acquired immunodeficiency syndrome with a cough and reported temperature of 101°F
- ○ **B.** A client with peripheral vascular disease with an ulcer on the left lower leg
- ○ **C.** A client with diabetes mellitus who needs a diabetic control index drawn
- ○ **D.** A client with an autograft to burns of the chest and trunk

159. The glycosylated hemoglobin of a 40-year-old client with diabetes mellitus is 2.5%. The nurse understands that:

Quick Answer: **140**
Detailed Answer: **156**

- ○ **A.** The client can have a higher-calorie diet.
- ○ **B.** The client has good control of her diabetes.
- ○ **C.** The client requires adjustment in her insulin dose.
- ○ **D.** The client has poor control of her diabetes.

160. A dexamethasone-suppression test has been ordered for a client with severe depression. The purpose of the dexamethasone suppression test is to:

Quick Answer: **140**
Detailed Answer: **156**

- ○ **A.** Determine which social intervention will be best for the client
- ○ **B.** Help diagnose the seriousness of the client's clinical symptoms
- ○ **C.** Determine whether the client will benefit from electroconvulsive therapy
- ○ **D.** Reverse the depressive symptoms the client is experiencing

161. The physician has ordered Stadol (butorphanol) for a post-operative client. The nurse knows that the medication is having its intended effect if the client:

Quick Answer: **140**
Detailed Answer: **157**

- ○ **A.** Is asleep 30 minutes after the injection
- ○ **B.** Asks for extra servings on his meal tray
- ○ **C.** Has an increased urinary output
- ○ **D.** States that he is feeling less nauseated

162. The mother of a child with cystic fibrosis tells the nurse that her child makes "snoring" sounds when breathing. The nurse is aware that many children with cystic fibrosis have:

Quick Answer: **140**
Detailed Answer: **157**

- ○ **A.** Choanal atresia
- ○ **B.** Nasal polyps
- ○ **C.** Septal deviations
- ○ **D.** Enlarged adenoids

163. The nurse is caring for a client with full thickness burns to the lower half of the torso and lower extremities. During the emergent phase of injury, the primary nursing diagnosis would focus on:

Quick Answer: **140**
Detailed Answer: **157**

- ○ **A.** Imbalanced nutrition less than body requirements related to hypermetabolic state
- ○ **B.** Risk for infection related to altered skin integrity
- ○ **C.** Risk for fluid volume imbalance related to intracompartmental fluid shift
- ○ **D.** Acute pain related to burn injury

164. A client is hospitalized with hepatitis A. Which of the client's regular medications is contraindicated due to the current illness?

Quick Answer: **140**
Detailed Answer: **157**

- ○ **A.** Prilosec (omeprazole)
- ○ **B.** Synthroid (levothyroxine)
- ○ **C.** Premarin (conjugated estrogens)
- ○ **D.** Lipitor (atorvastatin)

165. Which activity is suitable for a client who suffered an uncomplicated myocardial infarction (MI) two days ago?

Quick Answer: **140**
Detailed Answer: **157**

- ○ **A.** Sitting in the bedside chair for 15 minutes three times a day
- ○ **B.** Remaining on strict bed rest with bedside commode privileges
- ○ **C.** Ambulating in the room and hall as tolerated
- ○ **D.** Sitting on the bedside for five minutes three times a day with assistance

166. The nurse has been teaching the role of diet in regulating blood pressure to a client with hypertension. Which meal selection indicates the client understands his new diet?

   ○ **A.** Cornflakes, whole milk, banana, and coffee

   ○ **B.** Scrambled eggs, bacon, toast, and coffee

   ○ **C.** Oatmeal, apple juice, dry toast, and coffee

   ○ **D.** Pancakes, ham, tomato juice, and coffee

167. An 18-month-old is being discharged following hypospadias repair. Which instruction should be included in the nurse's discharge teaching?

   ○ **A.** The child should not play on his rocking horse.

   ○ **B.** Applying warm compresses will decrease pain.

   ○ **C.** Diapering should be avoided for 1–2 weeks.

   ○ **D.** The child will need a special diet to promote healing.

168. An obstetrical client calls the clinic with complaints of morning sickness. The nurse should tell the client to:

   ○ **A.** Keep crackers at the bedside for eating before she arises

   ○ **B.** Drink a glass of whole milk before going to sleep at night

   ○ **C.** Skip breakfast but eat a larger lunch and dinner

   ○ **D.** Drink a glass of orange juice after adding a couple of teaspoons of sugar

169. The nurse is making assignments for the day. The staff consists of an RN, a novice RN, an LPN, and a nursing assistant. Which client should be assigned to the RN?

   ○ **A.** A client with peptic ulcer disease

   ○ **B.** A client with skeletal traction for a fractured femur

   ○ **C.** A client with an abdominal cholecystectomy

   ○ **D.** A client with an esophageal tamponade

170. A child with Tetralogy of Fallot is scheduled for a modified Blalock Taussig procedure. The nurse understands that the surgery will:

   ○ **A.** Reverse the direction of the blood flow

   ○ **B.** Allow better blood supply to the lungs

   ○ **C.** Relieve pressure on the ventricles

   ○ **D.** Prevent the need for further correction

171. The nurse has taken the blood pressure of a client hospitalized with methicillin-resistant staphylococcus aureus (MRSA). Which action by the nurse indicates an understanding regarding the care of clients with MRSA?

Quick Answer: **140**
Detailed Answer: **158**

- ○ **A.** The nurse leaves the stethoscope in the client's room for future use.
- ○ **B.** The nurse cleans the stethoscope with alcohol and returns it to the exam room.
- ○ **C.** The nurse uses the stethoscope to assess the blood pressure of other assigned clients.
- ○ **D.** The nurse cleans the stethoscope with water, dries it, and returns it to the nurse's station.

172. The physician has discussed the need for medication with the parents of an infant with congenital hypothyroidism. The nurse can reinforce the physician's teaching by telling the parents that:

Quick Answer: **140**
Detailed Answer: **158**

- ○ **A.** The medication will be needed only during times of rapid growth.
- ○ **B.** The medication will be needed throughout the child's lifetime.
- ○ **C.** The medication schedule can be arranged to allow for drug holidays.
- ○ **D.** The medication is given one time daily every other day.

173. A client with diabetes mellitus has a prescription for Glucotrol XL (glipizide). The client should be instructed to take the medication:

Quick Answer: **140**
Detailed Answer: **158**

- ○ **A.** At bedtime
- ○ **B.** With breakfast
- ○ **C.** Before lunch
- ○ **D.** After dinner

174. The nurse is caring for a client admitted with suspected myasthenia gravis. Which finding is usually associated with a diagnosis of myasthenia gravis?

Quick Answer: **140**
Detailed Answer: **158**

- ○ **A.** Visual disturbances, including diplopia
- ○ **B.** Ascending paralysis and loss of motor function
- ○ **C.** Cogwheel rigidity and loss of coordination
- ○ **D.** Progressive weakness that is worse at the day's end

175. A preterm infant with sepsis is receiving Gentamycin (garamycin). Which physiological alteration places the preterm infant at increased risk for toxicity related to aminoglycoside therapy?

Quick Answer: **140**
Detailed Answer: **158**

- ○ **A.** Lack of subcutaneous fat deposits
- ○ **B.** Immature central nervous system
- ○ **C.** Presence of fetal hemoglobin
- ○ **D.** Immaturity of the renal system

176. The nurse is teaching the parents of an infant with osteogenesis imperfecta. The nurse should tell the parents:

Quick Answer: **140**
Detailed Answer: **158**

- ○ **A.** That the infant will need daily calcium supplements
- ○ **B.** That it is best to lift the infant by the buttocks when diapering
- ○ **C.** That the condition is a temporary one
- ○ **D.** That only the bones of the infant are affected by the disease

177. The home health nurse is visiting an elderly client following a hip replacement. Which finding requires further teaching?

Quick Answer: **140**
Detailed Answer: **158**

- ○ **A.** The client shares her apartment with a cat.
- ○ **B.** The client has a grab bar near the commode.
- ○ **C.** The client usually sits on a soft, low sofa.
- ○ **D.** The client wears supportive shoes with nonskid soles.

178. Physician's orders for a client with acute pancreatitis include the following: strict NPO and nasogastric tube to low intermittent suction. The nurse recognizes that withholding oral intake will:

Quick Answer: **140**
Detailed Answer: **158**

- ○ **A.** Reduce the secretion of pancreatic enzymes
- ○ **B.** Decrease the client's need for insulin
- ○ **C.** Prevent the secretion of gastric acid
- ○ **D.** Eliminate the need for pain medication

179. A client with diverticulitis is admitted with nausea, vomiting, and dehydration. Which finding suggests a complication of diverticulitis?

Quick Answer: **140**
Detailed Answer: **158**

- ○ **A.** Pain in the left lower quadrant
- ○ **B.** Boardlike abdomen
- ○ **C.** Low-grade fever
- ○ **D.** Abdominal distention

180. The physician has ordered Vancocin (vancomycin) 500mg IV
every six hours for a client with MRSA. The medication should be
administered:

Quick Answer: **140**
Detailed Answer: **158**

- ○ **A.** IV push
- ○ **B.** Over 15 minutes
- ○ **C.** Over 30 minutes
- ○ **D.** Over 60 minutes

181. The diagnostic work-up of a client hospitalized with complaints of
progressive weakness and fatigue confirm a diagnosis of myasthenia gravis. The medication used to treat myasthenia gravis is:

Quick Answer: **140**
Detailed Answer: **158**

- ○ **A.** Prostigmine (neostigmine)
- ○ **B.** Atropine (atropine sulfate)
- ○ **C.** Didronel (etidronate)
- ○ **D.** Tensilon (edrophonium)

182. A client with AIDS complains of a weight loss of 20 pounds in the
past month. Which diet is suggested for the client with AIDS?

Quick Answer: **140**
Detailed Answer: **159**

- ○ **A.** High calorie, high protein, high fat
- ○ **B.** High calorie, high carbohydrate, low protein
- ○ **C.** High calorie, low carbohydrate, high fat
- ○ **D.** High calorie, high protein, low fat

183. The nurse is caring for a four-year-old with cerebral palsy. Which
nursing intervention will help ready the child for rehabilitative
services?

Quick Answer: **140**
Detailed Answer: **159**

- ○ **A.** Patching one of the eyes to help strengthen the ocular
  muscles
- ○ **B.** Providing suckers and pinwheels to help strengthen
  tongue movement
- ○ **C.** Providing musical tapes to provide auditory training
- ○ **D.** Encouraging play with a video game to improve muscle coordination

184. A client is admitted with a diagnosis of duodenal ulcer. A common
complaint of the client with a duodenal ulcer is:

Quick Answer: **140**
Detailed Answer: **159**

- ○ **A.** Epigastric pain that is relieved by eating
- ○ **B.** Weight loss
- ○ **C.** Epigastric pain that is worse after eating
- ○ **D.** Vomiting after eating

185. A client with otosclerosis is scheduled for a stapedectomy. Which finding suggests a complication involving the seventh cranial nerve?

    ○ **A.** Diminished hearing
    ○ **B.** Sensation of fullness in the ear
    ○ **C.** Inability to move the tongue side to side
    ○ **D.** Changes in facial sensation

Quick Answer: **140**
Detailed Answer: **159**

186. At the six-week check-up, the mother asks when she can expect the baby to sleep all night. The nurse should tell the mother that most infants begin to sleep all night by age:

    ○ **A.** One month
    ○ **B.** Two months
    ○ **C.** 3–4 months
    ○ **D.** 5–6 months

Quick Answer: **140**
Detailed Answer: **159**

187. A client with emphysema has been receiving oxygen at 3L per minute by nasal cannula. The nurse knows that the goal of the client's oxygen therapy is achieved when the client's PaO_2 reading is:

    ○ **A.** 50–60mm Hg
    ○ **B.** 70–80mm Hg
    ○ **C.** 80–90mm Hg
    ○ **D.** 90–98mm Hg

Quick Answer: **140**
Detailed Answer: **159**

188. A client with diabetes insipidus is receiving DDAVP (desmopressin acetate). Which lab finding indicates that the medication is having its intended effect?

    ○ **A.** Blood glucose 92mg/dL
    ○ **B.** Urine specific gravity 1.020
    ○ **C.** White blood count of 7,500
    ○ **D.** Glycosylated hemoglobin 3.5mg/dL

Quick Answer: **140**
Detailed Answer: **159**

189. Which of the following pediatric clients is at greatest risk for latex allergy?

    ○ **A.** The child with a myelomeningocele
    ○ **B.** The child with epispadias
    ○ **C.** The child with coxa plana
    ○ **D.** The child with rheumatic fever

Quick Answer: **140**
Detailed Answer: **159**

190. The physician has ordered a serum aminophylline level for a client with chronic obstructive lung disease. The nurse knows that the therapeutic range for aminophylline is:

- ○ **A.** 1–3 micrograms/mL
- ○ **B.** 4–6 micrograms/mL
- ○ **C.** 7–9 micrograms/mL
- ○ **D.** 10–20 micrograms/mL

Quick Answer: **140**
Detailed Answer: **159**

191. The nurse is developing a plan of care for a client with acromegaly. Which nursing diagnosis should receive priority?

- ○ **A.** Alteration in body image related to change in facial features
- ○ **B.** Risk for immobility related to joint pain
- ○ **C.** Risk for ineffective airway clearance related to obstruction of airway by tongue
- ○ **D.** Sexual dysfunction related to altered hormone secretion

Quick Answer: **140**
Detailed Answer: **159**

192. A client with acute respiratory distress syndrome (ARDS) is placed on mechanical ventilation. To increase ventilation and perfusion to all areas of the lungs, the nurse should:

- ○ **A.** Tell the client to inhale deeply during the inspiratory cycle.
- ○ **B.** Increase the positive end expiratory pressure (PEEP).
- ○ **C.** Turn the client every hour.
- ○ **D.** Administer medication to prevent the client from fighting the ventilator.

Quick Answer: **140**
Detailed Answer: **160**

193. The nurse is teaching the mother of a child with cystic fibrosis how to do chest percussion. The nurse should tell the mother to:

- ○ **A.** Use the heel of her hand during percussion.
- ○ **B.** Change the child's position every 20 minutes during percussion sessions.
- ○ **C.** Do percussion after the child eats and at bedtime.
- ○ **D.** Use cupped hands during percussion.

Quick Answer: **140**
Detailed Answer: **160**

194. A client with Addison's disease asks the nurse what he needs to know to manage his condition. The nurse should give priority to:

Quick Answer: **140**
Detailed Answer: **160**

- ○ **A.** Emphasizing the need for strict adherence to his medication regimen
- ○ **B.** Teaching the client to avoid lotions and skin preparations containing alcohol
- ○ **C.** Explaining the need to avoid extremes of temperature
- ○ **D.** Assisting the client to choose a diet that contains adequate protein, fat, and carbohydrates

195. The nurse is caring for a client following the removal of a central line catheter when the client suddenly develops dyspnea and complains of substernal chest pain. The client is noticeably confused and fearful. Based on the client's symptoms, the nurse should suspect which complication of central line use?

Quick Answer: **140**
Detailed Answer: **160**

- ○ **A.** Myocardial infarction
- ○ **B.** Air embolus
- ○ **C.** Intrathoracic bleeding
- ○ **D.** Vagal response

196. The nurse calculates the amount of an antibiotic for injection to be given to an infant. The amount of medication to be administered is 1.25mL. The nurse should:

Quick Answer: **140**
Detailed Answer: **160**

- ○ **A.** Divide the amount into two injections and administer in each vastus lateralis muscle.
- ○ **B.** Give the medication in one injection in the dorsogluteal muscle.
- ○ **C.** Divide the amount in two injections and give one in the ventrogluteal muscle and one in the vastus lateralis muscle.
- ○ **D.** Give the medication in one injection in the ventrogluteal muscle.

197. A client with schizophrenia is receiving depot injections of Haldol Decanoate (haloperidol decanoate). The client should be told to return for his next injection in:

Quick Answer: **140**
Detailed Answer: **160**

- ○ **A.** One week
- ○ **B.** Two weeks
- ○ **C.** Four weeks
- ○ **D.** Six weeks

198. The physician is preparing to remove a central line. The nurse should tell the client to:

Quick Answer: **140**
Detailed Answer: **160**

    ❍ **A.** Breathe normally

    ❍ **B.** Take slow, deep breaths

    ❍ **C.** Take a deep breath and hold it

    ❍ **D.** Breathe as quickly as possible

199. Cystic fibrosis is an exocrine disorder that affects several systems of the body. The earliest sign associated with a diagnosis of cystic fibrosis is:

Quick Answer: **140**
Detailed Answer: **160**

    ❍ **A.** Steatorrhea

    ❍ **B.** Frequent respiratory infections

    ❍ **C.** Increased sweating

    ❍ **D.** Meconium ileus

200. A three-year-old is immobilized in a hip spica cast. Which discharge instruction should be given to the parents?

Quick Answer: **140**
Detailed Answer: **160**

    ❍ **A.** Keep the bed flat, with a small pillow beneath the cast.

    ❍ **B.** Provide crayons and a coloring book for play activity.

    ❍ **C.** Increase her intake of high-calorie foods for healing.

    ❍ **D.** Tuck a disposable diaper beneath the cast at the perineal opening.

201. The nurse is caring for a client following the reimplantation of the thumb and index finger. Which finding should be reported to the physician immediately?

Quick Answer: **140**
Detailed Answer: **161**

    ❍ **A.** Temperature of 100°F

    ❍ **B.** Coolness and discoloration of the digits

    ❍ **C.** Complaints of pain

    ❍ **D.** Difficulty moving the digits

202. Which client is at greatest risk for a Caesarean section due to cephalopelvic disproportion (CPD)?

Quick Answer: **140**
Detailed Answer: **161**

    ❍ **A.** A 25-year-old gravida 2, para 1

    ❍ **B.** A 30-year-old gravida 3, para 2

    ❍ **C.** A 17-year-old gravida 1, para 0

    ❍ **D.** A 32-year-old gravida 1, para 0

203. The nurse is caring for a client with amyotrophic lateral sclerosis (ALS, Lou Gehrig's disease). The nurse should give priority to:

- ○ **A.** Assessing the client's respiratory status
- ○ **B.** Providing an alternate means of communication
- ○ **C.** Referring the client and family to community support groups
- ○ **D.** Instituting a routine of active range-of-motion exercises

Quick Answer: **140**
Detailed Answer: **161**

204. The physician has ordered Claforan (cefotaxime) 1g every six hours. The pharmacy sends the medication premixed in 100mL of D5W with instructions to infuse the medication over one hour. The IV set delivers 20 drops per milliliter. The nurse should set the IV rate at:

- ○ **A.** 50 drops per minute
- ○ **B.** 33 drops per minute
- ○ **C.** 25 drops per minute
- ○ **D.** 12 drops per minute

Quick Answer: **140**
Detailed Answer: **161**

205. When assessing the urinary output of a client who has had extracorporeal lithotripsy, the nurse can expect to find:

- ○ **A.** Cherry-red urine that gradually becomes clearer
- ○ **B.** Orange-tinged urine containing particles of calculi
- ○ **C.** Dark red urine that becomes cloudy in appearance
- ○ **D.** Dark, smoky-colored urine with high specific gravity

Quick Answer: **140**
Detailed Answer: **161**

206. A client scheduled for an atherectomy asks the nurse about the procedure. The nurse understands that:

- ○ **A.** Plaque will be removed by rotational or directional catheters.
- ○ **B.** Plaque will be destroyed by a laser.
- ○ **C.** A balloon-tipped catheter will compress fatty lesions against the vessel wall.
- ○ **D.** Medication will be used to dissolve the build-up of plaque.

Quick Answer: **140**
Detailed Answer: **161**

207. An elderly client has a stage II pressure ulcer on her sacrum. During assessment of the client's skin, the nurse would expect to find:

- ○ **A.** A deep crater with a nonpainful wound base
- ○ **B.** A craterous area with a nonpainful wound base
- ○ **C.** Cracks and blisters with redness and induration
- ○ **D.** Nonblanchable redness with tenderness and pain

208. The physician has prescribed Cognex (tacrine) for a client with dementia. The nurse should monitor the client for adverse reactions, which include:

- ○ **A.** Hypoglycemia
- ○ **B.** Jaundice
- ○ **C.** Urinary retention
- ○ **D.** Tinnitus

209. The suggested diet for a child with cystic fibrosis is one that contains:

- ○ **A.** High calories, high protein, moderate fat
- ○ **B.** High calories, moderate protein, low fat
- ○ **C.** Moderate calories, moderate protein, moderate fat
- ○ **D.** Low calories, high protein, low fat

210. The physician has ordered a low-potassium diet for a client with acute glomerulonephritis. Which snack is suitable for the client with potassium restrictions?

- ○ **A.** Raisins
- ○ **B.** Orange
- ○ **C.** Apple
- ○ **D.** Banana

211. A client with increased intracranial pressure is placed on mechanical ventilation with hyperventilation. The nurse knows that the purpose of the hyperventilation is to:

- ○ **A.** Prevent the development of acute respiratory failure
- ○ **B.** Decrease cerebral blood flow
- ○ **C.** Increase systemic tissue perfusion
- ○ **D.** Prevent cerebral anoxia

212. The physician has ordered a blood test for *H. pylori*. The nurse should prepare the client by:

- ○ **A.** Withholding oral intake after midnight
- ○ **B.** Telling the client that no special preparation is needed
- ○ **C.** Explaining that a small dose of radioactive isotope will be used
- ○ **D.** Giving an oral suspension of glucose one hour before the test

213. The nurse is preparing to give an oral potassium supplement. The nurse should give the medication:

- ○ **A.** Without diluting it
- ○ **B.** With 4oz. of juice
- ○ **C.** With water only
- ○ **D.** On an empty stomach

214. A client with acute alcohol intoxication is being treated for hypo-magnesemia. During assessment of the client, the nurse would expect to find:

- ○ **A.** Bradycardia
- ○ **B.** Negative Chvostek's sign
- ○ **C.** Hypertension
- ○ **D.** Positive Trousseau's sign

215. The physician has ordered cultures for cytomegalovirus (CMV). Which statement is true of the collection of cultures for cytomegalovirus?

- ○ **A.** Stool cultures are preferred for definitive diagnosis.
- ○ **B.** Pregnant caregivers may obtain cultures.
- ○ **C.** Collection of one specimen is sufficient.
- ○ **D.** Accurate diagnosis depends on fresh specimens.

216. A home health nurse has four clients assigned for morning visits. The nurse should give priority to visiting the client with:

- ○ **A.** Diabetes mellitus with a nongranulated ulcer of the right foot
- ○ **B.** Congestive heart failure who reports coughing up frothy sputum
- ○ **C.** Hemiplegia with tenderness in the right flank and cloudy urine
- ○ **D.** Rheumatoid arthritis with soft tissue swelling behind the right knee

217. Four clients are admitted to a medical unit. If only one private room is available, it should be assigned to:

- ○ **A.** The client with ulcerative colitis
- ○ **B.** The client with neutropenia
- ○ **C.** The client with cholecystitis
- ○ **D.** The client with polycythemia vera

218. The RN is making assignments for the morning staff. Which client should be cared for by the RN?

- ○ **A.** A client with hemianopsia
- ○ **B.** A client with asterixis
- ○ **C.** A client with akathesia
- ○ **D.** A client with hemoptysis

219. The nurse is reviewing the lab reports on several clients. Which one should be reported to the physician immediately?

- ○ **A.** A serum creatinine of 5.2mg/dL in a client with chronic renal failure
- ○ **B.** A positive C reactive protein in a client with rheumatic fever
- ○ **C.** A hematocrit of 52% in a client with gastroenteritis
- ○ **D.** A white cell count of 2,200cu/mm in a client taking Dilantin (phenytoin)

220. The following clients are to be assigned for daily care. The newly licensed nurse should not be assigned to provide primary care for the client with:

- ○ **A.** Full-thickness burns of the abdomen and upper thighs
- ○ **B.** A fractured hip scheduled for hip replacement
- ○ **C.** Ileal reservoir following a cystectomy
- ○ **D.** Noncardiogenic pulmonary edema (ARDS)

221. The RN is making assignments for clients hospitalized on a neurological unit. Which client should be assigned to the LPN?

- ○ **A.** A client with a C3 injury immobilized by Crutchfield tongs
- ○ **B.** A client with exacerbation of multiple sclerosis
- ○ **C.** A client with a lumbar laminectomy
- ○ **D.** A client with hemiplegia and a urinary tract infection

222. The nurse has just received the change of shift report. The nurse should give priority to assessing the client with:

Quick Answer: **140**
Detailed Answer: **163**

- ○ **A.** A thoracotomy with 110mL of drainage in the past hour
- ○ **B.** A cholecystectomy with an oral temperature of 100°F
- ○ **C.** A transurethral prostatectomy who complains of urgency to void
- ○ **D.** A stapedectomy who reports diminished hearing in the past hour

223. A client with primary sclerosing cholangitis has received a liver transplant. The nurse should give priority to assessing the client for complications. Which findings are associated with an acute rejection of the new liver?

Quick Answer: **140**
Detailed Answer: **163**

- ○ **A.** Increased jaundice and prolonged prothrombin time
- ○ **B.** Fever and foul-smelling bile drainage
- ○ **C.** Abdominal distention and clay-colored stools
- ○ **D.** Increased uric acid and increased creatinine

224. The nurse is planning care for a client with adrenal insufficiency. The nurse should give priority to:

Quick Answer: **140**
Detailed Answer: **163**

- ○ **A.** Monitoring the client for signs of dehydration
- ○ **B.** Promoting sleep and rest
- ○ **C.** Providing high-calorie snacks
- ○ **D.** Promoting a healthy body image

225. A pediatric client with burns to the hands and arms has dressing changes with Sulfamylon (mafenide acetate) cream. The nurse is aware that the medication:

Quick Answer: **140**
Detailed Answer: **163**

- ○ **A.** Will cause dark staining of the surrounding skin
- ○ **B.** Produces a cooling sensation when applied
- ○ **C.** Can alter the function of the thyroid
- ○ **D.** Produces a burning sensation when applied

226. The physician has ordered Dilantin (phenytoin) for a client with generalized seizures. When planning the client's care, the nurse should:

Quick Answer: **140**
Detailed Answer: **163**

- ○ **A.** Maintain strict intake and output.
- ○ **B.** Check the pulse before giving the medication.
- ○ **C.** Administer the medication 30 minutes before meals.
- ○ **D.** Provide oral hygiene and gum care every shift.

Quick Check

227. The nurse is caring for a client receiving Capoten (captopril). The nurse should be alert for adverse reactions to the drug, which include:

    Quick Answer: **140**
    Detailed Answer: **163**

    ○ **A.** Increased red cell count

    ○ **B.** Decreased sodium level

    ○ **C.** Decreased white cell count

    ○ **D.** Increased calcium level

228. A client receiving chemotherapy for breast cancer has an order for Zofran (ondansetron) 8mg PO to be given 30 minutes before induction of the chemotherapy. The purpose of the medication is to:

    Quick Answer: **140**
    Detailed Answer: **163**

    ○ **A.** Prevent anemia

    ○ **B.** Promote relaxation

    ○ **C.** Prevent nausea

    ○ **D.** Increase neutrophil counts

229. The physician has ordered Cortisporin ear drops for a two-year-old. To administer the ear drops, the nurse should:

    Quick Answer: **140**
    Detailed Answer: **163**

    ○ **A.** Pull the ear down and back.

    ○ **B.** Pull the ear straight out.

    ○ **C.** Pull the ear up and back.

    ○ **D.** Leave the ear undisturbed.

230. A client with Lyme's disease is being treated with Achromycin (tetracycline HCl). The nurse should tell the client that the medication will be rendered ineffective if taken with:

    Quick Answer: **140**
    Detailed Answer: **163**

    ○ **A.** Antacids

    ○ **B.** Salicylates

    ○ **C.** Antihistamines

    ○ **D.** Sedative-hypnotics

231. A client with schizophrenia has been taking Thorazine (chlorpromazine) 200mg four times a day. Which finding should be reported to the doctor immediately?

    Quick Answer: **140**
    Detailed Answer: **163**

    ○ **A.** The client complains of thirst.

    ○ **B.** The client has gained four pounds in the past two months.

    ○ **C.** The client complains of a sore throat and fever.

    ○ **D.** The client naps throughout the day.

232. The doctor has prescribed Claritin (loratidine) for a client with seasonal allergies. The feature that separates Claritin from other antihistamines such as Benadryl (diphenhydramine) is that the medication:

    ○ **A.** Is nonsedating

    ○ **B.** Stimulates appetite

    ○ **C.** Is used for motion sickness

    ○ **D.** Is less expensive

Quick Answer: **140**
Detailed Answer: **163**

233. A six-month-old is being treated for thrush with Nystatin (mycostatin) oral suspension. The nurse should administer the medication by:

    ○ **A.** Placing it in a small amount of applesauce

    ○ **B.** Using a cotton-tipped swab

    ○ **C.** Adding it to the infant's formula

    ○ **D.** Placing it in 2–3oz. of water

Quick Answer: **140**
Detailed Answer: **163**

234. A client with iron-deficiency anemia is taking an oral iron supplement. The nurse should tell the client to take the medication with:

    ○ **A.** Orange juice

    ○ **B.** Water only

    ○ **C.** Milk

    ○ **D.** Apple juice

Quick Answer: **140**
Detailed Answer: **164**

235. A child is admitted to the emergency room following ingestion of a bottle of medication containing acetaminophen. The antidote for acetaminophen is:

    ○ **A.** Acetylcysteine

    ○ **B.** Deferoxamine

    ○ **C.** Edetate calcium disodium

    ○ **D.** Activated charcoal

Quick Answer: **140**
Detailed Answer: **164**

236. The nurse knows that a client with right-sided hemiplegia understands teaching regarding ambulation with a cane if she states:

    ○ **A.** "I will hold the cane in my right hand."

    ○ **B.** "I will advance my cane and my right leg at the same time."

    ○ **C.** "I will be able to walk only by using a walker."

    ○ **D.** "I will hold the cane in my left hand."

Quick Answer: **140**
Detailed Answer: **164**

237. A nursing assistant assigned to care for a client receiving linear accelerator radium therapy for laryngeal cancer states, "I don't want to be assigned to that radioactive patient." The best response by the nurse is to:

- ○ **A.** Tell the nursing assistant that the client is not radio-active.
- ○ **B.** Tell the nursing assistant to wear a radiation badge to detect the amount of radiation that she is receiving.
- ○ **C.** Instruct her regarding the use of a lead-lined apron.
- ○ **D.** Ask a co-worker to care for the client.

238. The nurse caring for a client scheduled for an angiogram should prepare the client for the procedure by telling him to expect:

- ○ **A.** Dizziness as the dye is injected
- ○ **B.** Nausea and vomiting after the procedure is completed
- ○ **C.** A decreased heart rate for several hours after the procedure is completed
- ○ **D.** A warm sensation as the dye is injected

239. A client with Parkinson's disease complains of "choking" when he swallows. Which intervention will improve the client's ability to swallow?

- ○ **A.** Withholding liquids until after meals
- ○ **B.** Providing semi-liquids when possible
- ○ **C.** Providing a full liquid diet
- ○ **D.** Offering small, more frequent meals

240. Which of the following statements best explains the rationale for placing the client in Trendelenburg position during the insertion of a central line catheter?

- ○ **A.** It will facilitate catheter insertion.
- ○ **B.** It will make the client more comfortable during the insertion.
- ○ **C.** It will prevent the occurrence of ventricular tachy-cardia.
- ○ **D.** It will prevent the development of pulmonary embolus.

241. The doctor has ordered the removal of a Davol drain. Which of the following instructions should the nurse give to the client before removing the drain?

Quick Answer: **140**
Detailed Answer: **164**

- ○ **A.** The client should be told to breathe normally.
- ○ **B.** The client should be told to take two or three deep breaths as the drain is being removed.
- ○ **C.** The client should be told to hold his breath as the drain is being removed.
- ○ **D.** The client should breathe slowly as the drain is being removed.

242. Which of the following findings is associated with right-sided heart failure?

Quick Answer: **140**
Detailed Answer: **164**

- ○ **A.** Shortness of breath
- ○ **B.** Nocturnal polyuria
- ○ **C.** Daytime oliguria
- ○ **D.** Crackles in the lungs

243. A client returns from surgery with a total knee replacement. Which of the following findings requires immediate nursing intervention?

Quick Answer: **140**
Detailed Answer: **164**

- ○ **A.** Bloody drainage of 30mL from the Davol drain is present.
- ○ **B.** The CPM is set on 90° flexion.
- ○ **C.** The client is unable to ambulate to the bathroom.
- ○ **D.** The client is complaining of muscle spasms.

244. Which of the following postpartal clients is at greatest risk for hemorrhage?

Quick Answer: **140**
Detailed Answer: **164**

- ○ **A.** A gravida 1 para 1 with an uncomplicated delivery of a 7-pound infant
- ○ **B.** A gravida 1 para 0 with a history of polycystic ovarian disease
- ○ **C.** A gravida 3 para 3 with a history of low–birth weight infants
- ○ **D.** A gravida 4 para 3 with a Caesarean section

245. An infant with a ventricular septal defect is discharged with a prescription for Lanoxin (digoxin) elixir 0.01mg PO q 12hrs. The bottle is labeled 0.10mg per 1/2 tsp. The nurse should instruct the mother to:

Quick Answer: **140**
Detailed Answer: **165**

- ○ **A.** Administer the medication using a nipple.
- ○ **B.** Administer the medication using the calibrated dropper in the bottle.
- ○ **C.** Administer the medication using a plastic baby spoon.
- ○ **D.** Administer the medication in a baby bottle with 1oz. of water.

246. An elderly client with glaucoma is scheduled for a cholecystectomy. Which medication order should the nurse question?

Quick Answer: **140**
Detailed Answer: **165**

- ○ **A.** Demerol (meperidine)
- ○ **B.** Tagamet (cimetadine)
- ○ **C.** Atropine (atropine)
- ○ **D.** Phenergan (promethazine)

247. Which instruction would *not* be included in the discharge teaching of the client receiving Thorazine (chlorpromazine)?

Quick Answer: **140**
Detailed Answer: **165**

- ○ **A.** "You will need to wear protective clothing or a sunscreen when you are outside."
- ○ **B.** "You will need to avoid eating aged cheese."
- ○ **C.** "You should carry hard candy with you to decrease dryness of the mouth."
- ○ **D.** "You should report a sign of infection immediately."

248. An elderly client who experiences nighttime confusion wanders from his room into the room of another client. The nurse can best help with decreasing the client's confusion by:

Quick Answer: **140**
Detailed Answer: **165**

- ○ **A.** Assigning a nursing assistant to sit with him until he falls asleep
- ○ **B.** Allowing the client to room with another elderly client
- ○ **C.** Administering a bedtime sedative
- ○ **D.** Leaving a nightlight on during the evening and night shifts

249. A four-year-old is scheduled for a routine tonsillectomy. Which of the following lab findings should be reported to the doctor?

Quick Answer: **140**
Detailed Answer: **165**

- ○ **A.** A hemoglobin of 12Gm
- ○ **B.** A platelet count of 200,000
- ○ **C.** A white blood cell count of 16,000
- ○ **D.** A urine specific gravity of 1.010

250. A client with psychotic depression is receiving Haldol (haloperidol). Which one of the following adverse effects is associated with the use of haloperidol?

Quick Answer: **140**
Detailed Answer: **165**

- ○ **A.** Akathisia
- ○ **B.** Cataracts
- ○ **C.** Diaphoresis
- ○ **D.** Polyuria

Quick Answers

1. A	31. D	61. B	91. C
2. A	32. A	62. B	92. A
3. D	33. A	63. D	93. A
4. C	34. B	64. D	94. D
5. B	35. B	65. D	95. C
6. A	36. D	66. C	96. B
7. D	37. B	67. A	97. B
8. A	38. C	68. C	98. D
9. A	39. C	69. D	99. A
10. D	40. A	70. B	100. C
11. A	41. D	71. A	101. B
12. C	42. C	72. C	102. D
13. B	43. B	73. B	103. A
14. A	44. D	74. C	104. A
15. B	45. B	75. C	105. B
16. A	46. B	76. A	106. C
17. D	47. C	77. C	107. D
18. B	48. C	78. A	108. C
19. A	49. D	79. B	109. A
20. B	50. D	80. B	110. B
21. D	51. C	81. D	111. D
22. C	52. A	82. C	112. A
23. C	53. D	83. D	113. B
24. D	54. A	84. B	114. C
25. A	55. B	85. B	115. B
26. C	56. C	86. A	116. A
27. A	57. B	87. A	117. A
28. B	58. A	88. D	118. B
29. C	59. C	89. C	119. D
30. A	60. C	90. B	120. C

121. D	154. D	187. A	220. D
122. D	155. C	188. B	221. C
123. B	156. A	189. A	222. A
124. A	157. B	190. D	223. A
125. D	158. A	191. C	224. A
126. B	159. B	192. C	225. D
127. A	160. C	193. D	226. D
128. C	161. A	194. A	227. C
129. D	162. B	195. B	228. C
130. B	163. C	196. A	229. A
131. C	164. D	197. C	230. A
132. B	165. D	198. C	231. C
133. C	166. C	199. D	232. A
134. A	167. A	200. D	233. B
135. C	168. A	201. B	234. A
136. D	169. D	202. C	235. A
137. D	170. B	203. A	236. D
138. B	171. A	204. B	237. A
139. D	172. B	205. A	238. D
140. A	173. B	206. A	239. B
141. D	174. D	207. C	240. A
142. B	175. D	208. B	241. B
143. D	176. B	209. A	242. B
144. C	177. C	210. C	243. B
145. A	178. A	211. B	244. D
146. B	179. B	212. B	245. B
147. B	180. D	213. B	246. C
148. A	181. A	214. D	247. B
149. A	182. D	215. D	248. D
150. B	183. B	216. B	249. C
151. A	184. A	217. B	250. A
152. B	185. D	218. B	
153. D	186. C	219. D	

Answers and Rationales

1. **Answer A is correct.** The major complication of SLE is lupus nephritis, which results in end-stage renal disease. SLE affects the musculoskeletal, integumentary, renal, nervous, and cardiovascular systems, but the major complication is renal involvement; therefore, answers B and D are incorrect. Answer C is incorrect because the SLE produces a "butterfly" rash, not desquamation.

2. **Answer A is correct.** Finasteride is an androgen inhibitor; therefore, women who are pregnant or who might become pregnant should be told to avoid touching the tablets. Answer B is incorrect because there are no benefits to giving the medication with food. Answer C is incorrect because the medication can take six months to a year to be effective. Answer D is not an accurate statement; therefore, it is incorrect.

3. **Answer D is correct.** The nurse can expect to find the presence of Trendelenburg sign. (While bearing weight on the affected hip, the pelvis tilts downward on the unaffected side instead of tilting upward, as expected with normal stability.) Scarf sign is a characteristic of the preterm newborn; therefore, answer A is incorrect. Harlequin sign can be found in normal newborns and indicates transient changes in circulation; therefore, answer B is incorrect. Answer C is incorrect because Cullen's sign is an indication of intra-abdominal bleeding.

4. **Answer C is correct.** A diet that is high in fat and refined carbohydrates increases the risk of colorectal cancer. High fat content results in an increase in fecal bile acids, which facilitate carcinogenic changes. Refined carbohydrates increase the transit time of food through the gastrointestinal tract and increase the exposure time of the intestinal mucosa to cancer-causing substances. Answers A, B, and D do not relate to the question; therefore, they are incorrect.

5. **Answer B is correct.** The nurse should avoid giving the infant a pacifier or bottle because sucking is not permitted. Holding the infant cradled in the arms, providing a mobile, and offering sterile water using a Breck feeder are permitted; therefore, answers A, C, and D are incorrect.

6. **Answer A is correct.** The client with asterixis or "flapping tremors" will have irregular flexion and extension of the wrists when the arms are extended and the wrist is hyperextended with the fingers separated. Asterixis is associated with hepatic encephalopathy. Answers B, C, and D do not relate to asterixis; therefore, they are incorrect.

7. **Answer D is correct.** The client with esophageal varices might develop spontaneous bleeding from the mechanical irritation caused by taking capsules; therefore, the nurse should request the medication in an alternative form such as a suspension. Answer A is incorrect because it does not best meet the client's needs. Answer B is incorrect because it is not the best means of preventing bleeding. Answer C is incorrect because the medications should not be given with milk or antacids.

8. **Answer A is correct.** Surgical repair of an inguinal hernia is recommended to prevent strangulation of the bowel, which could result in intestinal obstruction and necrosis. Answer B does not relate to an inguinal hernia; therefore, it is incorrect. Bile salts, which are important to the digestion of fats, are produced by the liver, not the intestines; therefore, answer C is incorrect. Repair of the inguinal hernia will prevent swelling and obstruction associated with strangulation, but it will not increase intestinal motility; therefore, answer D is incorrect.

9. **Answer A is correct.** Tomatoes are a poor source of iron, although they are an excellent source of vitamin C, which increases iron absorption. Answers B, C, and D are good sources of iron; therefore, they are incorrect.

10. **Answer D is correct.** Serum amylase levels greater than 200 units/dL help confirm the diagnosis of acute pancreatitis. Elevations of blood glucose occur with conditions other than acute pancreatitis; therefore, answer A is incorrect. Elevations in WBC are associated with infection and are not specific to acute pancreatitis; therefore, answer B is incorrect. Answer C is within the normal range; therefore, it is incorrect.

11. **Answer A is correct.** Periodically lying in a prone position without a pillow will help prevent the flexion of the spine that occurs with Parkinson's disease. Answers B and C flex the spine; therefore, they are incorrect. Answer D is not realistic because position changes during sleep; therefore, it is incorrect.

12. **Answer C is correct.** The medication should be administered slowly (no more than 50mg per minute); otherwise, cardiac arrhythmias can occur. Answer A is incorrect because the medication must be given slowly. Dextrose solutions cause the medication to crystallize in the line and the medication should be given through a large vein to prevent "purple glove" syndrome; therefore, answers B and D are incorrect.

13. **Answer B is correct.** The client recovering from acute pancreatitis needs a diet that is high in calories and low in fat. Answers A, C, and D are incorrect because they can increase the client's discomfort.

14. **Answer A is correct.** The client with polycythemia vera has an abnormal increase in the number of circulating red blood cells that results in increased viscosity of the blood. Increases in blood pressure further tax the overworked heart. Answers B, C, and D do not directly relate to the condition; therefore, they are incorrect.

15. **Answer B is correct.** Dressing in extra layers of clothing will help decrease the feeling of being cold that is experienced by the client with hypothyroidism. Decreased sensation and decreased alertness are common in the client with hypothyroidism. The use of electric blankets and heating pads can result in burns, making answers A and C incorrect. Answer D is incorrect because the client with hypothyroidism has dry skin, and a hot bath morning and evening would make her condition worse.

16. **Answer A is correct.** An ICP of 17mmHg should be reported to the doctor because it is elevated. (The ICP normally ranges from 4mmHg to 10mmHg, with upper limits of 15mmHg.) Answer B is incorrect because the pressure is not normal. Answer C is incorrect because the pressure is not low. Answer D is incorrect because the ICP reading provides a more reliable measurement than the Glascow coma scale.

17. **Answer D is correct.** A history of frequent alcohol and tobacco use is the most significant factor in the development of cancer of the larynx. Answers A, B, and C are also factors in the development of laryngeal cancer but they are not the most significant; therefore, they are incorrect.

18. **Answer B is correct.** Numbness and tingling in the extremities is common in the client with pernicious anemia, but not those with other types of anemia. Answers A, C, and D are incorrect because they are symptoms of all types of anemia.

19. **Answer A is correct.** Lying prone and allowing the feet to hang over the end of the mattress will help prevent flexion contractures. The client should be told to do this several times a day. Answers B, C, and D do not help prevent flexion contractures; therefore, they are incorrect.

20. **Answer B is correct.** The client with echolalia will repeat words or phrases used by others. Answer A is incorrect because it refers to clang association. Answer C is incorrect because it refers to circumstantiality. Answer D is incorrect because it refers to neologisms.

21. **Answer D is correct.** The presence of fetal hemoglobin until about six months of age protects affected infants from episodes of sickling. Answer A is incorrect because it is an untrue statement. Answer B is incorrect because infants do have insensible fluid loss. Answer C is incorrect because respiratory infections such as bronchiolitis and otitis media can cause fever and dehydration, which cause sickle cell crisis.

22. **Answer C is correct.** The warmth from holding a cup of coffee or hot chocolate helps to relieve the pain and stiffness in the hands of the client with rheumatoid arthritis. Answers A, B, and D do not relieve the symptoms of rheumatoid arthritis; therefore, they are incorrect.

23. **Answer C is correct.** If the client's own blood type and Rh are not available, the safest transfusion is O negative blood. Answers A, B, and D are incorrect because they can cause reactions that can prove fatal to the client.

24. **Answer D is correct.** Narcan is a narcotic antagonist that blocks the effects of the client's pain medication; therefore, the client will experience sudden, intense pain. Answers A, B, and C do not relate to the client's condition and the administration of Narcan; therefore, they are incorrect.

25. **Answer A is correct.** The infant's birth weight should double by six months of age. Answers B, C, and D are incorrect because they are greater than the expected weight gain by six months of age.

26. **Answer C is correct.** The symptoms of nontropical sprue as well as those of celiac are caused by the ingestion of gluten, found in wheat, oats, barley, and rye. Creamed soup and crackers as well as some cold cuts contain gluten. Answers A, B, and D do not contain gluten; therefore, they are incorrect.

27. **Answer A is correct.** Lanoxin slows and strengthens the contraction of the heart. An increase in urinary output shows that the medication is having a desired effect by eliminating excess fluid from the body. Answer B is incorrect because the weight would decrease. Answer C is not related to the medication; therefore, it is incorrect. Answer D is incorrect because pedal edema would decrease, not increase.

28. **Answer B is correct.** The toddler has gross motor skills suited to playing with a ball, which can be kicked forward or thrown overhand. Answers A and C are incorrect because they require fine motor skills. Answer D is incorrect because the toddler lacks gross motor skills for play on the swing set.

29. **Answer C is correct.** Jitteriness and irritability are signs of alcohol withdrawal in the newborn. Answer A is incorrect because it would be associated with use more recent than one day ago. Answers B and D are characteristics of a newborn with fetal alcohol syndrome, but they are not a priority at this time; therefore, they are incorrect.

30. **Answer A is correct.** Antacids containing aluminum tend to cause constipation. Answers B, C, and D are not common side effects of the medication.

31. **Answer D is correct.** The client with an abdominal aortic aneurysm frequently complains of pulsations or feeling the heart beat in the abdomen. Answers A and C are incorrect because they are not associated with abdominal aortic aneurysm. Answer B is incorrect because back pain is not affected by changes in position.

32. **Answer A is correct.** The client with nephotic syndrome will be treated with immunosuppressive drugs. Limiting visitors will decrease the chance of infection. Answer B is incorrect because the client needs additional protein. Answer C is incorrect because dialysis is not indicated for the client with nephrotic syndrome. Answer D is incorrect because additional fluids are not needed until the client begins diuresis.

33. **Answer A is correct.** The client with acute adrenal crisis has symptoms of hypovolemia and shock; therefore, the blood pressure would be low. Answer B is incorrect because the pulse would be rapid and irregular. Answer C is incorrect because the skin would be cool and pale. Answer D is incorrect because the urinary output would be decreased.

34. **Answer B is correct.** Tenseness of the anterior fontanel indicates an increase in intracranial pressure. Answer A is incorrect because periorbital edema is not associated with meningitis. Answer C is incorrect because a positive Babinski reflex is normal in the infant. Answer D is incorrect because it relates to the preterm infant, not the infant with meningitis.

35. **Answer B is correct.** The nurse should give priority to checking the client's blood pressure since pentamidine, if infused too rapidly, can cause severe hypotension and hypoglycemia. Answers A, C, and D do not relate specifically to the medication; therefore, they are incorrect choices.

36. **Answer D is correct.** The recommended dose ranges from 175mg to 350mg per day based on the infant's weight. The order as written calls for 400mg per day for an infant weighing 7kg; therefore, the nurse should check the order with the doctor before giving the medication. Answer A is incorrect because the dosage exceeds the recommended amount. Answers B and C are incorrect choices because they involve changing the doctor's order.

37. **Answer B is correct.** Bright red bleeding with many clots indicates arterial bleeding that requires surgical intervention. Answer A is within normal limits, answer C indicates venous bleeding, which can be managed by nursing intervention, and answer D does not indicate excessive need for pain management that requires the doctor's attention; therefore, they are incorrect.

38. **Answer C is correct.** The child will need additional fluids in summer to prevent dehydration that could lead to a sickle cell crises. Answer A is not a true statement; therefore, it is incorrect. Answer B is incorrect because the activity will create a greater oxygen demand and precipitate sickle cell crises. Answer D is not a true statement; therefore, it is incorrect.

39. **Answer C is correct.** The client should be assessed following completion of antibiotic therapy to determine whether the infection has cleared. Answer A would be done if there are repeated instances of otitis media, answer B is incorrect because it will not determine whether the child has completed the medication, and answer D is incorrect because the purpose of the recheck is to determine whether the infection is gone.

40. **Answer A is correct.** The child with Sydenham's chorea will exhibit irregular movements of the extremities, facial grimacing, and labile moods. Answer B is incorrect because it describes subcutaneous nodules. Answer C is incorrect because it describes erythema marginatum. Answer D is incorrect because it describes polymigratory arthritis.

41. **Answer D is correct.** The primary reason for placing a child with croup under a high humidity mist tent is to liquefy secretions and relieve laryngeal spasms. Answers A, B, and C are inaccurate statements; therefore, they are incorrect.

42. **Answer C is correct.** The recommended setting for performing tracheostomy suctioning on the adult client is 80–120mmHg. Answers A and B are incorrect because the amount of suction is too low. Answer D is incorrect because the amount of suction is excessive.

43. **Answer B is correct.** Symptoms of myxedema include weight gain, lethargy, slow speech, and decreased respirations. Answers A and D do not describe symptoms associated with myxedema; therefore, they are incorrect. Answer C describes symptoms associated with Graves disease.

44. **Answer D is correct.** The contagious stage of varicella begins 24 hours before the onset of the rash and lasts until all the lesions are crusted. Answers A, B, and C are inaccurate regarding the time of contagion.

45. **Answer B is correct.** The child with cystic fibrosis has sweat concentrations of chloride greater than 60mEq/L. Answers A and C are incorrect because they refer to potassium concentrations that are not used in making a diagnosis of cystic fibrosis. Answer D is incorrect because the sweat concentration of chloride is too low to be diagnostic.

46. **Answer B is correct.** The nurse should question the order because administering a narcotic so close to the time of delivery can result in respiratory depression in the newborn. Answers A, C, and D are incorrect because giving the medication prior to or during delivery can cause respiratory depression in the newborn.

47. **Answer C is correct.** During concrete operations, the child's thought processes become more logical and coherent. Answers A, B, and D are incorrect because they describe other types of development: sensorimotor, intuitive, and formal.

48. **Answer C is correct.** Delusions of grandeur are associated with feelings of low self-esteem. Answer A is incorrect because reaction formation, a defense mechanism, is characterized by outward emotions that are the opposite of internal feelings. Answers B and D can cause an increase in the client's delusions but do not explain their purpose; therefore, they are incorrect.

49. **Answer D is correct.** According to Kohlberg, in the preconventional stage of development, the behavior of the preschool child is determined by the consequences of the behavior. Answers A, B, and C describe other stages of moral development; therefore, they are incorrect.

50. **Answer D is correct.** Respiratory stridor is a symptom of partial airway obstruction. Answers A, B, and C are expected with a tonsillectomy; therefore, they are incorrect.

51. **Answer C is correct.** Pain associated with duodenal ulcers is lessened if the client eats a meal or snack. Answer A is incorrect because it makes the pain worse. Answer B lessens the discomfort of dumping syndrome; therefore, it is incorrect. Answer D lessens the discomfort of gastroesophageal reflux; therefore, it is incorrect.

52. **Answer A is correct.** Diminished femoral pulses are a sign of coarctation of the aorta. Answers B, C, and D are found in normal newborns and are not associated with cardiac anomaly.

53. **Answer D is correct.** A severe complication associated with Kawasaki's disease is the development of a giant aneurysm. Answers A, B, and C are incorrect because they have no relationship to Kawasaki's disease.

54. **Answer A is correct.** A nosebleed in the client with mild preeclampsia may indicate that the client's blood pressure is elevated. Answers B, C, and D are incorrect because the client will not need strict bed rest, pedal edema is common in the client with preeclampsia, and the client does not need to avoid sodium, although the client should limit or avoid high-sodium foods.

55. **Answer B is correct.** The client taking an MAO inhibitor should avoid over-the-counter medications for colds and hay fever because many contain pseudoephedrine. Combining an MAO inhibitor with pseudoephedrine can result in extreme elevations in blood pressure. Answer A is incorrect because it refers to the client taking an antipsychotic medication such as Thorazine. Answer C is not specific to the client taking an MAO inhibitor, and answer D does not apply to the question.

56. **Answer C is correct.** Foods containing rice or millet are permitted in the diet of the client with celiac disease. Answers A, B, and D are not permitted because they contain gluten, which exacerbates the symptoms of celiac disease; therefore, they are incorrect.

57. **Answer B is correct.** Increased thirst and increased urination are signs of lithium toxicity. Answers A and D are not associated with the use of lithium; therefore, they are incorrect. Answer C is an expected side effect of the medication; therefore, it is incorrect.

58. **Answer A is correct.** During dehydration, the kidneys compensate for electrolyte imbalance by retaining potassium. The nurse should check for urinary output before adding potassium to the IV fluid. Answer B is incorrect because it measures respiratory compensation caused by dehydration. Answers C and D do not apply to the use of intravenous fluid with potassium; therefore, they are incorrect.

59. **Answer C is correct.** The immunization protects the child against diphtheria, pertussis, tetanus, and H. influenzae b. Answer A is incorrect because a second injection is given before four years of age. Answer B is not a true statement, and answer D is not a one-time injection, nor does it protect against measles, mumps, rubella, or varicella.

60. **Answer C is correct.** A weight gain of six pounds in a week in the client taking glucocorticoids indicates that the dosage should be modified. Answers A and B are not specific to the question; therefore, they are incorrect. Answer D is an expected side effect of the medication; therefore, it is incorrect.

61. **Answer B is correct.** Assessing fetal heart tones reveals whether fetal distress occurred with rupture of the membranes. Answers A, C, and D are later interventions; therefore, they are incorrect.

62. **Answer B is correct.** Synthroid (levothyroxine) increases metabolic rate and cardiac output. Adverse reactions include tachycardia and dysrhythmias; therefore, the client should be taught to check her heart rate before taking the medication. Answer A is incorrect because the client does not have to take the medication after breakfast. Answer C does not relate to the medication; therefore, it is incorrect. The medication should not be stopped because of gastric upset; therefore, answer D is incorrect.

63. **Answer D is correct.** The nurse should wear a special badge when taking care of the client with a radioactive implant to measure the amount of time spent in the room. The nurse should limit the time of radiation exposure; therefore, answer A is incorrect. Standing at the foot of the bed of a client with a radioactive cervical implant increases the nurse's exposure to radiation; therefore, answer B is incorrect. The nurse does not have to avoid handling items used by the client; therefore, answer C is incorrect.

64. **Answer D is correct.** The milkshake will provide needed calories and nutrients for the client with mania. Answers A, B, and C are incorrect choices because they do not provide as many calories or nutrients as the milkshake.

65. **Answer D is correct.** The maximal effects from tricyclic antidepressants might not be achieved for up to six months after the medication is started. Answers A and B are incorrect because the time for maximal effects is too brief. Answer C is incorrect because it refers to the initial symptomatic relief rather than maximal effects.

66. **Answer C is correct.** Beta blockers such as timolol (Timoptic) can cause bronchospasms in the client with chronic obstructive lung disease. Timoptic is not contraindicated for use in the client with diabetes, gastric ulcers, or pancreatitis; therefore, answers A, B, and D are incorrect.

67. **Answer A is correct.** The child with intussusception has stools that contain blood and mucus, which are described as "currant jelly" stools. Answer B is a symptom of pyloric stenosis; therefore, it is incorrect. Answer C is a symptom of Hirschsprungs, therefore, it is incorrect. Answer D is a symptom of Wilms tumor; therefore, it is incorrect.

68. **Answer C is correct.** The infant with biliary atresia has abdominal distention, poor weight gain, and clay-colored stools. Answers A, B, and D do describe the symptoms associated with biliary atresia; therefore, they are incorrect.

69. **Answer D is correct.** The nurse should not use water, soap, or lotion on the area marked for radiation therapy. Answer A is incorrect because it would remove the marking. Answers B and C are not necessary for the client receiving radiation; therefore, they are incorrect.

70. **Answer B is correct.** Blood alcohol concentrations of 400–600mg/dL are associated with respiratory depression, coma, and death. Answer A occurs with blood alcohol concentrations of 50mg/dL, which affects coordination and speech but does not cause respiratory depression; therefore, it is incorrect. Answers C and D are associated with alcohol withdrawal, not overdose; therefore, they are incorrect.

71. **Answer A is correct.** Following a hypophysectomy, the nurse should check the client's blood sugar because insulin levels may rise rapidly resulting in hypoglycemia. Answer B is incorrect because suctioning should be avoided. Answer C is incorrect because the client's head should be elevated to reduce pressure on the operative site. Answer D is incorrect because coughing increases pressure on the operative site that can lead to a leak of cerebral spinal fluid.

72. **Answer C is correct.** Acarbose is to be taken with the first bite of a meal. Answers A, B, and D are incorrect because they specify the wrong schedule for taking the medication.

73. **Answer B is correct.** The client going for therapy in the hyperbaric oxygen chamber requires no special skin care; therefore, washing the skin with water and patting it dry are suitable. Lotions, petroleum products, perfumes, and occlusive dressings interfere with oxygenation of the skin; therefore, answers A, C, and D are incorrect.

74. **Answer C is correct.** Diabetes insipidus is characterized by excessive production of dilute urine. A decline in urinary output shows that the medication is having its intended effect. Answers A and D do not relate to the question; therefore, they are incorrect. Answer B refers to diabetes mellitus; therefore, it is incorrect.

75. **Answer C is correct.** Positioning the client on her left side will take pressure off the vena cava and allow better oxygenation of the fetus. Answers A and B do not relieve pressure on the vena cava; therefore, they are incorrect. Answer D is the preferred position for the client with a prolapsed cord; therefore, it is incorrect for this situation.

76. **Answer A is correct.** Prothrombin time measures the therapeutic level of Coumadin. Answer B is incorrect because it measures the quantity of each specific clotting factor. Answer C is incorrect because it measures the therapeutic level of heparin. Answer D is incorrect because it evaluates the vascular and platelet factors associated with hemostasis.

77. **Answer C is correct.** Accutane is made from concentrated vitamin A, a fat-soluble vitamin. Fat-soluble vitamins have the potential of being hepatotoxic, so a liver panel is needed. Answers A, B, and D do not relate to therapy with Accutane; therefore, they are incorrect.

78. **Answer A is correct.** The client's WBC is only slightly elevated and is most likely due to the birth process. Answer B is incorrect because the WBC would be more elevated if an acute bacterial infection was present. Answer C is incorrect because viral infections usually do not cause elevations in WBC. Answer D is incorrect because dehydration is not reflected by changes in the WBC.

79. **Answer B is correct.** PKU screening is usually done on the third day of life. Answer A is incorrect because the baby will not have had sufficient time to ingest protein sources of phenylalanine. Answer C is incorrect because blood is obtained from a heel stick, not from cord blood. Answer D is incorrect because the first immunizations are done at six weeks of age, and by that time, brain damage will already have occurred if the baby has PKU.

80. **Answer B is correct.** The client's blood gases indicate respiratory alkalosis. Answers A, C, and D are not reflected by the client's blood gases or present condition; therefore, they are incorrect.

81. **Answer D is correct.** Cor pulmonale, or right-sided heart failure, is characterized by edema of the legs and feet, enlarged liver, and distended neck veins. Answer A is incorrect because the symptoms are those of left-sided heart failure and pulmonary edema. Answer B is not specific to the question; therefore, it is incorrect. Answer C is incorrect because it does not relate to cor pulmonale.

82. **Answer C is correct.** The primary reason for the NG to is to allow for nourishment without contamination of the suture line. Answer A is not a true statement; therefore, it is incorrect. Answer B is incorrect because there is no mention of suction. Answer D is incorrect because the oral mucosa was not involved in the laryngectomy.

83. **Answer D is correct.** The client's complaints are due to swelling associated with surgery and catheter placement. Answer A is incorrect because it will not relieve the client's symptoms of pain and dribbling. Answer B is incorrect because perineal exercises will not help relieve the post-operative pain. Answer C is incorrect because the client's complaints do not indicate the need for catheter reinsertion.

84. **Answer B is correct.** The chest-drainage system can be disconnected from suction, but the chest tube should remain unclamped to prevent a tension pneumothorax. Answer A is incorrect because it could result in a tension pneumothorax. Answer C is not a true statement; therefore, it is not correct. Answer D is incorrect because the chest-drainage system should be kept lower than the client's chest and shoulders.

85. **Answer B is correct.** Cardiac dysrhythmias are the most common complication for the client with a myocardial infarction. Answers A and C do not relate to myocardial infarction; therefore, they are incorrect. Answer D is incorrect because it is not the most common complication following a myocardial infarction.

86. **Answer A is correct.** Elevations in temperature increase the cardiac output. Answer B is incorrect because temperature elevations are not associated with cardiac tamponade. Answer C is incorrect because temperature elevation does not decrease cardiac output. Answer D is incorrect because elevations in temperature in the client with a coronary artery bypass graft indicate inflammation, not necessarily graft rejection.

87. **Answer A is correct.** The client with expressive aphasia has trouble forming words that are understandable. Answer B is incorrect because it describes receptive aphasia. Answer C refers to apraxia and answer D refers to agnosia, so they are incorrect.

88. **Answer D is correct.** The client taking MAOI, including Parnate, should avoid eating aged cheeses, such as cheddar cheese, because a hypertensive crisis can result. Answer A is incorrect because processed cheese is less likely to produce a hypertensive crisis. Answers B and C do not cause a hypertensive crisis in the client taking an MAOI; therefore, they are incorrect.

89. **Answer C is correct.** The client with rheumatoid arthritis needs to continue moving affected joints within the limits of pain. Answer A and D are incorrect because they will increase stiffness and joint disuse. Answer B is incorrect because, if done correctly, passive range-of-motion exercises will improve the use of affected joints.

90. **Answer B is correct.** Exposed abdominal viscera should be covered with a sterile saline-soaked gauze, and the doctor should be notified immediately. Answer A is incorrect because the dressing should be sterile, not clean. Answer C is incorrect because attempting to replace abdominal contents can cause greater injury and should be done only surgically. Answer D is incorrect because the area is kept moist only with sterile normal saline.

91. **Answer C is correct.** Using the ABCD approach to the client with multiple trauma, the nurse in the ER would: establish an airway, determine whether the client is breathing, check circulation (control hemorrhage), and check for deficits (head injuries). Answers A, B, and D are incorrect because they are not in the appropriate sequence for maintaining life.

92. **Answer A is correct.** Stimulant medications such as Ritalin tend to cause anorexia and weight loss in some children with ADHD. Providing high-calorie snacks will help the child maintain an appropriate weight. Answer B is incorrect because the medication does not mask infection. Answer C is incorrect because the medication is a central nervous system stimulant, not a depressant. Answer D has no relationship to the medication; therefore, it is incorrect.

93. **Answer A is correct.** The most likely victim of elder abuse is the elderly female with a chronic, debilitating illness such as Alzheimer's dementia. Answers B, C, and D are less likely to be victims of elder abuse; therefore, they are incorrect.

94. **Answer D is correct.** Sunscreens of at least an SPF of 15 should be applied 20–30 minutes before going into the sun. Answers A, B, and C are incorrect because they do not allow sufficient time for sun protection.

95. **Answer C is correct.** Retinal hemorrhages are characteristically found in the child who has been violently shaken. Answers A, B, and D may result from trauma other than that related to abuse; therefore, they are incorrect.

96. **Answer B is correct.** The combination of the two medications produces a synergistic effect (an effect greater than that of either drug used alone). Agonist effects are similar to those produced by chemicals normally present in the body; therefore, answer A is incorrect. Antagonist effects are those in which the actions of the drugs oppose one another; therefore, answer C is incorrect. Answer D is incorrect because the drugs would have a combined depressing, not excitatory effect.

97. **Answer B is correct.** The client with a history of diabetes is most likely to deliver a preterm large for gestational age newborn. These newborns often lack sufficient surfactant levels to prevent respiratory distress syndrome. Answers A, C, and D are less likely to have newborns with respiratory distress syndrome, so they are incorrect choices.

98. **Answer D is correct.** Nursing care of the client with cervical tongs includes performance of sterile pin care and assessment of the site. Answers A, B, and C alter the traction and could result in serious injury or death of the client; therefore, they are incorrect.

99. **Answer A is correct.** Chest drainage greater than 100mL per hour is excessive, and the doctor should be notified regarding possible hemorrhage. Confusion and restlessness could be in response to pain, changes in oxygenation, or the emergence from anesthesia; therefore, answer B is incorrect. Answer C is incorrect because it is an expected finding in the client recently returning from a CABG. Answer D is within normal limits; therefore, it is incorrect.

100. **Answer C is correct.** The medication should be withheld and the doctor should be notified. Answers A, B, and D are incorrect because they do not provide for the client's safety.

101. **Answer B is correct.** Solid foods should be added to the diet one at a time, with intervals of 4–7 days between new foods. The extrusion reflex fades at 3–4 months of age; therefore, answer A is incorrect. Answer C is incorrect because solids should not be added to the bottle and the use of infant feeders is discouraged. Answer D is incorrect because the first food added to the infant's diet is rice cereal.

102. **Answer D is correct.** At 32 weeks gestation, the fetus can be expected to be active. Answers A, B, and C are not typical findings during the Leopold maneuver of a client who is 32 weeks gestation; therefore, they are incorrect.

103. **Answer A is correct.** The client needs to avoid using sweeteners containing aspartame. Answers B, C, and D indicate that the client understands the nurse's teaching; therefore, they are incorrect.

104. **Answer A is correct.** The treatment of galactosemia consists of eliminating all milk and lactose-containing foods, including breast milk. Answers B and D contain inaccurate information; therefore, they are incorrect. Galactosemia is inherited as an autosomal recessive disorder. There is a one-in-four chance that future children will be affected; therefore, answer C is incorrect.

105. **Answer B is correct.** The child with Tay Sachs disease has cherry-red spots on the macula of the eye. Answer A is incorrect because it is associated with anemia. Answer C is incorrect because it is associated with osteogenesis imperfecta. Answer D is incorrect because it is associated with Down syndrome.

106. **Answer C is correct.** The client's symptoms suggest an adverse reaction to the medication known as neuroleptic malignant syndrome. Answers A, B, and D are not appropriate interventions for the client; therefore, they are incorrect.

107. **Answer D is correct.** The client with HIV should adhere to a low-bacteria diet by avoiding raw fruits and vegetables. Answers A, B, and C are incorrect because they are permitted in the client's diet.

108. **Answer C is correct.** The child with leukemia has low platelet counts, which contribute to spontaneous bleeding. Answers A, B, and D, common in the child with leukemia, are not life-threatening.

109. **Answer A is correct.** The nurse should prevent the infant with atopic dermatitis (eczema) from scratching, which can lead to skin infections. Answer B is incorrect because fever is not associated with atopic dermatitis. Answers C and D are incorrect because they increase dryness of the skin, which worsens the symptoms of atopic dermatitis.

110. **Answer B is correct.** Pavulon is a neuromuscular blocking agent that paralyzes skeletal muscles, making it impossible for the client to fight the ventilator. Sublimaze is an analgesic used to control operative pain; therefore, answer A is incorrect. Versed is a benzodiazepine used to produce conscious sedation; therefore, answer C is incorrect. Answer D is wrong because Atarax is used to treat post-operative nausea.

111. **Answer D is correct.** Symptoms associated with diverticulitis are usually reported after eating foods like popcorn, celery, raw vegetables, whole grains, and nuts. Answers A, B, and C are incorrect because they are allowed in the diet of the client with diverticulitis.

112. **Answer A is correct.** The client with Paget's disease has problems with mobility. Keeping the environment free of clutter will help prevent falls. Answers B, C, and D will improve the client's overall health but are not specific to Paget's disease; therefore, they are incorrect.

113. **Answer B is correct.** The Whipple procedure is performed for cancer located in the head of the pancreas. Answers A, C, and D are not correct because of the location of the cancer.

114. **Answer C is correct.** Side effects of Pulmozyme include sore throat, hoarseness, and laryngitis. Answers A, B, and D are not associated with Pulmozyme; therefore, they are incorrect.

115. **Answer B is correct.** Retained placental fragments are the major cause of late postpartal hemorrhage. Uterine atony is the major cause of early postpartal hemorrhage; therefore, answer A is incorrect. Answers C and D result in slow, steady bleeding; therefore, they are incorrect.

116. **Answer A is correct.** The nurse has a legal responsibility to report suspected abuse and neglect. The nurse does not have the authority to remove the children from the home; therefore, answers B and C are incorrect. Answer D is incorrect because it is unrealistic.

117. **Answer A is correct.** Providing a caring attitude and supportive environment will make the client feel safe. Answer B is incorrect because the client needs to feel free to express anger. Answer C is incorrect because it will increase the client's anxiety. Answer D is incorrect because it is not the most important aspect of care for the client with PTSD.

118. **Answer B is correct.** The nurse should be concerned with alleviating the client's pain. Answers A, C, and D are not primary objectives in the care of the client receiving an opiate analgesic; therefore, they are incorrect.

119. **Answer D is correct.** The therapeutic range for aminophylline is 10–20 micrograms/mL. Levels greater than 20 micrograms/mL can produce signs of toxicity. Answer A is incorrect because it is too low to be therapeutic. Answers B and C are within the therapeutic range; therefore, they are incorrect.

120. **Answer C is correct.** Changes in breath sounds are the best indication of the need for suctioning in the client with ineffective airway clearance. Answers A, B, and D are incorrect because they can be altered by other conditions.

121. **Answer D is correct.** An adverse reaction to Myambutol is changes in visual acuity or color vision. Answer A is incorrect because it does not relate to the medication. Answer B is incorrect because it is an adverse reaction to Streptomycin. Answer C is incorrect because it is a side effect of Rifampin.

122. **Answer D is correct.** Insufficient erythropoietin production is the primary cause of anemia in the client with chronic renal failure. Answers A, B, and C do not relate to the anemia seen in clients with chronic renal failure; therefore, they are incorrect.

123. **Answer B is correct.** The nurse's highest priority should be asking the client about allergies to shellfish and iodine. The contrast media used during an intravenous pyelogram contains iodine, which can result in an anaphylactic reaction. Answers A, C, and D do not relate specifically to the test; therefore, they are incorrect.

124. **Answer A is correct.** Ataxia affects the client's mobility, making falls more likely. Answers B, C, and D are incorrect because they do not relate to the problem of ataxia.

125. **Answer D is correct.** Aspirin decreases platelet aggregation or clumping, thereby preventing clots. Answer A is incorrect because the low-dose aspirin will not prevent headaches. Answers B and C are untrue statements; therefore, they are incorrect.

126. **Answer B is correct.** Insulin molecules adhere to glass and plastic; therefore, the IV set and entire tubing should be flushed and 50mL discarded before administering the infusion to the client. Answers A and D are incorrect because insulin is mixed using 0.9% or 0.45% normal saline. Answer C is incorrect because the infusion is given using a pump or controller.

127. **Answer A is correct.** A serologic marker of HB8 AG that is present six months after acute infection with hepatitis B indicates that the client is a carrier or has chronic hepatitis. Answer B is incorrect because the HB8 AG would normally decline and disappear. Answer C is incorrect because the client can still be infected with hepatitis c. Answer D is incorrect because the client is a carrier.

128. **Answer C is correct.** The usual course of treatment using combined therapy with isoniazid and rifampin is six months. Two other medications, pyrazinamide and ethambutol, are usually given along with isoniazid and rifampin for 2 months. Answers A and D are incorrect because the treatment time is too brief. Answer B is incorrect because the medication is not needed for life.

129. **Answer D is correct.** At four months of age, the infant can roll over, which makes it vulnerable to falls from dressing tables or beds without rails. Answer A is incorrect because it does not prove a threat to safety. Answers B and C are incorrect choices because the four-month-old is not capable of crawling or standing.

130. **Answer B is correct.** Rhinitis, maculopapular rash, and hepatosplenomegaly are associated with congenital syphilis. Answer A is incorrect because it describes symptoms of scarlet fever. Answer C is incorrect because it describes symptoms of Fifth's disease. Answer D is incorrect because it describes the symptoms of Down syndrome.

131. **Answer C is correct.** It is recommended that infants up to 20 pounds be restrained in a car seat in a semi-reclining position facing the rear of the car. Answers A and B are incorrect because the child is young enough to require the rear-facing position. Answer D is incorrect because the child can be placed in an upright position in an approved safety seat facing forward.

132. **Answer B is correct.** The client with irritable bowel syndrome has bouts of constipation and diarrhea. Answer A is incorrect because it describes changes associated with diverticulosis. Answer C is incorrect because it describes changes associated with Crohn's disease. Answer D is incorrect because it describes findings associated with ulcerative colitis.

133. **Answer C is correct.** Adverse side effects of Dilantin include agranulocytosis and aplastic anemia; therefore, the client will need regularly scheduled blood work. Answer A is incorrect because the medication does not cause dental staining. Answer B is incorrect because the medication does not interfere with the metabolism of carbohydrates. Answer D is incorrect because the medication does not cause drowsiness.

134. **Answer A is correct.** The infant with hypospadias should not be circumcised because the foreskin is used in reconstruction. Answers B and C are incorrect because surgical correction is done when the infant is 16 to 18 months of age. Answer D is incorrect because the infant with hypospadias should not be circumcised.

135. **Answer C is correct.** Coconut oil is high in saturated fat and is not appropriate for the client on a low-cholesterol diet. Answers A, B, and D are incorrect because they are suggested for the client with elevated cholesterol levels.

136. **Answer D is correct.** Increased blood pressure following a renal transplant is an early sign of transplant failure. Answers A, B, and C are expected with successful renal transplant; therefore, they are incorrect.

137. **Answer D is correct.** The time it takes for alcohol to be fully metabolized is calculated by dividing the blood alcohol level on admission by 20mg/dL (amount metabolized in an hour). Answers A, B, and C are incorrect because there has not been sufficient time for the alcohol to be fully metabolized.

138. **Answer B is correct.** In stage III of Alzheimer's disease, the client develops agnosia, or failure to recognize familiar objects. Answer A is incorrect because it appears in stage I. Answer C is incorrect because it appears in stage II. Answer D is incorrect because it appears in stage IV.

139. **Answer D is correct.** The client taking steroid medication should receive an annual influenza vaccine. Answer A is incorrect because the medication should be taken with food. Answer B is incorrect because increased appetite and weight gain are expected side effects of the medication. Answer C is incorrect because wearing sunglasses will not prevent the development of cataracts in the client taking steroids.

140. **Answer A is correct.** The client with an above-the-knee amputation should be placed in a prone position 15–30 minutes twice a day to prevent hip flexion contractures. Answers B and D are incorrect choices because elevation of the extremity one day post amputation promotes the development of contractures. Use of a trochanter roll will prevent rotation of the extremity but will not prevent contracture; therefore, answer C is incorrect.

141. **Answer D is correct.** All 20 primary, or deciduous, teeth should be present by age 30 months. Answers A, B, and C are incorrect because the ages are wrong.

142. **Answer B is correct.** Displacement of the esophageal balloon is the most likely cause of respiratory distress in the client with an esophageal tamponade. The nurse should deflate both the gastric and esophageal balloons before removing the tube. Answers A and C are incorrect because applying nasal oxygen and elevating the head will not relieve airway obstruction. Answer D is incorrect because it would cause further obstruction of the airway.

143. **Answer D is correct.** The mitral valve is heard loudest at the fourth intercostal space midclavicular line, which is the apex of the heart. Answer A is incorrect because it is the location for the aortic valve. Answer B is incorrect because it is the location for the pulmonic valve. Answer C is wrong because it is the location for the tricuspid valve.

144. **Answer C is correct.** The radioactive implant should be picked up with tongs and returned to the lead-lined container. Answer A is incorrect because radioactive materials are placed in lead-lined containers, not plastic ones, and they are returned to the radiation department, not the lab. Answer B is incorrect because the client should not touch the implant or try to reinsert it. Answer D is incorrect because the implant should not be placed in the commode for disposal.

145. **Answer A is correct.** Following a laparoscopic cholecystectomy, the client should avoid a tub bath for 48 hours. Answer B is incorrect because the stools should not be clay colored. Answer C is incorrect because pain is usually located in the shoulders. Answer D is incorrect because pain in the back and shoulders is expected following laparoscopic surgery.

146. **Answer B is correct.** The client recovering from mononeucleosis should avoid contact sports and other activities that could result in injury or rupture of the spleen. Answer A is incorrect because the client does not need additional fluids. Hypoglycemia is not associated with mononeucleosis; therefore, answer C is incorrect. Answer D is incorrect because antibiotics are not usually indicated in the treatment of mononeucleosis.

147. **Answer B is correct.** Pancreatic enzyme replacement is given with meals and snacks. Answers A, C, and D do not specify a relationship to meals; therefore, they are incorrect.

148. **Answer A is correct.** Meat, eggs, and dairy products are the best sources of vitamin B12. Answer B is incorrect because peanut butter, raisins, and molasses are good sources of iron. Answer C is incorrect because broccoli, cauliflower, and cabbage are good sources of vitamin K. Answer D is incorrect because shrimp, legumes, and bran cereals are good sources of magnesium.

149. **Answer A is correct.** The client's aerobic workout should be 20–30 minutes long three times a week. Answers B, C, and D exceed the recommended time for the client beginning an aerobic program; therefore, they are incorrect.

150. **Answer B is correct.** Demadex is a loop diuretic that depletes potassium. Answers A, C, and D are incorrect because they are potassium-sparing diuretics.

151. **Answer A is correct.** Following a total mastectomy, the client's right arm should be elevated on pillows to facilitate lymph drainage. Answers B, C, and D are incorrect because they would not help facilitate lymph drainage and would create increased edema in the affected extremity.

152. **Answer B is correct.** Nitroglycerin is used to dilate coronary blood vessels, which provides improved circulation to the myocardium. Answers A, C, and D describe the effects of digoxin, not nitroglycerin; therefore, they are incorrect.

153. **Answer D is correct.** The client with flail chest will exhibit paradoxical respirations. (With inspiration, the affected side will move inward; with expiration, the affected side will move outward. Flail chest is frequently associated with high-speed motor vehicle accidents.) Answer A is incorrect because air or blood would be present in the thoracic cavity. Answer B is incorrect because the trachea would be shifted to the affected side. Answer C is incorrect because interstitial edema would be present.

154. **Answer D is correct.** Absence seizures, formerly known as petit mal seizures, are characterized by brief lapses in consciousness accompanied by rapid eye blinking, lip smacking, and minor myoclonus of the upper extremities. Answer A refers to myoclonic seizures; therefore, it is incorrect. Answer B refers to tonic clonic seizures, formerly known as grand mal seizures; therefore, it is incorrect. Answer C refers to atonic seizures; therefore, it is incorrect.

155. **Answer C is correct.** Keeping the room quiet and the lights dimmed will decrease sensory stimulation and help keep the client oriented during withdrawal from alcohol. Answer A is incorrect because darkness would increase confusion and disorientation in the client during withdrawal. Answers B and D are incorrect because they can contribute to the development of seizures.

156. **Answer A is correct.** A side effect of antipsychotic medication is the development of Parkinsonian symptoms. Answers B and C are incorrect choices because they are used to reverse Parkinsonian symptoms in the client taking antipsychotic medication. Answer D is incorrect because the medication is an anticonvulsant used to stabilize mood. Parkinsonian symptoms are not associated with anticonvulsant medication.

157. **Answer B is correct.** Exercises, such as swimming, that provide light passive resistance are best for the child with juvenile rheumatoid arthritis. Answers A and C require movement of the hands and fingers that could be too painful for the child with juvenile rheumatoid arthritis; therefore, they are incorrect. Answer D is incorrect because it requires the use of larger joints affected by the disease.

158. **Answer A is correct.** Reports of cough and fever in the client with AIDS suggest infection with pneumocystis carinii, which requires immediate intervention. Answers B, C, and D have conditions with more predictable outcomes; therefore, they are incorrect.

159. **Answer B is correct.** The client's diabetes is well under control. Answer A is incorrect because it will lead to elevated glucose levels. Answer C is incorrect because the diet and insulin dose are appropriate for the client. Answer D is incorrect because the desired range for glycosylated hemoglobin in the adult client is 2.5%–5.9%.

160. **Answer C is correct.** The purpose of the dexamethasone-suppression test is to identify clients who will benefit from therapy with antidepressants and electroconvulsive therapy rather than psychological or social interventions. Answers A, B, and D contain inaccurate statements; therefore, they are incorrect.

161. **Answer A is correct.** Stadol reduces the perception of pain, which allows the post-operative client to rest. Answers B and C are not affected by the medication; therefore, they are incorrect. Relief of pain generally results in less nausea, but it is not the intended effect of the medication; therefore, answer D is incorrect.

162. **Answer B is correct.** Children with cystic fibrosis are susceptible to chronic sinusitis and nasal polyps, which might require surgical removal. Answer A is incorrect because it is a congenital condition in which there is a bony obstruction between the nares and the pharynx. Answers C and D are not specific to the child with cystic fibrosis; therefore, they are incorrect.

163. **Answer C is correct.** During the emergent phase, the nursing priority for a client with burns confined to the lower body would focus on the risk for fluid volume imbalance. Answers A, B, and D are incorrect because they do not take priority over the risk for fluid volume imbalance or hypovolemia, during the emergent phase.

164. **Answer D is correct.** Lipid-lowering agents are contraindicated in the client with active liver disease. Answers A, B, and C are incorrect because they are not contraindicated in the client with active liver disease.

165. **Answer D is correct.** An appropriate activity for the client who has recently had an MI is sitting on the side of the bed for five minutes three times a day with assistance. Answers A and C are incorrect because they increase the workload on the heart too soon after the MI. Answer B is incorrect because it does not allow the client enough activity.

166. **Answer C is correct.** The client with hypertension should be placed on a low sodium, low cholesterol, high fiber diet. Oatmeal is low in sodium and high in fiber. Answer A is incorrect because cornflakes and whole milk are higher in sodium and are poor sources of fiber. Answers B and D are incorrect choices because they contain animal proteins that are high in both cholesterol and sodium.

167. **Answer A is correct.** Following hypospadias repair, the child will need to avoid straddle toys, such as a rocking horse, until allowed by the surgeon. Answers B, C, and D do not relate to the post-operative care of the child with hypospadias; therefore, they are incorrect.

168. **Answer A is correct.** Eating carbohydrates such as dry crackers or toast before arising helps to alleviate morning sickness. Answer B is incorrect because the additional fat might increase the client's nausea. Answer C is incorrect because the client does not need to skip meals. Answer D is the treatment of hypoglycemia, not morning sickness; therefore, it is incorrect.

169. **Answer D is correct.** An esophageal tamponade is used to control bleeding in the client with esophageal varices. Answers A, B, and C are incorrect because they can be assigned to either the novice RN or the LPN with assisted care by the nursing assistant.

170. **Answer B is correct.** The modified Blalock Taussig procedure is a palliative procedure in which the subclavian artery is joined to the pulmonary artery, thus allowing more blood to reach the lungs. Answers A, C, and D contain inaccurate statements; therefore, they are incorrect.

171. **Answer A is correct.** The stethoscope should be left in the client's room for future use. The stethoscope should not be returned to the exam room or the nurse's station; therefore, answers B and D are incorrect. The stethoscope should not be used to assess other clients; therefore, answer C is incorrect.

172. **Answer B is correct.** The medication will be needed throughout the child's lifetime. Answers A, C, and D contain inaccurate statements; therefore, they are incorrect.

173. **Answer B is correct.** Glucotrol XL is given once a day with breakfast. Answer A is incorrect because the client would develop hypoglycemia while sleeping. Answers C and D are incorrect choices because the client would develop hypoglycemia later in the day or evening.

174. **Answer D is correct.** The client with myasthenia develops progressive weakness that worsens during the day. Answer A is incorrect because it refers to symptoms of multiple sclerosis. Answer B is incorrect because it refers to symptoms of Guillain Barre syndrome. Answer C is incorrect because it refers to Parkinson's disease.

175. **Answer D is correct.** Immaturity of the kidneys places the preterm infant at greater risk for toxicity to aminoglycosides. Answers A, B, and C are true regarding the preterm infant, but they do not increase the risk for toxicity to the drug; therefore, they are incorrect.

176. **Answer B is correct.** To prevent fractures, the parents should lift the infant by the buttocks rather than the ankles when diapering. Answer A is incorrect because infants with osteogenesis imperfecta have normal calcium and phosphorus levels. Answer C is incorrect because the condition is not temporary. Answer D is incorrect because the teeth and the sclera are also affected.

177. **Answer C is correct.** Following a hip replacement, the client should avoid hip flexion. Sitting on a soft, low sofa permits hip flexion and increases the difficulty of standing. Having a pet is important to the client's emotional well-being; therefore, answer A is incorrect. Answers B and D indicate that the nurse's teaching has been effective; therefore, they are incorrect.

178. **Answer A is correct.** Withholding oral intake will help stop the inflammatory process by reducing the secretion of pancreatic enzymes. Answer B is incorrect because the client requires exogenous insulin. Answer C is incorrect because it does not prevent the secretion of gastric acid. Answer D is incorrect because it does not eliminate the need for pain medication.

179. **Answer B is correct.** A rigid or boardlike abdomen is suggestive of peritonitis, which is a complication of diverticulitis. Answers A, C, and D are common findings in diverticulitis; therefore, they are incorrect.

180. **Answer D is correct.** Vancomycin should be administered slowly to prevent "redman" syndrome. Answer A is incorrect because the medication is not given IV push. Answers B and C are incorrect choices because they allow the medication to be given too rapidly.

181. **Answer A is correct.** Prostigmine (neostigmine) is used to treat clients with myasthenia gravis. Answer B is incorrect because it is used to reverse the effects of neostigmine. Answer C is incorrect because the drug is unrelated to the treatment of myasthenia gravis. Answer D is incorrect because it is the test for myasthenia gravis.

182. **Answer D is correct.** The suggested diet for the client with AIDS is one that is high calorie, high protein, and low fat. Clients with AIDS have a reduced tolerance to fat because of the disease, as well as side effects from some antiviral medications; therefore, answers A and C are incorrect. Answer B is incorrect because the client needs a high-protein diet.

183. **Answer B is correct.** The nurse can help ready the child with cerebral palsy for speech therapy by providing activities that help the child develop tongue control. Most children with cerebral palsy have visual and auditory difficulties that require glasses or hearing devices rather than rehabilitative training; therefore, answers A and C are incorrect. Answer D is incorrect because video games are not appropriate to the age or developmental level for the child with cerebral palsy.

184. **Answer A is correct.** The client with duodenal ulcers commonly complains of epigastric pain that is relieved by eating a meal or snack. Answer B is incorrect because the client with a duodenal ulcer frequently reports weight gain. Answers C and D are incorrect because they describe symptoms associated with gastric ulcers.

185. **Answer D is correct.** Complications following a stapedectomy include damage to the seventh cranial nerve that results in changes in taste or facial sensation. Answers A and B are incorrect because they are expected immediately following a stapedectomy. Answer C is incorrect because it involves the twelfth cranial nerve (hypoglossal nerve).

186. **Answer C is correct.** Most infants begin nocturnal sleep lasting 9–11 hours by 3–4 months of age. Answers A and B are incorrect because the infant is still waking for nighttime feedings. Answer D is incorrect because most infants begin nocturnal sleep by 3–4 months of age.

187. **Answer A is correct.** The goal of oxygen therapy for the client with emphysema is maintaining a PaO2 of 50 to 60mmHg. Answers B, C, and D are incorrect because the PaO2 levels are too high.

188. **Answer B is correct.** The medication is having its intended effect when the client's urine specific gravity is within the normal range. Answers A and D refer to the client with diabetes mellitus not diabetes insipidus; therefore, they are incorrect. Answer C is incorrect because it is not related to diabetes insipidus.

189. **Answer A is correct.** The child with myelomeningocele is at greatest risk for the development of latex allergy because of repeated exposure to latex products during surgery and from numerous urinary catheterizations. The clients in answers B, C, and D are much less likely to be exposed to latex; therefore, they are incorrect.

190. **Answer D is correct.** The therapeutic range for aminophylline is 10–20 micrograms/mL. Answers A, B, and C are incorrect because they are too low to be therapeutic.

191. **Answer C is correct.** The priority nursing diagnosis for a client with acromegaly focuses on the risk for ineffective airway clearance. Answers A, B, and D apply to the client with acromegaly but do not take priority; therefore, they are incorrect.

192. **Answer C is correct.** The nurse can help increase ventilation and perfusion to all areas of the lungs by turning the client every hour. Rocking beds can also be used to keep the client in constant motion. Answer A is incorrect because the client with ARDS will have respirations controlled by the ventilator. Answer B is incorrect because the nurse must have a physician's order to increase the PEEP. Answer D is incorrect because it will not increase ventilation and perfusion.

193. **Answer D is correct.** The nurse or parent should use a cupped hand when performing chest percussion. Answer A is incorrect because the hand should be cupped. Answer B is incorrect because the child's position should be changed every 5–10 minutes, and the whole session should be limited to 20 minutes. Answer C is incorrect because chest percussion should be done before meals.

194. **Answer A is correct.** The client with Addison's disease requires lifetime management with steroids. The nurse should stress the importance of taking the medication exactly as directed by the physician, as well as reporting adverse reactions to the medication. The client should be cautioned not to skip doses or to abruptly discontinue the medication. Answers B, C, and D should be included in the client's teaching but do not pose life-threatening consequences; therefore, they are incorrect.

195. **Answer B is correct.** Air embolus can occur with insertion, maintenance, and removal of central line catheters. The client's history of recent removal of a central line and the development of dyspnea, substernal chest pain, confusion, and fear suggest an air embolus. Answer A is incorrect because it is not associated with central line use. Answer C is incorrect because the symptoms do not suggest bleeding. Answer D is incorrect because it is not a complication of central line use.

196. **Answer A is correct.** No more than 1mL should be given in the vastus lateralis of the infant. Answers B, C, and D are incorrect because the dorsogluteal and ventrogluteal muscles are not used for injections in the infant.

197. **Answer C is correct.** Depot injections of Haldol are administered every four weeks. Answers A and B are incorrect because the medication is still in the client's system. Answer D is incorrect because the medication has been eliminated from the client's system, which allows the symptoms of schizophrenia to return.

198. **Answer C is correct.** The client should take a deep breath and hold it (Valsalva maneuver) when the central line is being removed. This increases the intrathoracic pressure and decreases the likelihood of having an air embolus. Answers A and B do not increase intrathoracic pressure; therefore, they are incorrect for the situation. Answer D increases the likelihood of air embolus; therefore, it is incorrect.

199. **Answer D is correct.** The earliest sign of cystic fibrosis is meconium ileus, which may be present in the newborn with the disease. Answers A, B, and C are later manifestations; therefore, they are incorrect.

200. **Answer D is correct.** Tucking a disposable diaper at the perineal opening will help prevent soiling of the cast by urine and stool. Answer A is incorrect because the head of the bed should be elevated. Answer B is incorrect because the child can place the crayons beneath the cast, causing pressure areas to develop. Answer C is incorrect because the child does not need high-calorie foods that would cause weight gain while she is immobilized by the cast.

201. **Answer B is correct.** Coolness and discoloration of the reimplanted digits indicates compromised circulation, which should be reported immediately to the physician. The temperature should be monitored, but the client would receive antibiotics to prevent infection; therefore, answer A is incorrect. Answers C and D are expected following amputation and reimplantation; therefore, they are incorrect.

202. **Answer C is correct.** The obstetrical client under age 18 is at greatest risk for CPD because pelvic growth is not fully completed. Answers A, B, and D are incorrect because these clients are not as likely to have CPD.

203. **Answer A is correct.** Priority of care should focus on maintaining the client's airway. Answers B and C are important to the client's care, but they do not take priority over maintaining the client's airway; therefore, they are incorrect. Answer D is incorrect because the client will require a passive range of motion exercise.

204. **Answer B is correct.** Answers A, C, and D are incorrect because they are inaccurate amounts.

205. **Answer A is correct.** Following extracorporeal lithotripsy, the urine will appear cherry red in color but will gradually change to clear urine. Answer B is incorrect because the urine will be red, not orange. Answer C is incorrect because the urine will not be dark red or cloudy in appearance. Answer D is incorrect because it describes the urinary output of the client with acute glomerulonephritis.

206. **Answer A is correct.** Special rotational or directional catheters will be used to remove the plaque. Answer B is incorrect because it describes ablation. Answer C is incorrect because it describes percutaneous transluminal coronary angioplasty. Answer D is incorrect because it refers to lipid-lowering agents.

207. **Answer C is correct.** A stage II pressure ulcer has cracks and blisters with areas of redness and induration. Answer A is incorrect because it describes the appearance of a stage IV pressure ulcer. Answer B is incorrect because it describes the appearance of a stage III pressure ulcer. Answer D is incorrect because it describes the appearance of a stage I pressure ulcer.

208. **Answer B is correct.** An adverse reaction to Cognex is drug-induced hepatitis. The nurse should monitor the client for signs of jaundice. Answers A, C, and D are incorrect because they are not associated with the use of Cognex.

209. **Answer A is correct.** The child with cystic fibrosis needs a diet that is high in calories, with high protein and moderate amounts of fat. Answers B, C, and D are incorrect because they do not meet the nutritional requirements imposed by the disease.

210. **Answer C is correct.** Apples are low in potassium; therefore, this is a suitable snack for the client on a potassium-restricted diet. Raisins, oranges, and bananas are all high in potassium; therefore, answers A, B, and D are incorrect.

211. **Answer B is correct.** Hyperventilation reduces swelling and increased intracranial pressure by decreasing cerebral blood flow. Answers A, C, and D do not pertain to the situation; therefore, they are incorrect.

212. **Answer B is correct.** No special preparation is needed for the blood test for *H. pylori*. Answer A is incorrect because the client is not NPO before the test. Answer C is incorrect because it refers to preparation for the breath test. Answer D is incorrect because glucose is not administered before the test.

213. **Answer B is correct.** Oral potassium supplements should be given in at least 4oz of juice or other liquid such as fruit punch to disguise the unpleasant taste. Answers A, C, and D are incorrect because they cause gastric upset.

214. **Answer D is correct.** The client with hypomagnesemia will have a positive Trousseau's sign. Answer A is incorrect because the client would have tachycardia. Answer B is incorrect because the client would have a positive Chvostek's sign. Answer C is incorrect because the client would have hypotension.

215. **Answer D is correct.** Fresh specimens are essential for an accurate diagnosis of CMV. Answer A is incorrect because cultures of urine, sputum, and oral swab are preferred. Answer B is incorrect because pregnant caregivers should not be assigned to care for clients with suspected or known infection with CMV. Answer C is incorrect because a convalescent culture is obtained 2–4 weeks after diagnosis.

216. **Answer B is correct.** The client with congestive heart failure who reports coughing up frothy sputum should be carefully evaluated for increasing pulmonary edema, which requires immediate treatment. Answers A, C, and D involve chronic conditions with complications that require skilled nursing care and assessment, but they do not present immediate life-threatening situations; therefore, they are incorrect.

217. **Answer B is correct.** The client with neutropenia needs to be placed in a private room in protective isolation. The other clients can be placed in the room with other clients; therefore, answers A, C, and D are incorrect.

218. **Answer B is correct.** Asterixis is a symptom of impending liver failure, so the client should be cared for by the RN. The remaining clients can be cared for by the LPN; therefore, answers A, C, and D are incorrect.

219. **Answer D is correct.** Adverse reactions to phenytoin include agranulocytosis. The client's WBC is abnormally low and should be reported to the physician immediately. Answer A is incorrect because elevations in serum creatinine are expected in the client with chronic renal failure. Answer B is wrong because a positive C reactive protein is usually present in those with rheumatic fever. Answer C is wrong because a hematocrit of 52% in a client with gastroenteritis can be expected due to dehydration.

220. **Answer D is correct.** The newly licensed nurse should not be assigned to provide primary care for the client with noncardiogenic pulmonary edema (ARDS) because the client's condition warrants care by an experienced RN. Answers A, B, and C are incorrect because the newly licensed nurse could assume primary care for clients with those conditions.

221. **Answer C is correct.** The client with a lumbar laminectomy can be safely cared for by the LPN. Answer A is incorrect because the client with a high cervical injury immobilized by skeletal traction is best cared for by the RN. Answers B and D are incorrect choices because these clients have conditions that require intravenous medication, which requires the skill of the RN.

222. **Answer A is correct.** The client with a thoracotomy who has 110mL of drainage in the past hour has excessive bleeding that should be evaluated and reported to the physician immediately. A temperature of 100°F following a surgery is not unusual; therefore, answer B is incorrect. Feelings of urinary urgency are normal after a transurethral prostatectomy; therefore, answer C is incorrect. Diminished loss of hearing in the hours following a stapedectomy is expected due to the swelling and accumulation of blood in the inner ear; therefore, answer D is incorrect.

223. **Answer A is correct.** Increased jaundice and prolonged prothrombin time are indications that the liver is not working. Answer B is incorrect because the symptoms suggest infection. Answer C is incorrect because the symptoms suggest obstruction. Answer D is incorrect because the symptoms are associated with renal failure.

224. **Answer A is correct.** The client with adrenal insufficiency frequently suffers from fluid volume deficit and acidosis; therefore, the nurse should give priority to monitoring for signs of dehydration. Answers B, C, and D are incorrect because they do not pose a life-threatening situation; therefore, they do not take priority.

225. **Answer D is correct.** Sulfamylon produces a burning sensation when applied; therefore, the client should receive pain medication 30 minutes before application. Answer A is incorrect because it refers to therapy with silver nitrate. Answer B is incorrect because it refers to therapy with Silvadene. Answer C is incorrect because it refers to therapy with Betadine.

226. **Answer D is correct.** Gingival hyperplasia is a side effect of Dilantin, so the nurse should provide oral hygiene and gum care every shift. Answers A, B, and C do not apply to the medication; therefore, they are incorrect.

227. **Answer C is correct.** Adverse reactions to Capoten include a decreased white cell count. Answers A, B, and D are incorrect because they are associated with the medication.

228. **Answer C is correct.** Zofran is given before chemotherapy to prevent nausea. Answers A, B, and D are not associated with the medication; therefore, they are incorrect.

229. **Answer A is correct.** When administering ear drops to a child under three years of age, the nurse should pull the ear down and back to straighten the ear canal. Answers B and D are incorrect positions for administering ear drops. Answer C is used for administering ear drops to the adult client.

230. **Answer A is correct.** Antibiotics such as Achromycin should not be taken with antacids. Answers B, C, and D may be taken with antibiotics; therefore, they are incorrect.

231. **Answer C is correct.** The nurse should carefully monitor the client taking Thorazine for signs of infection that can quickly become overwhelming. Answers A, B, and D are incorrect because they are expected side effects of the medication.

232. **Answer A is correct.** Claratin does not produce sedation like other antihistamines. Answers B, C, and D are inaccurate statements; therefore, they are incorrect.

233. **Answer B is correct.** A cotton-tipped swab is used to apply the suspension to the affected areas. Answers A, C, and D are incorrect because they do not ensure that the medication reaches the affected areas.

234. **Answer A is correct.** Iron is better absorbed when taken with ascorbic acid. Orange juice is an excellent source of ascorbic acid. Answer B is incorrect because the medication should be taken with orange juice or tomato juice. Answer C is incorrect because iron should not be taken with milk because it interferes with absorption. Answer D is incorrect because apple juice does not contain high amounts of ascorbic acid.

235. **Answer A is correct.** Acetylcysteine is the antidote for acetaminophen overdose. Answer B is incorrect because it is the antidote for iron poisoning. Answer C is incorrect because it is the treatment for lead poisoning. Answer D is incorrect because it is used for noncorrosive poisonings.

236. **Answer D is correct.** The client should hold the cane on the unaffected side. Answer A is incorrect because this answer instructs the client to hold the cane on the affected side. It will not be necessary for the client to use a walker, and advancing the cane with the affected leg is not correct; thus, answers B and C are incorrect.

237. **Answer A is correct.** Linear accelerator therapy is done in the radium department and does not make the client radioactive. Answer B is incorrect because there is no radiation emitted from the client. Answer C is incorrect because it is not necessary for the nursing assistant to wear an apron when caring for this client. Answer D is incorrect because there is no need to reassign the nursing assistant.

238. **Answer D is correct.** The client undergoing an angiogram will experience a warm sensation as the dye is injected. Answers A, B, and C are not associated with an angiogram.

239. **Answer B is correct.** Semi-liquids are more easily swallowed by the client with dysphagia than either liquids or solids. Answers A, C, and D do not improve the client's ability to swallow, so they are incorrect choices.

240. **Answer A is correct.** Placing the client in the Trendelenburg position will engorge the vessels, make insertion of the catheter easier, and lessen the likelihood of air entering the central line. Answer B is incorrect because the client will not be more comfortable in the Trendelenburg position. Answers C and D are not correct statements.

241. **Answer B is correct.** Taking deep breaths will decrease the discomfort experienced during removal of the drain. Answers A, C, and D are incorrect statements because they do not decrease the discomfort during removal of the drain.

242. **Answer B is correct.** Increased voiding at night is a symptom of right-sided heart failure. Answers A, C, and D are incorrect because they are symptoms of left-sided heart failure.

243. **Answer B is correct.** The CPM machine should not be set at 90° flexion until the fifth post-operative day. Answers A, C, and D are expected findings and do not require immediate nursing intervention; therefore, they are incorrect.

244. **Answer D is correct.** The multiparous client with a large newborn has the greatest risk for postpartal hemorrhage. Answers A, B, and C are incorrect choices because they do not have a greater risk for postpartal hemorrhage.

245. **Answer B is correct.** The medication should be administered using the calibrated dropper that comes with the medication. Answers A and C are incorrect because part or all of the medication could be lost during administration. Answer D is incorrect because part or all of the medication will be lost if the child does not finish the bottle.

246. **Answer C is correct.** Atropine is contraindicated in the client with glaucoma because the medication increases intraocular pressure. Answers A, B, and D are not contraindicated in the client with glaucoma; therefore, they are incorrect answers.

247. **Answer B is correct.** Aged cheese, wine, and smoked or pickled meats should be avoided by the client taking an MAOI, not a phenothiazine. Answers A, C, and D are included in the discharge teaching of a client receiving chlorpromazine (Thorazine).

248. **Answer D is correct.** Leaving a nightlight on during the evening and night shifts helps the client remain oriented to the environment and fosters independence. Answers A and B will not decrease the client's confusion. Answer C will increase the likelihood of confusion in an elderly client.

249. **Answer C is correct.** Elevations in white cell count indicate the presence of infection, which requires treatment before surgery. Answers A, B, and D are within normal limits and require no intervention.

250. **Answer A is correct.** Akathisia is an adverse extrapyramidal side effect of many older antipsychotic medications such as Haldol (haloperidol) and Thorazine (chlorpromazine). Answers B, C, and D are not associated with the use of haloperidol.

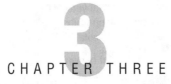

CHAPTER THREE

Practice Exam 3 and Rationales

1. The nurse is assessing the circulation of a patient in a long leg cast. Which of the following assessments indicate adequate circulation to the extremity?

   ○ **A.** Patient denies pain in the affected leg and foot.

   ○ **B.** Patient is able to wiggle the toes on command.

   ○ **C.** Sensation is reported when the soles of feet are touched.

   ○ **D.** Brisk capillary refill of less than three seconds.

Quick Answer: **220**
Detailed Answer: **223**

2. The amniocentesis reveals that the patient has a high AFP level. The nurse is aware that a high level of AFP is associated with which of the following?

   ○ **A.** Myelomeningocele

   ○ **B.** Esophageal atresia

   ○ **C.** Omphalocele

   ○ **D.** Trisomy 21

Quick Answer: **220**
Detailed Answer: **223**

3. Which nursing intervention would be of highest priority when caring for a patient admitted in sickle cell vaso-occlusive crisis?

   ○ **A.** Starting intravenous normal saline

   ○ **B.** Applying oxygen

   ○ **C.** Applying heat to the affected joints

   ○ **D.** Administering pain medication

Quick Answer: **220**
Detailed Answer: **223**

4. The physician has ordered an amniocentesis to determine the L/S ratio. The L/S ratio is a reliable indicator of:

   ○ **A.** Renal function

   ○ **B.** Rh isoimmunization

   ○ **C.** Fetal lung maturity

   ○ **D.** Anatomical abnormalities

Quick Answer: **220**
Detailed Answer: **223**

5. The nurse is caring for a patient hospitalized with leukopenia. Which of the following assessments should be reported to the physician immediately?

Quick Answer: **220**
Detailed Answer: **223**

   ○ **A.** The blood pressure is 110/62.

   ○ **B.** The apical pulse is 90.

   ○ **C.** The temperature has increased from 98.6°F to 99.8°F.

   ○ **D.** The respiratory rate is 24.

6. Which meal selection is most appropriate for a patient with iron deficiency anemia?

Quick Answer: **220**
Detailed Answer: **223**

   ○ **A.** Roast turkey, gelatin, green beans

   ○ **B.** Chicken salad sandwich, coleslaw, French fries

   ○ **C.** Egg salad on wheat bread, carrot sticks, spinach and kale salad

   ○ **D.** Pork chop, mashed potatoes, green peas

7. Which skin assessment in a newborn indicates a need for follow-up?

Quick Answer: **220**
Detailed Answer: **223**

   ○ **A.** Miliaria rubra

   ○ **B.** Erythema toxicum

   ○ **C.** Mongolian spots

   ○ **D.** Jaundice at birth

8. A two-year-old is being evaluated for hearing loss. Which finding in the child's history is likely to be a significant factor?

Quick Answer: **220**
Detailed Answer: **223**

   ○ **A.** Birth at 36 weeks gestation

   ○ **B.** Maternal history of hypertension

   ○ **C.** Birth weight of 6 pounds 6 ounces

   ○ **D.** Meningitis treated with intravenous garamycin

9. A vaginal exam of a laboring client reveals that the fetus is at 0 station. This assessment means that:

Quick Answer: **220**
Detailed Answer: **223**

   ○ **A.** The fetus has not descended into the birth canal.

   ○ **B.** The fetus is in a transverse lie.

   ○ **C.** The fetus is level with the ischial spines.

   ○ **D.** The fetus is at increased risk for precipitate delivery.

10. The nurse is conducting a physical assessment on a client with mild anemia. Which of the following would the nurse expect to observe?

Quick Answer: **220**
Detailed Answer: **223**

     ○ **A.** Heart murmur

     ○ **B.** Increased respiratory rate

     ○ **C.** Activity intolerance

     ○ **D.** Frequent respiratory infections

11. The nurse is teaching the client with polycythemia vera about prevention of complications of the disease. Which of the following statements by the client indicates a need for further teaching?

Quick Answer: **220**
Detailed Answer: **223**

     ○ **A.** "I will restrict my fluid intake to 1 liter per day."

     ○ **B.** "I will apply support hose before arising in the morning."

     ○ **C.** "I will elevate my legs when sitting."

     ○ **D.** "I will use an electric razor for shaving."

12. Which finding is considered a risk factor in the development of leukemia?

Quick Answer: **220**
Detailed Answer: **223**

     ○ **A.** The client is an avid stamp collector.

     ○ **B.** The client works as a computer programmer.

     ○ **C.** The client had radiation for Hodgkin's lymphoma.

     ○ **D.** The client's grandmother had stomach cancer.

13. The nurse is caring for an older client hospitalized with dehydration. Which site should be used to check for skin turgor?

Quick Answer: **220**
Detailed Answer: **224**

     ○ **A.** Hand

     ○ **B.** Arm

     ○ **C.** Abdomen

     ○ **D.** Forehead

14. Assessment of the client's skin reveals numerous café au lait spots over the trunk. These changes are associated with which diagnosis?

Quick Answer: **220**
Detailed Answer: **224**

     ○ **A.** Polycythemia vera

     ○ **B.** Neurofibromatosis

     ○ **C.** Thalassemia major

     ○ **D.** Acoustic neuroma

Quick Check

15. Which of the following interventions will be useful for the patient with Alzheimer's dementia who exhibits prosopagnosia?

Quick Answer: **220**
Detailed Answer: **224**

   ○ **A.** Provide the patient with a picture board for identifying familiar objects.

   ○ **B.** Encourage the family to bring pictures of the patient, family, and friends that are labeled.

   ○ **C.** Ensure adequate non-glare lighting.

   ○ **D.** Provide a large clock and calendar at the nurse's station.

16. Which of the following electrolyte imbalances is likely to result in a shortened QT interval?

Quick Answer: **220**
Detailed Answer: **224**

   ○ **A.** Hypercalcemia

   ○ **B.** Hyponatremia

   ○ **C.** Hypomagnesemia

   ○ **D.** Hyperphosphatemia

17. A client with thrombocytopenic purpura is being treated with Neumega (oprelvekin). Which of the following indicates a favorable response to the medication?

Quick Answer: **220**
Detailed Answer: **224**

   ○ **A.** Platelet count of 150,000/cu.mm

   ○ **B.** WBC 7,500/cu.mm

   ○ **C.** MCV 80–96 fL/red cell

   ○ **D.** MCHC 33–36 g/dL

18. A patient with thrombocytopenia has a platelet count of 80,000. It will be most important to teach the client about:

Quick Answer: **220**
Detailed Answer: **224**

   ○ **A.** Measures to reduce the risk of bleeding

   ○ **B.** Increasing the fluid intake

   ○ **C.** Activities to improve oxygenation

   ○ **D.** Ways to conserve energy

19. The client has surgery for removal of a prolactinoma. Which of the following interventions would be appropriate for this client?

Quick Answer: **220**
Detailed Answer: **224**

   ○ **A.** Place the client in Trendelenburg position for postural drainage.

   ○ **B.** Encourage coughing and deep breathing every two hours.

   ○ **C.** Elevate the head of the bed 30°.

   ○ **D.** Encourage the client to gently blow the nose every two hours to remove secretions.

20. The client with a history of diabetes insipidus is admitted with polyuria, polydipsia, and mental confusion. The priority intervention for this client is:

Quick Answer: **220**
Detailed Answer: **224**

- ○ **A.** Measuring the urinary output
- ○ **B.** Checking the vital signs
- ○ **C.** Encouraging increased fluid intake
- ○ **D.** Weighing the client

21. Which ECG finding is most likely to be present in the client with a potassium of 6.0 mEq/L?

Quick Answer: **220**
Detailed Answer: **224**

- ○ **A.** Depressed S-T segments
- ○ **B.** Presence of U wave
- ○ **C.** Peaked T waves
- ○ **D.** Fusion of the T and U waves

22. A client has had a unilateral adrenalectomy to remove a tumor. The most important measurement in the immediate post-operative period for the nurse to take is:

Quick Answer: **220**
Detailed Answer: **224**

- ○ **A.** The blood pressure
- ○ **B.** The temperature
- ○ **C.** The urinary output
- ○ **D.** The specific gravity of the urine

23. A client with Addison's disease is receiving Solu-Medrol (methylprednisolone). Which of the following interventions would the nurse implement?

Quick Answer: **220**
Detailed Answer: **224**

- ○ **A.** Glucometer readings as ordered
- ○ **B.** Intake/output measurements
- ○ **C.** Evaluating the sodium and potassium levels
- ○ **D.** Daily weights

24. A client had a total thyroidectomy yesterday. The client is complaining of tingling around the mouth and in the fingers and toes. What do the client's symptoms indicate?

Quick Answer: **220**
Detailed Answer: **224**

- ○ **A.** Hypernatremia
- ○ **B.** Hypocalcemia
- ○ **C.** Hypermagnesemia
- ○ **D.** Hypokalemia

25. Which of the following nursing diagnoses is of highest priority for the patient with hypothyroidism?

○ **A.** Impaired physical mobility

○ **B.** Hypothermia

○ **C.** Disturbed thought processes

○ **D.** Decreased cardiac output

26. The client presents to the clinic with a serum cholesterol of 275mg/dL and is placed on rosuvastatin (Crestor). Which instruction should be given to the client taking rosuvastatin (Crestor)?

○ **A.** Report unexplained muscle weakness to the physician

○ **B.** Allow six months for the drug to take effect

○ **C.** Take the medication with fruit juice

○ **D.** Report difficulty sleeping

27. Hyperstat (diazoxide) is ordered for a patient with hypertension. Which side effect is associated with the medication?

○ **A.** Photophobia

○ **B.** Numbness of the hands

○ **C.** Urinary frequency

○ **D.** Alopecia

28. A six-month-old is receiving Lanoxin elixir (digoxin) following the repair of a VSD. Which finding should be reported to the physician?

○ **A.** Blood pressure of 80/52

○ **B.** Blood glucose of 100 mg/dL

○ **C.** Heart rate of 80 beats per minute

○ **D.** Respiratory rate of 30 per minute

29. The client admitted with angina is given a prescription for nitro-glycerine. The client should be instructed to:

○ **A.** Replenish his supply every three months

○ **B.** Take one tablet every 15 minutes if pain occurs

○ **C.** Leave the medication in the brown bottle

○ **D.** Crush the medication and take with water

30. The client is instructed regarding foods that are low in fat and cholesterol. Which diet selection is lowest in saturated fats?

Quick Answer: **220**
Detailed Answer: **225**

- ○ **A.** Macaroni and cheese
- ○ **B.** Shrimp with rice
- ○ **C.** Turkey breast
- ○ **D.** Spaghetti with meat sauce

31. The nurse is preparing to check a client for Trousseau's sign. Which equipment should the nurse obtain?

Quick Answer: **220**
Detailed Answer: **225**

- ○ **A.** Tongue blade
- ○ **B.** Blood pressure cuff
- ○ **C.** Reflex hammer
- ○ **D.** Stethoscope

32. The nurse is checking the client's central venous pressure. The nurse should place the zero of the manometer at the:

Quick Answer: **220**
Detailed Answer: **225**

- ○ **A.** Phlebostatic axis
- ○ **B.** Point of maximal impulse
- ○ **C.** Erb's point
- ○ **D.** Tail of Spence

33. The physician orders Zestril (lisinopril) and Lasix (furosemide) to be administered at the same time to a client with hypertension. The nurse should:

Quick Answer: **220**
Detailed Answer: **225**

- ○ **A.** Question the order
- ○ **B.** Administer the medications as ordered
- ○ **C.** Administer the medications separately
- ○ **D.** Contact the pharmacy

34. The best indicator of peripheral edema is determined by:

Quick Answer: **220**
Detailed Answer: **225**

- ○ **A.** Weighing the client daily
- ○ **B.** Measuring the extremity
- ○ **C.** Measuring the intake and output
- ○ **D.** Checking for pitting

35. A client with vaginal cancer is being treated with a radioactive vaginal implant. The client's husband asks the nurse if he can spend the night with his wife. The nurse should explain that:

   ○ **A.** Overnight stays by family members is against hospital policy.

   ○ **B.** There is no need for him to stay because staffing is adequate.

   ○ **C.** His wife will rest much better knowing that he is at home.

   ○ **D.** Visitation is limited to 30 minutes when the implant is in place.

Quick Answer: **220**
Detailed Answer: **226**

36. The nurse is caring for a client hospitalized with a facial stroke. Which diet selection would be suited to the client?

   ○ **A.** Roast beef sandwich, potato chips, pickle spear, iced tea

   ○ **B.** Split pea soup, mashed potatoes, pudding, milk

   ○ **C.** Tomato soup, cheese toast, gelatin, coffee

   ○ **D.** Hamburger, baked beans, fruit cup, iced tea

Quick Answer: **220**
Detailed Answer: **226**

37. The physician has prescribed NovoLog (as part) insulin for a client with diabetes mellitus. Which statement indicates that the client knows when the onset of the insulin occurs?

   ○ **A.** "I will make sure I eat breakfast within 10 minutes of taking my insulin."

   ○ **B.** "I will need to carry candy or some form of sugar with me all the time."

   ○ **C.** "I will eat a snack around three o'clock each afternoon."

   ○ **D.** "I can save my dessert from supper for a bedtime snack."

Quick Answer: **220**
Detailed Answer: **226**

38. The nurse is teaching basic newborn care to a group of first-time parents. The nurse should explain that a sponge bath is recommended for the first two weeks of life because:

   ○ **A.** New parents need time to learn how to hold the newborn.

   ○ **B.** The umbilical cord needs time to separate.

   ○ **C.** Newborn skin is easily traumatized by washing.

   ○ **D.** The chance of chilling the newborn outweighs the benefits of bathing.

Quick Answer: **220**
Detailed Answer: **226**

39. A client with leukemia who has been receiving Trimetrexate (methotrexate) has an order for Wellcovorin (leucovorin). The rationale for administering Wellcovorin is to:

Quick Answer: **220**
Detailed Answer: **226**

- ○ **A.** Treat anemia caused by the methotrexate
- ○ **B.** Create a synergistic effect that shortens treatment time
- ○ **C.** Increase the number of circulating neutrophils
- ○ **D.** Reverse drug toxicity and prevent tissue damage

40. The well child assessment of a one-year-old reveals orange discoloration of the nasolabial folds. Based on this finding the nurse should:

Quick Answer: **220**
Detailed Answer: **226**

- ○ **A.** Obtain a diet history from the mother
- ○ **B.** Inquire about the passage of clay-colored stools
- ○ **C.** Measure the abdominal girth
- ○ **D.** Assess the sclera for the presence of jaundice

41. The physician has prescribed Nexium (esomeprazole) for a client with erosive gastritis. The nurse should administer the medication:

Quick Answer: **220**
Detailed Answer: **226**

- ○ **A.** Thirty minutes before breakfast
- ○ **B.** With each meal
- ○ **C.** In a single dose at bedtime
- ○ **D.** Thirty minutes after meals

42. A client on the psychiatric unit is threatening other clients and staff, and interventions to distract him have not been successful. What action should the nurse take?

Quick Answer: **220**
Detailed Answer: **226**

- ○ **A.** Call security for assistance and administer PRN medication to calm the client
- ○ **B.** Tell the client to calm down and ask him again if he would like to play cards
- ○ **C.** Tell the client that if he continues this behavior he will lose recreational privileges
- ○ **D.** Ignore the client since it is unlikely he will actually harm anyone

43. When the nurse checks the fundus of a client on the first postpartum day, she notes that the fundus is firm, level with the umbilicus, and displaced to the side. The next action the nurse should take is to:

   ○ **A.** Check for bladder distention

   ○ **B.** Assess the blood pressure for hypotension

   ○ **C.** Determine whether an oxytocic drug was given

   ○ **D.** Check for the expulsion of small clots

Quick Answer: **220**
Detailed Answer: **226**

44. Which of the following side effects is associated with androgen therapy?

   ○ **A.** Gynecomastia

   ○ **B.** Increased appetite

   ○ **C.** Virilization

   ○ **D.** Euphoria

Quick Answer: **220**
Detailed Answer: **226**

45. Which finding in the patient's history contraindicates the use of Imitrex (sumatriptan) for the prevention of migraine headaches?

   ○ **A.** Diabetes

   ○ **B.** Angina

   ○ **C.** Renal calculi

   ○ **D.** Peptic ulcer disease

Quick Answer: **220**
Detailed Answer: **227**

46. Which of the following describes a positive Kernig's sign?

   ○ **A.** Pain on flexion of the hip and knee

   ○ **B.** Nuchal rigidity on flexion of the neck

   ○ **C.** Pain when the head is turned to the left side

   ○ **D.** Dizziness when changing positions

Quick Answer: **220**
Detailed Answer: **227**

47. The client with Alzheimer's disease is being assisted with activities of daily living when the nurse notes that the client uses her toothbrush to brush her hair. The nurse is aware that the client is exhibiting:

   ○ **A.** Agnosia

   ○ **B.** Apraxia

   ○ **C.** Anomia

   ○ **D.** Aphasia

Quick Answer: **220**
Detailed Answer: **227**

48. An elderly client has been noted to have increasing confusion late in the afternoon and before bedtime. The nurse is aware that the client is experiencing:

- ○ **A.** Proprioception
- ○ **B.** Agnosia
- ○ **C.** Sundowning
- ○ **D.** Confabulation

49. A terrorist attack has left hundreds of patients with injuries determined to be in the immediate category as defined by NATO. The color to designate this group is:

- ○ **A.** Black
- ○ **B.** Yellow
- ○ **C.** Red
- ○ **D.** Green

50. The doctor has prescribed Exelon (rivastigmine) for the client with Alzheimer's disease. Which side effect is most often associated with this drug?

- ○ **A.** Urinary incontinence
- ○ **B.** Headaches
- ○ **C.** Confusion
- ○ **D.** Nausea

51. An obstetrical client is admitted in active labor. During examination, the nurse notes a papular lesion on the perineum. Which initial action is most appropriate?

- ○ **A.** Document the finding
- ○ **B.** Report the finding to the physician
- ○ **C.** Prepare the client for a C-section
- ○ **D.** Continue primary care as prescribed

52. A client with a diagnosis of HPV is at increased risk for which of the following?

- ○ **A.** Hodgkin's lymphoma
- ○ **B.** Cervical cancer
- ○ **C.** Multiple myeloma
- ○ **D.** Ovarian cancer

53. During the intake assessment, a client reports that she has a painful blister on the labia. The client's symptoms are likely the result of infection with:

- ○ **A.** Syphilis
- ○ **B.** HSV II
- ○ **C.** Gonorrhea
- ○ **D.** Condylomata

54. The best diagnostic test for treponema pallidum is:

- ○ **A.** Venereal Disease Research Lab (VDRL)
- ○ **B.** Rapid plasma reagin (RPR)
- ○ **C.** Fluorescent treponemal antibody (FTA)
- ○ **D.** Thayer-Martin culture (TMC)

55. A 15-year-old primigravida is admitted with a tentative diagnosis of HELLP syndrome. Which laboratory finding is associated with HELLP syndrome?

- ○ **A.** Elevated blood glucose
- ○ **B.** Elevated platelet count
- ○ **C.** Elevated creatinine clearance
- ○ **D.** Elevated liver enzymes

56. The nurse is assessing the deep tendon reflexes of a client with preeclampsia. Which method is used to elicit the biceps reflex?

- ○ **A.** The nurse places her thumb on the muscle inset in the antecubital space and taps the thumb briskly with the reflex hammer.
- ○ **B.** The nurse loosely suspends the client's arm in an open hand while tapping the back of the client's elbow.
- ○ **C.** The nurse instructs the client to dangle her legs as the nurse strikes the area below the patella with the blunt side of the reflex hammer.
- ○ **D.** The nurse instructs the client to place her arms loosely at her side as the nurse strikes the muscle insert just above the wrist.

57. A primigravida with diabetes is admitted to the labor and delivery unit at 34 weeks gestation. Which physician's order should the nurse question?

   ○ **A.** Magnesium sulfate 4gm (25%) IV

   ○ **B.** Brethine (terbutaline) 10mcg IV

   ○ **C.** Stadol (butorphanol)1mg IV push every four hours as needed PRN for pain

   ○ **D.** Ancef (cefazolin) 2gm IVPB every six hours

58. An amniocentesis at 32 weeks gestation reveals that a multigravida with diabetes has an L/S ratio of 1:1 with the presence of phosphatidylglycerol. Based on the amniocentesis, the nurse knows that if delivered now:

   ○ **A.** The newborn is at low risk for congenital anomalies.

   ○ **B.** The newborn is at high risk for intrauterine growth retardation.

   ○ **C.** The newborn is at high risk for respiratory distress syndrome.

   ○ **D.** The newborn is at high risk for birth trauma.

59. Which newborn assessment is considered an abnormal finding that requires immediate attention?

   ○ **A.** Cyanosis of the hands and feet

   ○ **B.** Umbilical stump with three vessels

   ○ **C.** Jitteriness and shaking

   ○ **D.** Presence of harlequin sign

60. The nurse caring for a client receiving intravenous magnesium sulfate must closely observe for side effects associated with drug therapy. An expected side effect of magnesium sulfate is:

   ○ **A.** Decreased urinary output

   ○ **B.** Hypersomnolence

   ○ **C.** Absence of knee jerk reflex

   ○ **D.** Decreased respiratory rate

61. The client has elected to have epidural anesthesia to relieve labor pain. If the client experiences hypotension, the nurse should:

   ○ **A.** Place her in Trendelenburg position

   ○ **B.** Decrease the rate of the IV infusion

   ○ **C.** Administer oxygen via nasal cannula

   ○ **D.** Increase the rate of the IV infusion

62. The nurse is caring for a client with cancer of the pancreas. Which finding indicates involvement of the bile ducts?

Quick Answer: **220**
Detailed Answer: **228**

- ○ **A.** Dark urine
- ○ **B.** Petechiae
- ○ **C.** Dark stools
- ○ **D.** Steatorrhea

63. A patient with renal disease has developed uremic frost. Which nursing intervention helps to decrease the risk of tissue damage related to uremic frost?

Quick Answer: **220**
Detailed Answer: **228**

- ○ **A.** Cleansing the client's skin with warm water
- ○ **B.** Changing the client's position every hour
- ○ **C.** Keeping the client's fingernails trimmed
- ○ **D.** Applying padded protection over the client's heels and elbows

64. Which of the following is *not* a step in primary assessment of a client presenting to the emergency department after being involved in a motor vehicle accident?

Quick Answer: **220**
Detailed Answer: **228**

- ○ **A.** Assessing and maintaining a patent airway
- ○ **B.** Obtaining vital signs
- ○ **C.** Using the Glasgow Coma Scale to check responsiveness
- ○ **D.** Controlling bleeding

65. Which of the following is an expected finding in a child with osteogenesis imperfecta?

Quick Answer: **220**
Detailed Answer: **228**

- ○ **A.** Blue sclera
- ○ **B.** Hutchinson's teeth
- ○ **C.** Anisocoria
- ○ **D.** Pectus excavatum

66. Which statement is true regarding a patient with a Sengstaken-Blakemore tube?

Quick Answer: **220**
Detailed Answer: **229**

- ○ **A.** The smaller balloon will provide direct pressure to control bleeding from the esophagus.
- ○ **B.** The tube has four lumens, one of which drains esophageal secretions.
- ○ **C.** The esophageal balloon should be inflated to a pressure between 30–35 mmHg.
- ○ **D.** Scissors should be kept at the patient's bedside.

67. The nurse is caring for a postoperative client when the client becomes nonresponsive and pale, with a BP of 90/40. The nurse recognizes that the necessary intervention at this time is to:

Quick Answer: **220**
Detailed Answer: **229**

- ○ **A.** Place the client in Trendelenburg position
- ○ **B.** Increase the IV infusion rate
- ○ **C.** Administer atropine intravenously
- ○ **D.** Move the emergency cart to the bedside

68. A client is scheduled for a biologic heart valve replacement. The nurse is aware that the client will require:

Quick Answer: **220**
Detailed Answer: **229**

- ○ **A.** Lifelong anticoagulant therapy
- ○ B. Valve replacement every two years
- ○ **C.** Strict dental hygiene to prevent bacterial infection
- ○ **D.** Use of electric razor instead of safety razor

69. A client being treated with sodium warfarin (Coumadin) has a prothrombin time of 120 seconds. The nurse recognizes that:

Quick Answer: **220**
Detailed Answer: **229**

- ○ **A.** Close assessment for signs of bleeding is needed.
- ○ **B.** The dosage of Coumadin is inadequate to prevent thrombi.
- ○ **C.** The client should limit the intake of foods rich in vitamin K.
- ○ **D.** Skipped doses should be made up by taking an additional dose.

70. Which food selection would provide the most calcium for a client who is four months pregnant?

Quick Answer: **220**
Detailed Answer: **229**

- ○ **A.** Bowl of oatmeal
- ○ **B.** Bran muffin
- ○ **C.** One cup of yogurt
- ○ **D.** Large orange

71. A client with preeclampsia is admitted with an order for magnesium sulfate. Which action by the nurse indicates an understanding of magnesium toxicity?

Quick Answer: **220**
Detailed Answer: **229**

- ○ **A.** The nurse lowers the temperature of the room.
- ○ **B.** The nurse places an airway at the bedside.
- ○ **C.** The nurse inserts an indwelling catheter and obtains an hourly intake and output.
- ○ **D.** The nurse darkens the room to reduce environmental stimuli.

72. The best size cathlon for administration of a blood transfusion to a six-year-old is:

Quick Answer: 220
Detailed Answer: 229

   - ○ **A.** 18 gauge
   - ○ **B.** 19 gauge
   - ○ **C.** 22 gauge
   - ○ **D.** 20 gauge

73. A client is admitted to the unit two hours after an explosion causes burns to the face. The nurse would be most concerned with the client developing which of the following?

Quick Answer: 220
Detailed Answer: 229

   - ○ **A.** Hypovolemia
   - ○ **B.** Laryngeal edema
   - ○ **C.** Hypernatremia
   - ○ **D.** Hyperkalemia

74. The nurse is caring for a client with diabetes mellitus. Which instruction should be given to the client?

Quick Answer: 220
Detailed Answer: 229

   - ○ **A.** Tell the client to avoid stairs
   - ○ B. Tell the client to decrease her intake of sodium
   - ○ **C.** Instruct the client to weigh daily
   - ○ **D.** Tell the client to report numbness and tingling in her feet and toes

75. The nurse is caring for a client following cast application for a fractured ulna. Which finding should be reported to the doctor?

Quick Answer: 220
Detailed Answer: 229

   - ○ **A.** Pain beneath the cast
   - ○ **B.** Warm fingers
   - ○ **C.** Pulse is present
   - ○ **D.** Paresthesia of the fingers

76. A client with AIDS is being treated with Genvoya (elvitegravir/emtricitabine/tenofovir alafenamide/cobicistat). The client should be taught to:

Quick Answer: 220
Detailed Answer: 229

   - ○ **A.** Avoid warm climates
   - ○ **B.** Refrain from taking herbals
   - ○ **C.** Avoid routine exercising
   - ○ **D.** Report any changes in skin color

77. Which action by the healthcare worker indicates a need for further teaching?

Quick Answer: **220**
Detailed Answer: **229**

- ○ **A.** The nursing assistant ambulates the elderly client using a gait belt.

- ○ **B.** The nurse wears goggles while performing a venipuncture.

- ○ **C.** The nurse washes his hands after changing a dressing.

- ○ **D.** The nurse wears gloves to monitor the IV infusion rate.

78. The client is having electroconvulsive therapy for treatment of severe depression. Prior to the ECT, the nurse should:

Quick Answer: **220**
Detailed Answer: **229**

- ○ **A.** Apply a tourniquet to the client's arm

- ○ **B.** Administer an anticonvulsant medication

- ○ **C.** Ask the client if he is allergic to shellfish

- ○ **D.** Apply a blood pressure cuff to the arm

79. The five-year-old is being tested for enterobiasis (pinworms). Which symptom is associated with enterobiasis?

Quick Answer: **220**
Detailed Answer: **230**

- ○ **A.** Rectal itching

- ○ **B.** Nausea

- ○ **C.** Oral ulcerations

- ○ **D.** Scalp itching

80. The nurse is teaching a mother regarding treatment for pediculosis capitis. Which information should be given to the mother?

Quick Answer: **220**
Detailed Answer: **230**

- ○ **A.** Treatment is not recommended for children less than 10 years of age.

- ○ **B.** Bed linens should be washed in hot water.

- ○ **C.** Medication therapy will continue for one year.

- ○ **D.** Intravenous antibiotic therapy will be ordered.

81. The registered nurse is making assignments for the day. Which client should be assigned to the nurse who is pregnant?

Quick Answer: **220**
Detailed Answer: **230**

- ○ **A.** The client with HIV treated with Pentam (pentamidine)

- ○ **B.** The client with cervical cancer treated with a radium implant

- ○ **C.** The client with RSV treated with Virazole (ribavirin)

- ○ **D.** The client with cytomegalovirus treated with Valcyte (valganciclovir)

82. The nurse is planning room assignments for the day. Which client should be assigned to a private room if only one is available?

Quick Answer: **220**
Detailed Answer: **230**

  ○ **A.** The client with MRSA

  ○ **B.** The client with diabetes

  ○ **C.** The client with pancreatitis

  ○ **D.** The client with Addison's disease

83. Which term applies to the misconduct by a healthcare provider that results in harm to the patient?

Quick Answer: **220**
Detailed Answer: **230**

  ○ **A.** Negligence

  ○ **B.** Tort

  ○ **C.** Assault

  ○ **D.** Malpractice

84. The nurse is preparing to administer oral potassium chloride to an elderly client. Which action should the nurse take before administering the medication?

Quick Answer: **220**
Detailed Answer: **230**

  ○ **A.** Perform a fingerstick for morning glucose

  ○ B. Assess for signs of hypocalcemia

  ○ **C.** Withhold food for thirty minutes

  ○ **D.** Check the creatinine level

85. A mother calls the clinic to report that her otherwise healthy newborn has a rash on his forehead and face. The nurse should tell the mother:

Quick Answer: **220**
Detailed Answer: **230**

  ○ **A.** To use a mild soap when washing the newborn's face

  ○ **B.** That many newborns have a rash that will go away by one month of life

  ○ **C.** That the rash indicates illness and she needs to bring the newborn in immediately

  ○ **D.** To check for signs of illness among family members

86. A client is admitted with kidney disease. Which type of intravenous fluid is likely to be ordered for this client?

Quick Answer: **220**
Detailed Answer: **230**

  ○ **A.** Hypertonic

  ○ **B.** Isotonic

  ○ **C.** Colloid

  ○ **D.** Hypotonic

87. Which situation would be reportable to the state board of nursing?

   ○ **A.** The facility fails to provide literature in both Spanish and English.

   ○ **B.** The narcotic count has been incorrect on the unit for the past three days.

   ○ **C.** The client fails to receive an itemized account of his bills and services received during his hospital stay.

   ○ **D.** Needles and sharps are found in the client's waste can.

88. A client with SIADH is admitted with severe hyponatremia. Which type of intravenous solution would the nurse expect to be ordered?

   ○ **A.** Isotonic (0.9% normal saline)

   ○ **B.** Hypertonic (3% sodium chloride)

   ○ **C.** Colloid (Dextran)

   ○ **D.** Hypotonic (5% dextrose in water)

89. The home health nurse is planning for the day's visits. Which client should be seen first?

   ○ **A.** The 78-year-old with dysphagia following a stroke

   ○ **B.** The 55-year-old diabetic with above-the-knee amputation

   ○ **C.** The 50-year-old with MRSA being treated with Vancocin (vancomycin) via a PICC line

   ○ **D.** The 30-year-old with relapsing-remitting multiple sclerosis being treated with intravenous corticosteroids

90. Which clients can be assigned to share a room in the emergency department during a disaster?

   ○ **A.** A client having auditory hallucinations and a client with ulcerative colitis

   ○ **B.** A client who is pregnant and a client with a fractured arm

   ○ **C.** A child who is cyanotic with severe dyspnea and a client with a frontal head injury

   ○ **D.** A client who arrives with a large puncture wound to the abdomen and a client with chest pain

91. Before administering eardrops to a toddler, the nurse should recognize that it is essential to consider which of the following?

   ○ **A.** Age

   ○ **B.** Weight

   ○ **C.** Developmental level

   ○ **D.** Ability to understand

Quick Answer: **220**
Detailed Answer: **230**

92. The nurse is discussing meal planning with the mother of a two-year-old. Which of the following statements, if made by the mother, would require a need for further instruction?

   ○ **A.** "It is okay to give my child white grape juice for breakfast."

   ○ **B.** "My child can have a grilled cheese sandwich for lunch."

   ○ **C.** "We are going on a camping trip this weekend, and I have bought hot dogs to grill for his lunch."

   ○ **D.** "For a snack, my child can have ice cream."

Quick Answer: **220**
Detailed Answer: **231**

93. A client with AIDS has a viral load of 200 copies per mL. The nurse should interpret this finding as:

   ○ **A.** The client is at risk for opportunistic diseases.

   ○ **B.** The client is no longer communicable.

   ○ **C.** The client's viral load is extremely low so he is relatively free of circulating virus.

   ○ **D.** The client's T-cell count is extremely low.

Quick Answer: **220**
Detailed Answer: **231**

94. The client has an order for sliding scale insulin at 1900 hours and Lantus (glargine) insulin at the same hour. The nurse should:

   ○ **A.** Administer the two medications together.

   ○ **B.** Administer the medications in two injections.

   ○ **C.** Draw up the Lantus insulin and then the regular insulin and administer them together.

   ○ **D.** Contact the doctor because these medications should not be given to the same client.

Quick Answer: **220**
Detailed Answer: **231**

95. A priority nursing diagnosis for a child following a tonsillectomy is:

   ○ **A.** Altered nutrition

   ○ **B.** Impaired communication

   ○ **C.** Risk for injury/aspiration

   ○ **D.** Altered urinary elimination

Quick Answer: **220**
Detailed Answer: **231**

96. Which of the following is a classic manifestation of glomeru-lonephritis?

   ○ **A.** Hypertension

   ○ **B.** Lassitude

   ○ **C.** Fatigue

   ○ **D.** Vomiting and diarrhea

Quick Answer: **220**
Detailed Answer: **231**

97. A child is admitted with suspected epiglottitis. Which action is *not* a part of the nursing care?

   ○ **A.** Checking the vital signs

   ○ **B.** Assessing the throat with a tongue blade

   ○ **C.** Administering oxygen as needed

   ○ **D.** Administering IV antibiotics

Quick Answer: **220**
Detailed Answer: **231**

98. The physician has ordered synthetic thyroid medication for a patient with hypothyroidism. The nurse should instruct the client to:

   ○ **A.** Take the medication with food to prevent nausea

   ○ **B.** Take the medication at bedtime

   ○ **C.** Take the medication in the morning with water

   ○ **D.** Take the medication with the evening meal

Quick Answer: **220**
Detailed Answer: **231**

99. Which of the following foods, if selected by the mother of a child with celiac disease, would indicate her understanding of the dietary instructions?

   ○ **A.** Whole-wheat toast

   ○ **B.** Angel hair pasta

   ○ **C.** Reuben on rye

   ○ **D.** Rice cereal

Quick Answer: **220**
Detailed Answer: **231**

100. The first action that the nurse should take if she finds the client has an O_2 saturation of 68% is:

   ○ **A.** Elevate the head of the bed

   ○ **B.** Recheck the O_2 saturation in 30 minutes

   ○ **C.** Apply oxygen by mask

   ○ **D.** Assess the heart rate

Quick Answer: **220**
Detailed Answer: **231**

101. Which observation would the nurse expect to make after an amniotomy?

   ○ **A.** Dark yellow amniotic fluid

   ○ **B.** Clear amniotic fluid

   ○ **C.** Greenish amniotic fluid

   ○ **D.** Red amniotic fluid

Quick Answer: **221**
Detailed Answer: **231**

102. The client taking glyburide (Diabeta) should be cautioned to:

   ○ **A.** Avoid eating sweets

   ○ **B.** Report changes in urinary pattern

   ○ **C.** Allow three hours for onset

   ○ **D.** Check the glucose daily

Quick Answer: **221**
Detailed Answer: **231**

103. The obstetric client's fetal heart rate is 80–90 during the contractions. The first action the nurse should take is:

   ○ **A.** Reposition the monitor

   ○ **B.** Turn the client to her left side

   ○ **C.** Ask the client to ambulate

   ○ **D.** Prepare the client for delivery

Quick Answer: **221**
Detailed Answer: **231**

104. Arterial ulcers are best described as ulcers that:

   ○ **A.** Are smooth in texture

   ○ **B.** Have irregular borders

   ○ **C.** Are cool to touch

   ○ **D.** Are painful to touch

Quick Answer: **221**
Detailed Answer: **231**

105. A vaginal exam reveals a footling breech presentation. The nurse should take which of the following actions at this time?

   ○ **A.** Anticipate the need for a Caesarean section

   ○ **B.** Apply an internal fetal monitor

   ○ **C.** Place the client in genupectoral position

   ○ **D.** Perform an ultrasound

Quick Answer: **221**
Detailed Answer: **232**

106. A vaginal exam reveals that the cervix is 4 cm dilated, with intact membranes and a fetal heart tone rate of 160–170bpm. The nurse decides to apply an external fetal monitor. The rationale for this implementation is:

   ○ **A.** The cervix is closed.

   ○ **B.** The membranes are still intact.

Quick Answer: **221**
Detailed Answer: **232**

○ **C.** The fetal heart tones are within normal limits.

○ **D.** The contractions are intense enough for insertion of an internal monitor.

107. The following are all nursing diagnoses appropriate for a gravida 1 para 0 in labor. Which one would be most appropriate for the primigravida as she completes the early phase of labor?

Quick Answer: **221**
Detailed Answer: **232**

○ **A.** Impaired gas exchange related to hyperventilation

○ **B.** Alteration in placental perfusion related to maternal position

○ **C.** Impaired physical mobility related to fetal-monitoring equipment

○ **D.** Potential fluid volume deficit related to decreased fluid intake

108. As the client reaches 6cm dilation, the nurse notes late decelerations on the fetal monitor. What is the most likely explanation of this pattern?

Quick Answer: **221**
Detailed Answer: **232**

○ **A.** The baby is sleeping.

○ **B.** The umbilical cord is compressed.

○ **C.** There is head compression.

○ **D.** There is uteroplacental insufficiency.

109. The nurse notes variable decelerations on the fetal monitor strip. The most appropriate initial action would be to:

Quick Answer: **221**
Detailed Answer: **232**

○ **A.** Notify her doctor

○ **B.** Start an IV

○ **C.** Reposition the client

○ **D.** Readjust the monitor

110. Which of the following is a characteristic of an ominous periodic change in the fetal heart rate?

Quick Answer: **221**
Detailed Answer: **232**

○ **A.** A fetal heart rate of 120–130bpm

○ **B.** A baseline variability of 6–10bpm

○ **C.** Accelerations in FHR with fetal movement

○ **D.** A recurrent rate of 90–100bpm at the end of the contractions

111. The rationale for inserting a French catheter every hour for the client with epidural anesthesia is:

Quick Answer: **221**
Detailed Answer: **232**

 ○ **A.** The bladder fills more rapidly because of the medication used for the epidural.

 ○ **B.** Her level of consciousness is such that she is in a trancelike state.

 ○ **C.** The sensation of the bladder filling is diminished or lost.

 ○ **D.** She is embarrassed to ask for the bedpan that frequently.

112. A client in the family planning clinic asks the nurse about the most likely time for her to conceive. The nurse explains that conception is most likely to occur when:

Quick Answer: **221**
Detailed Answer: **232**

 ○ **A.** Estrogen levels are low.

 ○ **B.** Luteinizing hormone is high.

 ○ **C.** The endometrial lining is thin.

 ○ **D.** The progesterone level is low.

113. A client tells the nurse that she plans to use the rhythm method of birth control. The nurse is aware that the success of the rhythm method depends on the:

Quick Answer: **221**
Detailed Answer: **232**

 ○ **A.** Age of the client

 ○ **B.** Frequency of intercourse

 ○ **C.** Regularity of the menses

 ○ **D.** Range of the client's temperature

114. A client with diabetes asks the nurse for advice regarding methods of birth control. Which method of birth control is most suitable for the client with diabetes?

Quick Answer: **221**
Detailed Answer: **232**

 ○ **A.** Intrauterine device

 ○ **B.** Oral contraceptives

 ○ **C.** Diaphragm

 ○ **D.** Contraceptive sponge

115. The doctor suspects that the client has an ectopic pregnancy. Which symptom is consistent with a diagnosis of a ruptured ectopic pregnancy?

Quick Answer: **221**
Detailed Answer: **232**

 ○ **A.** Painless vaginal bleeding

 ○ **B.** Abdominal cramping

 ○ **C.** Throbbing pain in the upper quadrant

 ○ **D.** Sudden, stabbing pain in the lower quadrant

116. The nurse is teaching a pregnant client about nutritional needs during pregnancy. Which menu selection will best meet the nutritional needs of the pregnant client?

Quick Answer: 221
Detailed Answer: 233

- ○ **A.** Hamburger patty, green beans, French fries, and iced tea
- ○ **B.** Roast beef sandwich, potato chips, baked beans, and cola
- ○ **C.** Baked chicken, fruit cup, potato salad, coleslaw, yogurt, and iced tea
- ○ **D.** Fish sandwich, gelatin with fruit, and coffee

117. The client with hyperemesis gravidarum is at risk for developing:

Quick Answer: 221
Detailed Answer: 233

- ○ **A.** Respiratory alkalosis without dehydration
- ○ **B.** Metabolic acidosis with dehydration
- ○ **C.** Respiratory acidosis without dehydration
- ○ **D.** Metabolic alkalosis with dehydration

118. A client tells the doctor that she is about 20 weeks pregnant. The most definitive sign of pregnancy is:

Quick Answer: 221
Detailed Answer: 233

- ○ **A.** Elevated human chorionic gonadatropin
- ○ **B.** The presence of fetal heart tones
- ○ **C.** Uterine enlargement
- ○ **D.** Breast enlargement and tenderness

119. The nurse is caring for a neonate whose mother is diabetic. The nurse will expect the neonate to be:

Quick Answer: 221
Detailed Answer: 233

- ○ **A.** Hypoglycemic, small for gestational age
- ○ **B.** Hyperglycemic, large for gestational age
- ○ **C.** Hypoglycemic, large for gestational age
- ○ **D.** Hyperglycemic, small for gestational age

120. Which of the following instructions should be included in the nurse's teaching regarding oral contraceptives?

Quick Answer: 221
Detailed Answer: 233

- ○ **A.** Weight gain should be reported to the physician.
- ○ **B.** An alternate method of birth control is needed when taking antibiotics.
- ○ **C.** If the client misses one or more pills, two pills should be taken per day for one week.
- ○ **D.** Changes in the menstrual flow should be reported to the physician.

121. The nurse is discussing breastfeeding with a postpartum client. Breastfeeding is contraindicated in the postpartum client with:

Quick Answer: **221**
Detailed Answer: **233**

- ○ **A.** Diabetes
- ○ **B.** HIV
- ○ **C.** Hypertension
- ○ **D.** Thyroid disease

122. A client is admitted to the labor and delivery unit complaining of vaginal bleeding with very little discomfort. The nurse's first action should be to:

Quick Answer: **221**
Detailed Answer: **233**

- ○ **A.** Assess the fetal heart tones
- ○ **B.** Check for cervical dilation
- ○ **C.** Check for firmness of the uterus
- ○ **D.** Obtain a detailed history

123. A client telephones the emergency room stating that she thinks that she is in labor. The nurse should tell the client that labor has probably begun when:

Quick Answer: **221**
Detailed Answer: **233**

- ○ **A.** Her contractions are two minutes apart.
- ○ **B.** She has back pain and a bloody discharge.
- ○ **C.** She experiences abdominal pain and frequent urination.
- ○ **D.** Her contractions are five minutes apart.

124. The nurse is teaching a group of prenatal clients about the effects of cigarette smoke on fetal development. Which characteristic is associated with babies born to mothers who smoked during pregnancy?

Quick Answer: **221**
Detailed Answer: **233**

- ○ **A.** Low birth weight
- ○ **B.** Large for gestational age
- ○ **C.** Preterm birth, but appropriate size for gestation
- ○ **D.** Growth retardation in weight and length

125. The physician has ordered an injection of RhoGAM (Rho[D]immune globulin) for the postpartum client whose blood type is A negative and whose baby is O positive. To provide postpartum prophylaxis, RhoGAM should be administered:

Quick Answer: **221**
Detailed Answer: **234**

- ○ **A.** Within 72 hours of delivery
- ○ **B.** Within one week of delivery
- ○ **C.** Within two weeks of delivery
- ○ **D.** Within one month of delivery

126. After the physician performs an amniotomy, the nurse's first action should be to assess the:

   ○ **A.** Degree of cervical dilation

   ○ **B.** Fetal heart tones

   ○ **C.** Client's vital signs

   ○ **D.** Client's level of discomfort

Quick Answer: **221**
Detailed Answer: **234**

127. A client is admitted to the labor and delivery unit. The nurse performs a vaginal exam and determines that the client's cervix is 5cm dilated with 75% effacement. Based on the nurse's assessment, the client is in which phase of labor?

   ○ **A.** Active

   ○ **B.** Latent

   ○ **C.** Transition

   ○ **D.** Early

Quick Answer: **221**
Detailed Answer: **234**

128. A newborn with narcotic abstinence syndrome is admitted to the nursery. Nursing care of the newborn should include:

   ○ **A.** Teaching the mother to provide tactile stimulation

   ○ **B.** Wrapping the newborn snugly in a blanket

   ○ **C.** Placing the newborn in the infant seat

   ○ **D.** Initiating an early infant-stimulation program

Quick Answer: **221**
Detailed Answer: **234**

129. A client elects to have epidural anesthesia to relieve the discomfort of labor. Following the initiation of epidural anesthesia, the nurse should give priority to:

   ○ **A.** Checking for cervical dilation

   ○ **B.** Placing the client in a supine position

   ○ **C.** Checking the client's blood pressure

   ○ **D.** Obtaining a fetal heart rate

Quick Answer: **221**
Detailed Answer: **234**

130. The nurse is aware that the best way to prevent post-operative wound infection in the surgical client is to:

   ○ **A.** Administer a prescribed antibiotic

   ○ **B.** Wash her hands for two minutes before care

   ○ **C.** Wear a mask when providing care

   ○ **D.** Ask the client to cover her mouth when she coughs

Quick Answer: **221**
Detailed Answer: **234**

131. The elderly client is admitted to the emergency room. Which symptom is the client with a fractured hip most likely to exhibit?

Quick Answer: 221
Detailed Answer: 234

   ○ **A.** Pain

   ○ **B.** Disalignment

   ○ **C.** Cool extremity

   ○ **D.** Absence of pedal pulses

132. The nurse knows that a 60-year-old female client's susceptibility to osteoporosis is most likely related to:

Quick Answer: 221
Detailed Answer: 234

   ○ **A.** Lack of exercise

   ○ **B.** Hormonal changes

   ○ **C.** Lack of calcium

   ○ **D.** Genetic predisposition

133. A two-year-old is admitted for repair of a fractured femur and is placed in Bryant's traction. Which finding by the nurse indicates that the traction is working properly?

Quick Answer: 221
Detailed Answer: 234

   ○ **A.** The infant no longer complains of pain.

   ○ **B.** The buttocks are 15° off the bed.

   ○ **C.** The legs are suspended in the traction.

   ○ **D.** The pins are secured within the pulley.

134. Which statement is true regarding balanced skeletal traction? Balanced skeletal traction:

Quick Answer: 221
Detailed Answer: 235

   ○ **A.** Uses a Steinman pin

   ○ **B.** Requires that both legs be secured

   ○ **C.** Utilizes Kirschner wires

   ○ **D.** Is used primarily to heal the fractured hips

135. The client is admitted for an open reduction internal fixation of a fractured hip. Immediately following surgery, the nurse should give priority to assessing the:

Quick Answer: 221
Detailed Answer: 235

   ○ **A.** Serum collection (Davol) drain

   ○ **B.** Client's pain

   ○ **C.** Nutritional status

   ○ **D.** Immobilizer

136. Which statement made by the family member caring for the client with a percutaneous gastrostomy tube indicates understanding of the nurse's teaching?

- ○ **A.** "I must flush the tube with water after feedings and clamp the tube."
- ○ **B.** "I must check placement four times per day."
- ○ **C.** "I will report to the doctor any signs of indigestion."
- ○ **D.** "If my father is unable to swallow, I will discontinue the feeding and call the clinic."

Quick Answer: **221**
Detailed Answer: **235**

137. The nurse is assessing the client with a total knee replacement two hours post-operative. Which information requires notification of the doctor?

- ○ **A.** Scant bleeding on the dressing
- ○ **B.** Low-grade temperature
- ○ **C.** Hemoglobin of 7gm/dL
- ○ **D.** Urine output of 120mL during the last hour

Quick Answer: **221**
Detailed Answer: **235**

138. Which information in the child's health history is likely related to the diagnosis of plumbism?

- ○ **A.** The child has traveled out of the country in the last six months.
- ○ **B.** The child's parents are skilled stained glass artists.
- ○ **C.** The child lives in a house built in 1990.
- ○ **D.** The child attends a public daycare facility.

Quick Answer: **221**
Detailed Answer: **235**

139. Which equipment would assist the client with a total hip replacement with activities of daily living?

- ○ **A.** Raised commode
- ○ **B.** Velcro fasteners
- ○ **C.** Hand grip utensils
- ○ **D.** Large button clothing

Quick Answer: **221**
Detailed Answer: **235**

140. Which complaint by the client raises the possibility of compartment syndrome following cast application to the leg?

- ○ **A.** Diffuse aching in the leg
- ○ **B.** Tight burning pain in the calf
- ○ **C.** Localized pain along the shin
- ○ **D.** Throbbing sensation in the toes

Quick Answer: **221**
Detailed Answer: **235**

141. Which roommate would be most suitable for the six-year-old male with a fractured femur in Russell's traction?

Quick Answer: **221**
Detailed Answer: **235**

- ○ **A.** Sixteen-year-old male with leukemia
- ○ **B.** Twelve-year-old male with a fractured humerus
- ○ **C.** Ten-year-old male with sarcoma
- ○ **D.** Six-year-old male with osteomyelitis

142. A client with osteoarthritis has a prescription for Celebrex (celecoxib). Which instruction should be included in the discharge teaching?

Quick Answer: **221**
Detailed Answer: **235**

- ○ **A.** Take the medication with milk
- ○ **B.** Report chest pain to the physician
- ○ **C.** Remain upright 30 minutes after taking the medication
- ○ **D.** Allow six weeks for optimal effects

143. Which action by the nurse indicates understanding of the care of a client with a fiberglass leg cast?

Quick Answer: **221**
Detailed Answer: **235**

- ○ **A.** The nurse handles the cast with the fingertips.
- ○ **B.** The nurse allows 24 hours for the cast to dry.
- ○ **C.** The nurse dries the cast with a blow dryer.
- ○ **D.** The nurse tells the client to wait 30 minutes before bearing weight.

144. The teenager with a fiberglass cast asks the nurse if it will be okay to allow his friends to autograph his cast. Which response would be best?

Quick Answer: **221**
Detailed Answer: **235**

- ○ **A.** "It will be alright for your friends to autograph the cast."
- ○ **B.** "Because the cast is made of plaster, autographing can weaken the cast."
- ○ **C.** "If they don't use chalk to autograph, it is okay."
- ○ **D.** "Autographing or writing on the cast in any form will harm the cast."

145. The nurse is assigned to care for the client with a Steinman pin. During pin care, she notes that the LPN uses sterile gloves and cotton tipped applicators to clean the pin. Which action should the nurse take at this time?

Quick Answer: **221**
Detailed Answer: **236**

- ○ **A.** Assist the LPN with opening sterile packages and peroxide
- ○ **B.** Tell the LPN that clean gloves are allowed

   ○   **C.** Tell the LPN that the registered nurse should perform pin care

   ○   **D.** Ask the LPN to clean the weights and pulleys with peroxide

146. Which nursing action is specific to the care of the client in a body cast?

   ○   **A.** Auscultating bowel sounds

   ○   **B.** Assessing the blood pressure

   ○   **C.** Offering pain medication as needed

   ○   **D.** Assessing for swelling in the upper extremities

Quick Answer: **221**
Detailed Answer: **236**

147. Which statement is true regarding the care of the patient in skeletal traction?

   ○   **A.** The nurse may remove the weights for bathing.

   ○   **B.** Blocks should be placed beneath the head of the bed.

   ○   **C.** The weights must hang freely to be effective.

   ○   **D.** The nurse should massage reddened areas to prevent skin breakdown.

Quick Answer: **221**
Detailed Answer: **236**

148. A client with a total knee replacement has a CPM (continuous passive motion) device applied during the post-operative period. Which statement made by the nurse indicates understanding of the care of the client with a CPM device?

   ○   **A.** "Use of the CPM device will permit the client to ambulate during the therapy."

   ○   **B.** "The CPM device controls should be positioned out of the client's reach."

   ○   **C.** "If the client complains of pain during therapy, I will discontinue use of the device and call the doctor."

   ○   **D.** "Use of the CPM device will eliminate the need for physical therapy after the client is discharged."

Quick Answer: **221**
Detailed Answer: **236**

149. A client with a fractured hip is being taught correct use of the walker. The nurse is aware that the correct use of the walker is achieved if the:

   ○   **A.** Palms of the hands rest lightly on the handles.

   ○   **B.** Elbows are extended 0°.

   ○   **C.** Client steps all the way forward to the front of the walker.

   ○   **D.** Client lifts and carries the walker while ambulating.

Quick Answer: **221**
Detailed Answer: **236**

150. When assessing a laboring client, the nurse finds a prolapsed cord. The nurse should:

Quick Answer: **221**
Detailed Answer: **236**

- ○ **A.** Attempt to replace the cord
- ○ **B.** Place the client on her left side
- ○ **C.** Elevate the client's hips
- ○ **D.** Cover the cord with a dry, sterile gauze

151. The nurse is caring for a 30-year-old male admitted with a stab wound. While in the emergency room, a chest tube is inserted. Which of the following explains the primary rationale for insertion of chest tubes?

Quick Answer: **221**
Detailed Answer: **236**

- ○ **A.** The tube will allow for equalization of the lung expansion.
- ○ **B.** Chest tubes serve as a method of draining blood and serous fluid and assist in reinflating the lungs.
- ○ **C.** Chest tubes relieve pain associated with a collapsed lung.
- ○ **D.** Chest tubes assist with cardiac function by stabilizing lung expansion.

152. A client who delivered this morning tells the nurse that she plans to breastfeed her baby. The nurse is aware that successful breast-feeding is most dependent on the:

Quick Answer: **221**
Detailed Answer: **236**

- ○ **A.** Mother's educational level
- ○ **B.** Infant's birth weight
- ○ **C.** Size of the mother's breast
- ○ **D.** Mother's desire to breastfeed

153. The nurse is monitoring the progress of a client in labor. Which finding should be reported to the physician immediately?

Quick Answer: **221**
Detailed Answer: **236**

- ○ **A.** The presence of scant bloody discharge
- ○ **B.** Frequent urination
- ○ **C.** The presence of green-tinged amniotic fluid
- ○ **D.** Moderate uterine contractions

Quick Check

154. The nurse is measuring the duration of the client's contractions. Which statement is true regarding the measurement of the duration of contractions?

Quick Answer: **221**
Detailed Answer: **236**

- ○ **A.** Duration is measured by timing from the beginning of one contraction to the beginning of the next contraction.
- ○ **B.** Duration is measured by timing from the end of one contraction to the beginning of the next contraction.
- ○ **C.** Duration is measured by timing from the beginning of one contraction to the end of the same contraction.
- ○ **D.** Duration is measured by timing from the peak of one contraction to the end of the same contraction.

155. The physician has ordered an intravenous infusion of Pitocin (oxytocin) for the induction of labor. When caring for the obstetric client receiving intravenous Pitocin (oxytocin), the nurse should monitor for:

Quick Answer: **221**
Detailed Answer: **236**

- ○ **A.** Maternal hypoglycemia
- ○ **B.** Fetal bradycardia
- ○ **C.** Maternal hyperreflexia
- ○ **D.** Fetal movement

156. A client with diabetes visits the prenatal clinic at 28 weeks gestation. Which statement is true regarding insulin needs during pregnancy?

Quick Answer: **221**
Detailed Answer: **236**

- ○ **A.** Insulin requirements moderate as the pregnancy progresses.
- ○ **B.** A decreased need for insulin occurs during the second trimester.
- ○ **C.** Elevations in human chorionic gonadotropin decrease the need for insulin.
- ○ **D.** Fetal development depends on adequate insulin regulation.

157. A client in the prenatal clinic is assessed to have a blood pressure of 180/96. The nurse should give priority to:

Quick Answer: **221**
Detailed Answer: **237**

- ○ **A.** Providing a calm environment
- ○ **B.** Obtaining a diet history
- ○ **C.** Administering an analgesic
- ○ **D.** Assessing fetal heart tones

158. A primigravida, age 42, is six weeks pregnant. Based on the client's age, her infant is at increased risk for:

Quick Answer: **221**
Detailed Answer: **237**

- ○ **A.** Down syndrome
- ○ **B.** Respiratory distress syndrome
- ○ **C.** Turner syndrome
- ○ **D.** Pathological jaundice

159. A client with a missed abortion at 29 weeks gestation is admitted to the hospital. The client will most likely be treated with:

Quick Answer: **221**
Detailed Answer: **237**

- ○ **A.** Magnesium sulfate
- ○ **B.** Calcium gluconate
- ○ **C.** Dinoprostone (Prostin E.)
- ○ **D.** Bromocriptine (Parlodel)

160. A client with preeclampsia has been receiving an infusion containing magnesium sulfate for a blood pressure that is 160/80. Deep tendon reflexes are 2 plus, and the urinary output for the past hour is 100mL. The nurse should:

Quick Answer: **221**
Detailed Answer: **237**

- ○ **A.** Continue the infusion of magnesium sulfate while monitoring the client's blood pressure.
- ○ **B.** Stop the infusion of magnesium sulfate and contact the physician.
- ○ **C.** Slow the infusion rate and turn the client on her left side.
- ○ **D.** Administer calcium gluconate IV push and continue to monitor the blood pressure.

161. Which statement made by the nurse describes the inheritance pattern of autosomal recessive disorders?

Quick Answer: **221**
Detailed Answer: **237**

- ○ **A.** An affected child has unaffected parents.
- ○ **B.** An affected child has one affected parent.
- ○ **C.** Affected parents have a one-in-four chance of passing on the defective gene.
- ○ **D.** Affected parents have unaffected children who are carriers.

162. A pregnant client, age 32, asks the nurse why her doctor has recommended a serum alpha fetoprotein. The nurse should explain that the doctor has recommended the test:

Quick Answer: **221**
Detailed Answer: **237**

- ○ **A.** Because it is a state law
- ○ **B.** To detect cardiovascular defects

○ **C.** Because of her age

○ **D.** To detect neurological defects

163. A client with hypothyroidism asks the nurse if she will still need to take thyroid medication during the pregnancy. The nurse's response is based on the knowledge that:

○ **A.** There is no need to take thyroid medication because the fetus's thyroid produces a thyroid-stimulating hormone.

○ **B.** Regulation of thyroid medication is more difficult because the thyroid gland increases in size during pregnancy.

○ **C.** It is more difficult to maintain thyroid regulation during pregnancy due to a slowing of metabolism.

○ **D.** Fetal growth is arrested if thyroid medication is continued during pregnancy.

Quick Answer: **221**
Detailed Answer: **237**

164. The nurse is responsible for performing a neonatal assessment on a full-term infant. At one minute, the nurse could expect to find:

○ **A.** An apical pulse of 100

○ **B.** An absence of tonus

○ **C.** Cyanosis of the feet and hands

○ **D.** Jaundice of the skin and sclera

Quick Answer: **221**
Detailed Answer: **237**

165. A client with sickle cell anemia is admitted to the labor and delivery unit during the first phase of labor. The nurse should anticipate the client's need for:

○ **A.** Supplemental oxygen

○ **B.** Fluid restriction

○ **C.** Blood transfusion

○ **D.** Delivery by Caesarean section

Quick Answer: **221**
Detailed Answer: **237**

166. A client with gestational diabetes has an order for ultrasonography. Preparation for an ultrasound includes:

○ **A.** Increasing fluid intake

○ **B.** Limiting ambulation

○ **C.** Administering an enema

○ **D.** Withholding food for eight hours

Quick Answer: **221**
Detailed Answer: **238**

167. An infant who weighs 8 pounds at birth would be expected to weigh how many pounds at six months?

Quick Answer: **221**
Detailed Answer: **238**

- ○ **A.** 14 pounds
- ○ **B.** 24 pounds
- ○ **C.** 18 pounds
- ○ **D.** 16 pounds

168. A pregnant client with a history of alcohol addiction is scheduled for a nonstress test. The nonstress test:

Quick Answer: **221**
Detailed Answer: **238**

- ○ **A.** Determines the lung maturity of the fetus
- ○ **B.** Measures the activity of the fetus
- ○ **C.** Shows the effect of contractions on the fetal heart rate
- ○ **D.** Measures the neurological well-being of the fetus

169. A client with ankylosing spondylitis is to begin treatment with Cosentyx (secukinumab). Prior to beginning the medication, the physician will most likely order which of the following?

Quick Answer: **221**
Detailed Answer: **238**

- ○ **A.** Chest x-ray
- ○ **B.** Pregnancy test
- ○ **C.** Allergy testing
- ○ **D.** TB skin test

170. A gravida 3 para 2 is admitted to the labor unit. Vaginal exam reveals that the client's cervix is 8cm dilated, with complete effacement. The priority nursing diagnosis at this time is:

Quick Answer: **221**
Detailed Answer: **238**

- ○ **A.** Alteration in coping related to pain
- ○ **B.** Potential for injury related to precipitate delivery
- ○ **C.** Alteration in elimination related to anesthesia
- ○ **D.** Potential for fluid volume deficit related to NPO status

171. A child receiving immunosuppressive medication has contracted varicella. The physician will most likely order which of the following medications?

Quick Answer: **221**
Detailed Answer: **238**

- ○ **A.** Dilantin (phenytoin)
- ○ **B.** ASA (aspirin)
- ○ **C.** Zovirax (acyclovir)
- ○ **D.** Motrin (ibuprofen)

172. A client is admitted complaining of chest pain. Which of the following medications is not indicated in the care of the client with chest pain?

- ○ **A.** Nitro-Stat (nitroglycerin)
- ○ **B.** Atropine
- ○ **C.** Inderal (propranolol)
- ○ **D.** Calan (verapamil)

173. Which of the following instructions should be included in the teaching for the client with rheumatoid arthritis?

- ○ **A.** Avoid exercise because it fatigues the joints
- ○ **B.** Take prescribed anti-inflammatory medications with meals
- ○ **C.** Alternate hot and cold packs to affected joints
- ○ **D.** Avoid weight-bearing activity

174. Which medication should be avoided by the client with acute pancreatitis?

- ○ **A.** Demerol (meperidine)
- ○ **B.** Pepcid (famotidine)
- ○ **C.** Zantac (ranitidine)
- ○ **D.** Duramorph (morphine sulfate)

175. The client is admitted for observation because of ingestion of a hallucinogenic drug. Which statement is true regarding hallucinogen drugs?

- ○ **A.** Hallucinogenic drugs create both stimulant and depressant effects.
- ○ **B.** Hallucinogenic drugs induce a state of altered perception.
- ○ **C.** Hallucinogenic drugs produce severe respiratory depression.
- ○ **D.** Hallucinogenic drugs induce rapid physical dependence.

176. A client has a history of abusing barbiturates. Which of the following is a sign of mild barbiturate intoxication?

- ○ **A.** Rapid speech
- ○ **B.** Nystagmus
- ○ **C.** Anisocoria
- ○ **D.** Polyphagia

177. During the assessment of a laboring client, the nurse notes that the FHT are loudest in the upper-right quadrant. The infant is most likely in which position?

Quick Answer: **221**
Detailed Answer: **238**

- ○ **A.** Right breech presentation
- ○ **B.** Right occipital anterior presentation
- ○ **C.** Left sacral anterior presentation
- ○ **D.** Left occipital transverse presentation

178. Which of the following is considered an intrinsic factor in the development of asthma?

Quick Answer: **221**
Detailed Answer: **239**

- ○ **A.** Sinusitis
- ○ **B.** Hormonal influences
- ○ **C.** Food additives
- ○ **D.** Psychological stress

179. A client with mania is unable to finish her dinner. To help her maintain sufficient nourishment, the nurse should:

Quick Answer: **221**
Detailed Answer: **239**

- ○ **A.** Serve high-calorie foods she can carry with her
- ○ **B.** Encourage her appetite by sending out for her favorite foods
- ○ **C.** Serve her small, attractively arranged portions
- ○ **D.** Allow her in the unit kitchen for extra food whenever she pleases

180. To maintain Bryant's traction, the nurse must make certain that the child's:

Quick Answer: **221**
Detailed Answer: **239**

- ○ **A.** Hips are resting on the bed with the legs suspended at a right angle to the bed.
- ○ **B.** Hips are slightly elevated above the bed and the legs are suspended at a right angle to the bed.
- ○ **C.** Hips are elevated above the level of the body on a pillow and the legs are suspended parallel to the bed.
- ○ **D.** Hips and legs are flat on the bed with the traction positioned at the foot of the bed.

181. Which nursing intervention is appropriate when caring for a client with herpes zoster?

Quick Answer: **221**
Detailed Answer: **239**

- ○ **A.** Covering the lesions with a sterile dressing
- ○ **B.** Wearing gloves when providing care
- ○ **C.** Administering aspirin for discomfort
- ○ **D.** Administering Zovirax (acyclovir) within 72 hours of the outbreak

182. There is an order for a trough level to be drawn on the client receiving Vancocin (vancomycin). The nurse is aware that the lab should collect the blood:

Quick Answer: **221**
Detailed Answer: **239**

- ○ **A.** 15 minutes after the infusion
- ○ **B.** Prior to the fourth infusion
- ○ **C.** One hour after the infusion
- ○ **D.** Two hours before the second infusion

183. The client using a diaphragm should be instructed to:

Quick Answer: **221**
Detailed Answer: **239**

- ○ **A.** Refrain from keeping the diaphragm in longer than four hours
- ○ **B.** Store the diaphragm in a cool place
- ○ **C.** Have the diaphragm resized if she gains five pounds
- ○ **D.** Have the diaphragm resized if she has any surgery

184. The nurse is providing postpartum teaching for a mother planning to breastfeed her infant. Which of the client's statements indicates the need for additional teaching?

Quick Answer: **221**
Detailed Answer: **239**

- ○ **A.** "I'm wearing a support bra."
- ○ **B.** "I'm expressing milk from my breast."
- ○ **C.** "I'm drinking four glasses of fluid during a 24-hour period."
- ○ **D.** "While I'm in the shower, I'll allow the water to run over my breasts."

185. Damage to the VII cranial nerve results in:

Quick Answer: **221**
Detailed Answer: **239**

- ○ **A.** Facial pain
- ○ **B.** Absence of ability to smell
- ○ **C.** Absence of eye movement
- ○ **D.** Tinnitus

186. A client is receiving Pyridium (phenazopyridine hydrochloride) for a urinary tract infection. The client should be taught that the medication may:

Quick Answer: **221**
Detailed Answer: **239**

- ○ **A.** Cause diarrhea
- ○ **B.** Change the color of her urine
- ○ **C.** Cause mental confusion
- ○ **D.** Cause changes in taste

187. Which of the following should be performed before beginning therapy with Accutane (isotretinoin)?

   ○ **A.** Calcium level

   ○ **B.** Pregnancy test

   ○ **C.** Potassium level

   ○ **D.** Creatinine level

Quick Answer: **221**
Detailed Answer: **239**

188. A client with HIV is taking Zovirax (acyclovir). Which instruction should the nurse give the client taking acyclovir?

   ○ **A.** "Limit your activity while taking the medication."

   ○ **B.** "Supplement your diet with high-carbohydrate sources."

   ○ **C.** "Use an incentive spirometer to improve respiratory function."

   ○ **D.** "Increase your fluid intake to eight glasses of water a day."

Quick Answer: **221**
Detailed Answer: **240**

189. A female client is admitted for a CAT scan with contrast medium. Which of the following findings would prevent the client from having the ordered test?

   ○ **A.** Pregnancy

   ○ **B.** A titanium hip replacement

   ○ **C.** Allergy to eggs

   ○ **D.** Inability to lie still for 30 minutes

Quick Answer: **221**
Detailed Answer: **240**

190. The nurse is caring for the client receiving Amphotericin B. Which of the following indicates that the client has experienced toxicity to this drug?

   ○ **A.** Changes in vision

   ○ **B.** Nausea

   ○ **C.** Urinary frequency

   ○ **D.** Changes in skin color

Quick Answer: **221**
Detailed Answer: **240**

191. The nurse should visit which of the following clients first?

   ○ **A.** The client with diabetes with a blood glucose of 95mg/dL

   ○ **B.** The client with hypertension being maintained on Zestril (lisinopril)

   ○ **C.** The client with chest pain and a history of angina

   ○ **D.** The client with Raynaud's disease

Quick Answer: **221**
Detailed Answer: **240**

192. A client with cystic fibrosis is taking pancreatic enzymes. The nurse should administer this medication:

    ○ **A.** Once per day in the morning

    ○ **B.** Three times per day with meals

    ○ **C.** Once per day at bedtime

    ○ **D.** Four times per day

Quick Answer: **221**
Detailed Answer: **240**

193. Cataracts result in opacity of the crystalline lens. Which of the following best explains the functions of the lens?

    ○ **A.** The lens controls stimulation of the retina.

    ○ **B.** The lens orchestrates eye movement.

    ○ **C.** The lens focuses light rays on the retina.

    ○ **D.** The lens magnifies small objects.

Quick Answer: **221**
Detailed Answer: **240**

194. A client who has glaucoma is to have miotic eye drops instilled in both eyes. The nurse knows that the purpose of the medication is to:

    ○ **A.** Anesthetize the cornea

    ○ **B.** Dilate the pupils

    ○ **C.** Constrict the pupils

    ○ **D.** Paralyze the muscles of accommodation

Quick Answer: **221**
Detailed Answer: **240**

195. A client with a corneal abrasion has an order for Garamycin (gentamicin) ophthalmic drops 1 bid and PredForte (prednisolone) ophthalmic drops 1 bid. Which of the following methods should be used when administering the medications?

    ○ **A.** Allow five minutes between the administration of the two medications

    ○ **B.** Administer the two medications at the same time

    ○ **C.** Allow 30 minutes between the administration of the two medications

    ○ **D.** Separate the administration of the medication by one to two hours

Quick Answer: **221**
Detailed Answer: **240**

196. The client with color blindness will have problems distinguishing which of the following colors?

    ○ **A.** Orange

    ○ **B.** Violet

    ○ **C.** Red

    ○ **D.** Yellow

Quick Answer: **221**
Detailed Answer: **240**

197. The client with a pacemaker should be taught to:

    ○ **A.** Report ankle edema

    ○ **B.** Check his blood pressure daily

    ○ **C.** Refrain from using a microwave oven

    ○ **D.** Monitor his pulse rate

198. The client with enuresis is being taught regarding bladder retraining. The nurse should advise the client to refrain from drinking after:

    ○ **A.** 1900

    ○ **B.** 1200

    ○ **C.** 1000

    ○ **D.** 0700

199. Which of the following diet instructions should be given to the client with recurring urinary tract infections?

    ○ **A.** Increase intake of red meats

    ○ **B.** Avoid citrus fruits

    ○ **C.** Limit the intake of dairy products

    ○ **D.** Drink a glass of cranberry juice every day

200. The physician has prescribed NPH insulin for a client with diabetes mellitus. Which statement indicates that the client knows when the peak action of the insulin occurs?

    ○ **A.** "I will make sure I eat breakfast within two hours of taking my insulin."

    ○ **B.** "I will need to carry candy or some form of sugar with me all the time."

    ○ **C.** "I will eat a snack around three o'clock each afternoon."

    ○ **D.** "I can save my dessert from supper for a bedtime snack."

201. The physician has ordered Zyvox (linezolid) for a patient diagnosed with vancomycin resistant enterococcus. Which food should be avoided?

    ○ **A.** Wheat bread

    ○ **B.** Honey

    ○ **C.** Oranges

    ○ **D.** Aged cheese

202. The nurse is preparing to administer a Meruvax II (rubella) vaccine to an adult client. Which one of the following allergies contraindicates the use of the vaccine?

Quick Answer: **221**
Detailed Answer: **241**

- ○ **A.** Penicillin
- ○ **B.** Neomycin
- ○ **C.** Acyclovir
- ○ **D.** Tetracycline

203. The physician has prescribed Zantac (ranitidine) for a client with reflux. The nurse should administer the medication:

Quick Answer: **221**
Detailed Answer: **241**

- ○ **A.** Mid afternoon
- ○ **B.** Thirty minutes before eating
- ○ **C.** In a single dose at bedtime
- ○ **D.** Mid-morning

204. A temporary colostomy is performed on the client with colon cancer. The nurse is aware that the proximal end of a double barrel colostomy:

Quick Answer: **221**
Detailed Answer: **241**

- ○ **A.** Opens on the left side of the abdomen
- ○ **B.** Will produce only mucus
- ○ **C.** Opens on the right side of the abdomen
- ○ **D.** Will be bluish colored in appearance

205. While assessing the postpartal client, the nurse notes that the fundus is displaced to the right. Based on this finding, the nurse should:

Quick Answer: **221**
Detailed Answer: **241**

- ○ **A.** Ask the client to void
- ○ **B.** Assess the blood pressure for hypotension
- ○ **C.** Administer oxytocin
- ○ **D.** Check for vaginal bleeding

206. The physician has ordered an MRI as a part of the client's diagnostic work-up. An MRI should not be done if the client has:

Quick Answer: **221**
Detailed Answer: **241**

- ○ **A.** The need for oxygen therapy
- ○ **B.** A history of claustrophobia
- ○ **C.** A permanent pacemaker
- ○ **D.** Sensory deafness

207. Which toy is best suited to the developmental skills of a one-year-old?

    ○ **A.** Pounding board

    ○ **B.** Pull toy

    ○ **C.** Soft books

    ○ **D.** Puzzle with large pieces

Quick Answer: **221**
Detailed Answer: **241**

208. Which of the following statements is true regarding management of the client with multiple sclerosis?

    ○ **A.** Taking a hot bath will decrease stiffness and spasticity.

    ○ **B.** A schedule of strenuous exercise will improve muscle strength.

    ○ **C.** Rest periods should be scheduled throughout the day.

    ○ **D.** Visual disturbances can be corrected with prescription glasses.

Quick Answer: **221**
Detailed Answer: **241**

209. A client on the postpartum unit has a proctoepisiotomy. The nurse should anticipate administering which medication?

    ○ **A.** Dulcolax suppository

    ○ **B.** Docusate sodium (Colace)

    ○ **C.** Methylergonovine maleate (Methergine)

    ○ **D.** Bromocriptine sulfate (Parlodel)

Quick Answer: **222**
Detailed Answer: **241**

210. A client with pancreatic cancer who is receiving TPN has an order for sliding-scale insulin. The reason for the ordered insulin is:

    ○ **A.** TPN leads to negative nitrogen balance and elevated glucose levels.

    ○ **B.** TPN cannot be managed with oral hypoglycemics.

    ○ **C.** TPN is a high-glucose solution that can elevate the blood glucose levels.

    ○ **D.** TPN use can depress the activity of the beta cells of the islets of Langerhans.

Quick Answer: **222**
Detailed Answer: **242**

211. An adolescent primigravida who is 10 weeks pregnant attends the antepartal clinic for a first check-up. To develop a teaching plan, the nurse should initially assess:

    ○ **A.** The client's knowledge of the signs of preterm labor

    ○ **B.** The client's feelings about the pregnancy

    ○ **C.** The client's method of birth control

    ○ **D.** The client's plans for continuing school

Quick Answer: **222**
Detailed Answer: **242**

212. A client is admitted with a two-day history of nausea and vomiting. Which IV fluid is appropriate for the client with moderate dehydration?

Quick Answer: **222**
Detailed Answer: **242**

   ○ **A.** Lactated Ringer's

   ○ **B.** Dextrose 1% in water

   ○ **C.** Three percent normal saline

   ○ **D.** Dextrose 5% /.45% normal saline

213. The physician has ordered a thyroid scan to confirm the diagnosis of a goiter. Before the procedure, the nurse should:

Quick Answer: **222**
Detailed Answer: **242**

   ○ **A.** Assess the client for allergies to iodine

   ○ **B.** Bolus the client with IV fluid

   ○ **C.** Administer an anxiolytic

   ○ **D.** Insert a urinary catheter

214. The physician has ordered an injection of RhoGAM for a client with blood type A negative. The nurse understands that RhoGAM is given to:

Quick Answer: **222**
Detailed Answer: **242**

   ○ **A.** Provide immunity against Rh isoenzymes

   ○ **B.** Prevent the formation of Rh antibodies

   ○ **C.** Eliminate circulating Rh antibodies

   ○ **D.** Convert the Rh factor from negative to positive

215. The nurse is caring for a client admitted to the emergency room after a fall. X-rays reveal that the client has several fractured bones in the foot. Which treatment should the nurse anticipate for the fractured foot?

Quick Answer: **222**
Detailed Answer: **242**

   ○ **A.** Application of a walking boot

   ○ **B.** Stabilization with a cast

   ○ **C.** Surgery with Kirschner wire implantation

   ○ **D.** Application of spica cast

216. A client with prostate cancer is being treated with iridium seed implants. The nurse's discharge teaching should include telling the client to:

Quick Answer: **222**
Detailed Answer: **242**

   ○ **A.** Strain his urine

   ○ **B.** Increase his fluid intake

   ○ **C.** Report urinary frequency

   ○ **D.** Avoid prolonged sitting

217. A patient with pulmonary tuberculosis is receiving combination therapy. To increase the effects of the medication, the patient may be given:

Quick Answer: **222**
Detailed Answer: **242**

- ○ **A.** Inderal (propranolol)
- ○ **B.** Dilantin (phenytoin)
- ○ **C.** Benemid (probenecid)
- ○ **D.** Neoral (cyclosporine)

218. The nurse is preparing a client for cataract surgery. The nurse is aware that:

Quick Answer: **222**
Detailed Answer: **242**

- ○ **A.** Mydriatics will be used to dilate the pupil.
- ○ **B.** Miotics will be used to constrict the pupil.
- ○ **C.** A laser will be used to smooth and reshape the lens.
- ○ **D.** Silicone oil injections will be used to hold the retina in place.

219. A client with Alzheimer's disease is in a skilled nursing facility. Which intervention is therapeutic for the client?

Quick Answer: **222**
Detailed Answer: **242**

- ○ **A.** Placing mirrors in several locations in the facility
- ○ **B.** Placing a picture of the client in her room
- ○ **C.** Placing simple signs to indicate the location of her room, the bathroom, and dining room
- ○ **D.** Alternating healthcare workers to prevent boredom

220. A client with an abdominal cholecystectomy returns from surgery with a Jackson-Pratt drain. The chief purpose of the Jackson-Pratt drain is to:

Quick Answer: **222**
Detailed Answer: **242**

- ○ **A.** Prevent the need for dressing changes
- ○ **B.** Reduce edema at the incision
- ○ **C.** Provide for wound drainage
- ○ **D.** Keep the common bile duct open

221. The nurse is performing an initial assessment of a newborn delivered at 32 weeks gestation. The nurse can expect to find the presence of:

Quick Answer: **222**
Detailed Answer: **243**

- ○ **A.** Vernix caseosa
- ○ **B.** Sucking pads
- ○ **C.** Head lag
- ○ **D.** Absence of scarf sign

222. The nurse is caring for a client admitted with multiple trauma. Fractures include the pelvis, femur, and ulna. Which finding should be reported to the physician immediately?

- ○ **A.** Hematuria
- ○ **B.** Muscle spasms
- ○ **C.** Dizziness
- ○ **D.** Nausea

223. A client with a history of cocaine abuse is experiencing tactile hallucinations. This symptom is known as:

- ○ **A.** Dyskinesia
- ○ **B.** Confabulation
- ○ **C.** Formication
- ○ **D.** Dystonia

224. The nurse is preparing to suction the client with a tracheotomy. The nurse notes a previously used bottle of normal saline on the client's bedside table. There is no label to indicate the date or time of initial use. The nurse should:

- ○ **A.** Lip the bottle and use a pack of sterile 4×4 for the dressing
- ○ **B.** Obtain a new bottle and label it with the date and time of first use
- ○ **C.** Ask the ward secretary when the solution was requested
- ○ **D.** Label the existing bottle with the current date and time

225. An infant's Apgar score is 9 at five minutes. The nurse is aware that the most likely cause for the deduction of one point is:

- ○ **A.** The newborn is hypothermic.
- ○ **B.** The newborn is experiencing bradycardia.
- ○ **C.** The newborn has acrocyanosis.
- ○ **D.** The newborn is lethargic.

226. The primary reason for rapid continuous rewarming of the area affected by frostbite is to:

- ○ **A.** Lessen the amount of cellular damage
- ○ **B.** Prevent the formation of blisters
- ○ **C.** Promote movement
- ○ **D.** Prevent pain and discomfort

227. A client recently started on hemodialysis wants to know how the dialysis will take the place of his kidneys. The nurse's response is based on the knowledge that hemodialysis works by:

   ○ **A.** Passing water through a dialyzing membrane

   ○ **B.** Eliminating plasma proteins from the blood

   ○ **C.** Lowering the pH by removing nonvolatile acids

   ○ **D.** Filtering waste through a dialyzing membrane

Quick Answer: **222**
Detailed Answer: **243**

228. A client hospitalized with AIDS tells the nurse that he has been exposed to measles. The nurse should contact the physician regarding an order for:

   ○ **A.** An antibiotic

   ○ **B.** Immune globulin

   ○ **C.** An antiviral

   ○ **D.** Airborne isolation

Quick Answer: **222**
Detailed Answer: **243**

229. A client hospitalized with MRSA is placed on contact precautions. Which statement is true regarding precautions for infections spread by contact?

   ○ **A.** The client should be placed in a room with negative pressure.

   ○ **B.** Infection requires close contact; therefore, the door may remain open.

   ○ **C.** Transmission is highly likely, so the client should wear a mask at all times.

   ○ **D.** Infection requires skin-to-skin contact and is prevented by hand washing, gloves, and a gown.

Quick Answer: **222**
Detailed Answer: **243**

230. A client who is admitted with an above-the-knee amputation tells the nurse that his foot hurts and itches. Which response by the nurse indicates understanding of phantom limb pain?

   ○ **A.** "The pain will go away in a few days."

   ○ **B.** "The pain is due to peripheral nervous system interruptions. I will get you some pain medication."

   ○ **C.** "The pain is psychological because your foot is no longer there."

   ○ **D.** "The pain and itching are due to the infection you had before the surgery."

Quick Answer: **222**
Detailed Answer: **243**

231. A client with cancer of the pancreas has undergone a Whipple procedure. The Whipple procedure includes the removal of:

   ○ **A.** The head of the pancreas

   ○ **B.** The proximal third of the small intestine

   ○ **C.** The stomach and duodenum

   ○ **D.** The esophagus and jejunum

Quick Answer: **222**
Detailed Answer: **244**

232. The physician has ordered a minimal-bacteria diet for a client with neutropenia. The client should be taught to avoid using which condiment?

   ○ **A.** Mustard

   ○ **B.** Salt

   ○ **C.** Pepper

   ○ **D.** Ketchup

Quick Answer: **222**
Detailed Answer: **244**

233. A client is discharged home with a prescription for Coumadin (sodium warfarin). The client should be instructed to:

   ○ **A.** Avoid antihistamines containing diphenhydramine

   ○ **B.** Increase the intake of all vegetables

   ○ **C.** Have a PTT checked monthly

   ○ **D.** Have a CBC drawn every six months

Quick Answer: **222**
Detailed Answer: **244**

234. The nurse is assisting the physician with removal of a central venous catheter. To facilitate removal, the nurse should instruct the client to:

   ○ **A.** Take a deep breath, hold it, and bear down as the catheter is withdrawn

   ○ **B.** Turn his head to the left side and hyperextend the neck

   ○ **C.** Take slow, deep breaths as the catheter is removed

   ○ **D.** Turn his head to the right while maintaining a sniffing position

Quick Answer: **222**
Detailed Answer: **244**

235. A client has an order for streptokinase. Before administering the medication, the nurse should assess the client for:

   ○ **A.** Allergies to pineapples and bananas

   ○ **B.** A history of streptococcal infections

   ○ **C.** Prior therapy with phenytoin

   ○ **D.** A history of alcohol abuse

Quick Answer: **222**
Detailed Answer: **244**

236. The nurse is providing discharge teaching for the client with leukemia. The client should be told to avoid:

    ○ **A.** Using oils or cream-based soaps

    ○ **B.** Flossing between the teeth

    ○ **C.** The intake of salt

    ○ **D.** Using an electric razor

237. The nurse is changing the ties of the client with a tracheostomy. The safest method of changing the tracheostomy ties is to:

    ○ **A.** Apply the new tie before removing the old one

    ○ **B.** Have a helper present in case assistance is needed

    ○ **C.** Hold the tracheostomy tie with the nondominant hand while removing the old tie

    ○ **D.** Ask the client to hold the tracheostomy in place as the ties are changed

238. The nurse is monitoring a client following a lung resection. The hourly output from the mediastinal tube was 300mL. The nurse should give priority to:

    ○ **A.** Turning the client to the left side

    ○ **B.** Milking the tube to ensure patency

    ○ **C.** Slowing the intravenous infusion

    ○ **D.** Notify the physician of the amount

239. An infant with congenital heart disease is admitted with symptoms of congestive heart failure. Which of the following is a sign of fluid overload in the infant?

    ○ **A.** Bulging fontanels

    ○ **B.** Bradycardia

    ○ **C.** Urine specific gravity of 1.015

    ○ **D.** Bradypnea

240. The nurse is educating the lady's club in self-breast exam. The nurse is aware that most malignant breast masses occur in the tail of Spence. On the diagram, place an X on the tail of Spence.

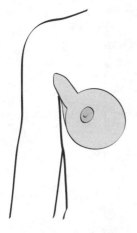

241. A toddler is admitted for the repair of a VSD. The nurse is aware that the child with a VSD will:

- ○ **A.** Tire more easily
- ○ **B.** Have normal patterns of growth and development
- ○ **C.** Require more calories
- ○ **D.** Need additional fluids to prevent thrombi

242. An obstetrical client with a history of stillbirths has an order for a nonstress test. The nurse is aware that a nonstress test is ordered to:

- ○ **A.** Determine lung maturity
- ○ **B.** Measure the fetal activity
- ○ **C.** Show the effect of contractions on fetal heart rate
- ○ **D.** Measure the well-being of the fetus

Quick Check

243. The nurse is evaluating the client who was admitted eight hours ago for induction of labor. The following graph is noted on the monitor. Which action should be taken first by the nurse?

Quick Answer: **222**
Detailed Answer: **245**

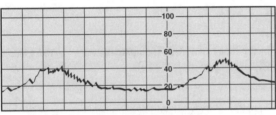

Fetal Heart Rate

Uterine Contractions

- ○ **A.** Instruct the client to push
- ○ **B.** Perform a vaginal exam
- ○ **C.** Stop the infusion of Pitocin (oxytocin)
- ○ **D.** Place the client in a semi-Fowler's position

244. The nurse notes the following on the ECG monitor. The nurse would evaluate the cardiac arrhythmia as:

Quick Answer: **222**
Detailed Answer: **245**

- ○ **A.** Atrial flutter
- ○ **B.** A sinus rhythm
- ○ **C.** Ventricular tachycardia
- ○ **D.** Atrial fibrillation

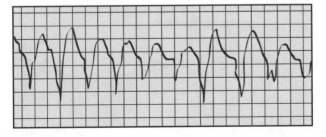

245. Which instruction should be given to the client who is self-administering Lovenox (enoxaparin)?

○ **A.** Inject the medication into the deltoid muscle

○ **B.** Inject the medication into the abdomen

○ **C.** Aspirate before administering the medication

○ **D.** Clear the air from the syringe before administering the medication

Quick Answer: **222**
Detailed Answer: **245**

246. The nurse has a preoperative order to administer Valium (diazepam) 10mg and Phenergan (promethazine) 25mg. The correct method of administering these medications is to:

○ **A.** Administer the medications together in one syringe

○ **B.** Administer the medications separately

○ **C.** Administer the Valium, wait five minutes, and then administer the Phenergan

○ **D.** Question the order because the medications should not be given to the same patient

Quick Answer: **222**
Detailed Answer: **246**

247. A female client with a history of frequent urinary tract infections asks the nurse how she can reduce the risk of recurrence. The nurse should tell the client to:

○ **A.** Douche after intercourse

○ **B.** Void every three hours

○ **C.** Increase her intake of foods containing vitamin C

○ **D.** Wipe from back to front after voiding

Quick Answer: **222**
Detailed Answer: **246**

248. Which task is within the scope of practice of the nursing assistant?

○ **A.** Obtaining vital signs on a patient following a craniotomy

○ **B.** Obtaining hourly intake and output on a client with preeclampsia

○ **C.** Feeding the client with depression

○ **D.** Ambulating the client following a hip replacement

Quick Answer: **222**
Detailed Answer: **246**

249. Which finding indicates a complication following a parathyroidectomy?

○ **A.** Two-inch circle of blood behind the neck

○ **B.** Eupnea

○ **C.** Absence of carpopedal spasms

○ **D.** Negative Chvostek's sign

Quick Answer: **222**
Detailed Answer: **246**

250. The physician has ordered amphotericin B for a client with histoplasmosis. In order to reduce the risk of nephrotoxicity, the nurse should:

○ **A.** Premedicate the patient with diphenhydramine and acetaminophen.

○ **B.** Test for hypersensitivity prior to administration.

○ **C.** Administer with heparin and hydrocortisone over four to six hours.

○ **D.** Hydrate with IV fluids before and after the drug is administered.

Quick Answer: **222**
Detailed Answer: **246**

Quick Answers

1. D	26. A	51. B	76. B
2. D	27. B	52. B	77. D
3. B	28. C	53. B	78. D
4. C	29. C	54. C	79. A
5. C	30. C	55. D	80. B
6. C	31. B	56. A	81. A
7. D	32. A	57. B	82. A
8. D	33. B	58. C	83. D
9. C	34. B	59. C	84. D
10. B	35. D	60. B	85. B
11. A	36. B	61. D	86. B
12. C	37. A	62. A	87. B
13. D	38. B	63. C	88. B
14. B	39. D	64. B	89. D
15. B	40. A	65. A	90. B
16. A	41. A	66. D	91. A
17. A	42. A	67. B	92. C
18. A	43. A	68. C	93. C
19. C	44. C	69. A	94. B
20. B	45. B	70. C	95. C
21. C	46. A	71. C	96. A
22. A	47. B	72. D	97. B
23. A	48. C	73. B	98. C
24. B	49. C	74. D	99. D
25. D	50. D	75. D	100. C

101. B	**128.** B	**155.** B	**182.** B
102. D	**129.** C	**156.** D	**183.** B
103. B	**130.** B	**157.** A	**184.** C
104. D	**131.** B	**158.** A	**185.** A
105. B	**132.** B	**159.** C	**186.** B
106. B	**133.** B	**160.** A	**187.** B
107. D	**134.** A	**161.** C	**188.** D
108. D	**135.** A	**162.** D	**189.** A
109. C	**136.** A	**163.** B	**190.** D
110. D	**137.** C	**164.** C	**191.** C
111. C	**138.** B	**165.** A	**192.** B
112. B	**139.** A	**166.** A	**193.** C
113. C	**140.** B	**167.** D	**194.** C
114. C	**141.** B	**168.** B	**195.** A
115. D	**142.** B	**169.** D	**196.** B
116. C	**143.** D	**170.** A	**197.** D
117. B	**144.** A	**171.** C	**198.** A
118. B	**145.** A	**172.** B	**199.** D
119. C	**146.** A	**173.** B	**200.** C
120. B	**147.** C	**174.** D	**201.** D
121. B	**148.** B	**175.** B	**202.** B
122. A	**149.** A	**176.** B	**203.** B
123. D	**150.** C	**177.** A	**204.** C
124. A	**151.** B	**178.** D	**205.** A
125. A	**152.** D	**179.** A	**206.** C
126. B	**153.** C	**180.** B	**207.** C
127. A	**154.** C	**181.** B	**208.** C

209. B

210. C

211. B

212. A

213. A

214. B

215. B

216. A

217. C

218. A

219. C

220. C

221. C

222. A

223. C

224. B

225. C

226. A

227. D

228. B

229. D

230. B

231. A

232. C

233. A

234. A

235. B

236. B

237. A

238. D

239. A

240. See diagram.

241. A

242. B

243. C

244. C

245. B

246. B

247. B

248. C

249. A

250. D

Answers and Rationales

1. **Answer D is correct.** Brisk capillary refill less than three seconds indicates adequate circulation to the extremity. Answers A, B, and C do not assess circulation; therefore, they are incorrect.

2. **Answer D is correct.** High levels of AFP are associated with Trisomy 21 (Down syndrome). Answers A, B, and C are associated with low levels of AFP; therefore, they are incorrect.

3. **Answer B is correct.** Applying oxygen is the highest nursing priority when caring for the patient in vaso-occlusive crisis. Answers A, C, and D are appropriate interventions but do not take priority over applying oxygen; therefore, they are incorrect choices.

4. **Answer C is correct.** L/S ratio is a reliable indicator of fetal lung maturity. Answers A, B, and D are not measured by L/S ratio so they are incorrect choices.

5. **Answer C is correct.** An increase in temperature of $1°$ or greater in the patient with leukopenia should be reported to the physician immediately. Answers A, B, and D are not significant; therefore, they are incorrect choices.

6. **Answer C is correct.** Eggs, wheat bread, carrots, and dark green leafy vegetables are rich in iron. The foods in Answers A, B, and D are not as rich in iron; therefore, these choices are incorrect.

7. **Answer D is correct.** Jaundice in a newborn at birth or within the first 24 hours of life is an abnormal assessment and indicates a need for follow-up. Answers A, B, and C are incorrect because they are findings in the normal newborn.

8. **Answer D is correct.** A history of meningitis and treatment with intravenous garamycin are likely factors in the two-year-old's loss of hearing. Answers A, B, and C are not significant factors associated with hearing loss, so they are incorrect choices.

9. **Answer C is correct.** 0 station indicates that the fetus is level with the ischial spines. Answers A, B, and D do not relate to the question; therefore, they are incorrect.

10. **Answer B is correct.** Increased respiratory rate is often observed in the patient with mild anemia. Answers A, C, and D are incorrect because they are observed in the patient with moderate to severe anemia.

11. **Answer A is correct.** A major complication of polycythemia vera is clotting. An intake of at least 3 liters per day is important in preventing clot formation, so the statement to limit intake to 1 liter a day indicates a need for further teaching. Answers B, C, and D are incorrect because they indicate an understanding regarding the prevention of complications.

12. **Answer C is correct.** Radiation treatment for other types of cancer such as Hodgkin's lymphoma is a risk factor in the development of leukemia. Answers A, B, and D are not considered risk factors for the development of leukemia; therefore, they are incorrect.

13. **Answer D is correct.** When checking skin turgor in an older client, the nurse should use the forehead or chest. Answers A, B, and C are incorrect because they are not sites to use when checking skin turgor of an older client.

14. **Answer B is correct.** The presence of café au lait spots is associated with a diagnosis of neurofibromatosis. Answers A, C, and D are incorrect because they are not associated with café au lait spots.

15. **Answer B is correct.** Prosopagnosia is the inability to recognize oneself and other familiar faces. The nurse should encourage the family to provide pictures of the patient, family members, and friends that are labeled. Answers A, C, and D are not interventions for the patient with prosopagnosia; therefore, they are incorrect.

16. **Answer A is correct.** Hypercalcemia is likely to result in shortened QT intervals. Answers B, C, and D are not associated with shortened QT intervals; therefore, they are incorrect.

17. **Answer A is correct.** A platelet count of 150,000 in the patient treated with Neumega (oprelvekin) indicates a favorable response. Answers B, C, and D are not associated with the use of Neumega; therefore, they are incorrect.

18. **Answer A is correct.** The normal platelet count is 200,000–400,000. Bleeding occurs in clients with low platelets. The priority is teaching measures to reduce the risk of bleeding. Answers B, C, and D are not as important as measures to reduce the risk of bleeding; therefore, they are incorrect.

19. **Answer C is correct.** A prolactinoma is a type of pituitary tumor. Elevating the head of the bed 30° decreases the intracranial pressure and reduces the risk of CSF leaks. Answers A, B, and D are incorrect choices because they increase intracranial pressure.

20. **Answer B is correct.** The loss of electrolytes would be reflected in the vital signs. Measuring the urinary output is important, but the question already states that the client has polyuria, so Answer A is incorrect. Encouraging fluid intake will not correct the problem, making Answer C incorrect. Answer D is incorrect because weighing the client is not necessary at this time.

21. **Answer C is correct.** Peaked T waves are most likely to be present in the ECG of a client with hyperkalemia. Answers A, B, and D are not associated with hyperkalemia.

22. **Answer A is correct.** Blood pressure is the best indicator of cardiovascular collapse in the client who has had a unilateral adrenalectomy. The remaining adrenal gland might have been suppressed due to the tumor activity. Temperature would be an indicator of infection, decreased output would be a clinical manifestation but would take longer to occur than blood pressure changes, and specific gravity changes occur with other disorders; therefore, Answers B, C, and D are incorrect.

23. **Answer A is correct.** IV glucocorticoids raise the glucose levels, and the client may require insulin. Answers B, C, and D are not priorities at this time.

24. **Answer B is correct.** Tingling around the mouth and in the fingers and toes is associated with hypocalcemia. Answers A, C, and D are not associated with the client's symptoms so they are incorrect choices.

25. **Answer D is correct.** The patient with hypothyroidism has a priority diagnosis of decreased cardiac output. Answers A, B, and C are appropriate for the patient with hypothyroidism but do not take priority over decreased cardiac output.

26. **Answer A is correct.** The client taking antilipidemics such as Crestor (rosuvastatin) should report unexplained muscle weakness to the physician. Answer B is incorrect because the medication usually takes effect within one month. The medication should be taken with water because fruit juice, particularly grapefruit, can cause interactions, making Answer C incorrect. Answer D is incorrect because difficulty sleeping is not associated with the medication.

27. **Answer B is correct.** Numbness in the hands is a side effect of Hyperstat (diazoxide). Answers A, C, and D are not associated with the medication, so they are incorrect.

28. **Answer C is correct.** A heart rate of 80 beats per minute in a six-month-old taking Lanoxin elixir should be reported to the physician immediately. Answers A, B, and C are within normal limits, so they are incorrect.

29. **Answer C is correct.** Nitroglycerine should be kept in a brown bottle (or even a special air-tight, water-tight, solid or plated silver or gold container) because of its instability and tendency to become less potent when exposed to air, light, or water. The supply should be replenished every six months, not three months, and one tablet should be taken every five minutes until pain subsides, so Answers A and B are incorrect. If the pain does not subside, the client should go immediately to the nearest emergency room. The medication should be taken sublingually and should not be crushed, as stated in Answer D.

30. **Answer C is correct.** Turkey contains the least amount of saturated fat. Answers A, B, and D are incorrect because cheese, shrimp, and beef contain more saturated fat.

31. **Answer B is correct.** A blood pressure cuff is needed to check for Trousseau's sign. Answers A, C, and D are not used to check Trousseau's sign, so they are incorrect.

32. **Answer A is correct.** The phlebostatic axis is located at the fifth intercostal space mid-axillary line and is the correct placement of the manometer. The PMI or point of maximal impulse is located at the fifth intercostal space mid-clavicular line, so answer B is incorrect. Erb's point is the location at which you can auscultate the valves closing simultaneously, making Answer C incorrect. The tail of Spence (the upper outer quadrant of the breast) is the area where most breast cancers are located and has nothing to do with placement of a manometer; thus, Answer D is incorrect.

33. **Answer B is correct.** The nurse should administer the medications as ordered. Zestril (lisinopril) is an ACE inhibitor and is frequently given with a diuretic such as Lasix (furosemide) for hypertension. Answers A, C, and D are incorrect because the order is accurate. There is no need to question the order, administer the medication separately, or contact the pharmacy.

34. **Answer B is correct.** The best indicator of peripheral edema is determined by measuring the extremity. A paper tape measure should be used rather than one made of plastic or cloth, and the area should be marked with a pen, providing the most objective

assessment. Answer A is incorrect because weighing the client will not indicate peripheral edema. Answer C is incorrect because checking the intake and output will not indicate peripheral edema. Answer D is incorrect because checking for pitting edema is less reliable than measuring with a paper tape measure.

35. **Answer D is correct.** The client with a vaginal radium implant should have close contact limited to 30 minutes per visit. Answers A, B, and C are not empathetic and do not address the question; therefore, they are incorrect.

36. **Answer B is correct.** The client with a facial stroke will have difficulty chewing and swallowing. The foods in Answer B require the least amount of chewing. Answers A, C, and D require more chewing and, therefore, are incorrect.

37. **Answer A is correct.** NovoLog (as part) insulin is a rapid-acting insulin with an onset of 10 to 20 minutes, so food should be available within 10–15 minutes of taking the insulin. Answer B does not address a particular type of insulin, so it is incorrect. Answer C is incorrect because it describes the peak for intermediate acting insulin such as NPH, which peaks in 6–14 hours. Answer D is incorrect because there is no need to save the dessert until bedtime.

38. **Answer B is correct.** A sponge bath is recommended for the newborn during the first two weeks of life in order for the umbilical cord to have time to separate. Answers A, C, and D are true statements; however, they are not the reason for using sponge baths for the newborn.

39. **Answer D is correct.** The rationale for administering Wellcovorin (leucovorin) is to reverse drug toxicity caused by methotrexate (leucovorin rescue). Answers A, B, and C are not associated with the use of leucovorin; therefore, they are incorrect choices.

40. **Answer A is correct.** The nurse should obtain a diet history from the mother. Orange discoloration of the nasolabial folds in a well child is associated with a high intake of carrots and other yellow or orange vegetables. Answers B, C, and D are not appropriate for the assessment findings; therefore, they are incorrect.

41. **Answer A is correct.** Nexium (esomeprazole) should be taken prior to breakfast. Answers B, C, and D are incorrect times for giving proton pump inhibitors such as Nexium.

42. **Answer A is correct.** If the client is a threat to the staff or others, the nurse should call for help and prepare to administer a PRN medication such as Haldol (haloperidol) to calm him. Answers B, C, and D are incorrect because they do not protect the client or others from injury.

43. **Answer A is correct.** The next action by the nurse should be to check for bladder distention and catheterize if necessary. Answers B, C, and D are actions for the client with postpartal hemorrhage so they are incorrect choices.

44. **Answer C is correct.** Virilization is a side effect of androgen therapy. Answers A, B, and D are not associated with androgen therapy, so they are incorrect choices.

45. **Answer B is correct.** Imitrex (sumatriptan) is contraindicated in the patient with a history of angina. Serotonin–selective drugs (known as triptans) can cause vasoconstriction and coronary spasms. There is no contraindication for taking triptan drugs in the patient with diabetes, renal calculi, or peptic ulcer disease, making Answers A, C, and D incorrect.

46. **Answer A is correct.** Kernig's sign is positive if pain occurs on flexion of the hip and knee. Answers B, C, and D do not describe a positive Kernig's sign, so they are incorrect.

47. **Answer B is correct.** Apraxia is the inability to use objects appropriately. Agnosia is loss of sensory comprehension, anomia is the inability to find words, and aphasia is the inability to speak or understand, so Answers A, C, and D are incorrect.

48. **Answer C is correct.** Increasing confusion late in the afternoon and before bedtime is known as sundowning. Answers A, B, and D are not associated with confusion; therefore, they are incorrect.

49. **Answer C is correct.** The color red is used to designate those with immediate injuries (life threatening but survivable with minimal care). Answer A refers to those with expectant injuries, Answer B refers to those with significant injuries, and Answer D refers to those with minor injuries. Therefore, answers A, B, and D are incorrect.

50. **Answer D is correct.** The most common side effect associated with Exelon (rivastigmine) is nausea. Answers A, B, and C are not common side effects, so they are incorrect.

51. **Answer B is correct.** Any lesion noted on the perineum of a laboring client should be reported to the physician. Clients with open lesions related to herpes are delivered by Cesarean section because there is a possibility of transmission of the infection to the fetus with direct contact to lesions. It is not enough to document the finding, so Answer A is incorrect. The physician must make the decision to perform a C-section, making Answer C incorrect. It is not enough to continue primary care, so Answer D is incorrect.

52. **Answer B is correct.** The client with HPV is at increased risk for cervical and vaginal cancer related to this STI. She is not at higher risk for the other cancers mentioned in Answers A, C, and D, so those are incorrect.

53. **Answer B is correct.** The client's symptoms are likely caused by HSV II. Answer A is incorrect because the lesion associated with syphilis is not painful. Answer C is incorrect because a lesion is not associated with gonorrhea. Answer D is incorrect because condylomata lesions are painless warts.

54. **Answer C is correct.** Fluorescent treponemal antibody (FTA) is the best diagnostic test for treponema pallidum. VDRL and RPR are screening tests done for syphilis, so Answers A and B are incorrect. The Thayer-Martin culture is done for gonorrhea, so Answer D is incorrect.

55. **Answer D is correct.** The criteria for HELLP is hemolysis, elevated liver enzymes, and low platelet count. An elevated blood glucose level is not associated with HELLP, so answer A is incorrect. Platelets are decreased, not elevated, in HELLP syndrome, as stated in Answer B. The creatinine levels are elevated in renal disease and are not associated with HELLP syndrome, so Answer C is incorrect.

56. **Answer A is correct.** Answer B elicits the triceps reflex, so it is incorrect. Answer C elicits the patella reflex, making it incorrect. Answer D elicits the radial reflex, so it is incorrect.

57. **Answer B is correct.** The nurse should question the order for Brethine (terbutaline) because the medication increases blood glucose levels. Answers A, C, and D are all medications that may be used in the care of the obstetrical client with diabetes, so they are incorrect.

58. **Answer C is correct.** The L/S ratio indicates that the newborn is at increased risk for respiratory distress syndrome due to fetal lung immaturity. Answers A, B, and D are not associated with L/S ratio; therefore, they are incorrect.

59. **Answer C is correct.** Jitteriness and shaking in the newborn are signs of seizure activity that require immediate intervention. Answers A, B, and D are incorrect because they are not abnormal findings.

60. **Answer B is correct.** An expected side effect of intravenous magnesium sulfate is hypersomnolence. Decreased urinary output, absence of the knee-jerk reflex, and decreased respiratory rate indicate drug toxicity, so Answers A, C, and D are incorrect.

61. **Answer D is correct.** If the client experiences hypotension during epidural anesthesia, the nurse should turn her to the left side, apply oxygen by facemask, and increase the rate of the IV infusion. Answers A, B, and C are incorrect interventions; therefore, they are wrong choices.

62. **Answer A is correct.** Dark urine, clay-colored stools, jaundice, and pruritis indicate involvement of the bile ducts in the client with pancreatic cancer. Answers B, C, and D are not associated with bile duct involvement, so they are incorrect choices.

63. **Answer C is correct.** The patient with uremic frost develops pruritis. Keeping the patient's fingernails trimmed helps reduce the risk of tissue damage. Answer A is incorrect because a warm bath increases pruritis. Answers B and D are incorrect because they do not specifically address the problem of pruritis caused by uremic frost.

64. **Answer B is correct.** Obtaining vital signs is not part of the primary assessment of the client presenting to the emergency department following a major event such as a motor vehicle accident. Vital signs are part of the secondary assessment. Answers A, C, and D are incorrect because they are part of the primary assessment.

65. **Answer A is correct.** Findings associated with osteogenesis imperfecta include blue sclera and a history of fractures with little or no trauma. Answers B, C, and D are not associated with osteogenesis imperfecta.

66. **Answer D is correct.** Scissors should be kept at the patient's bedside in case there is a need to deflate the balloons and remove the tube rapidly. Answers A, B, and C are incorrect statements.

67. **Answer B is correct.** The client is hypotensive, so the necessary intervention at this time is to increase the rate of the IV infusion. Answers A, C, and D are not initial interventions to take, so they are incorrect.

68. **Answer C is correct.** The client with a biologic heart valve replacement will need strict dental hygiene to prevent bacterial infections. Answers A, B, and D are not true regarding the client with a biologic heart valve replacement, so they are incorrect choices.

69. **Answer A is correct.** The client's prothrombin time is elevated, so the nurse should assess the client for signs of bleeding. Answers B, C, and D are incorrect statements.

70. **Answer C is correct.** The food selection with the most calcium is the yogurt. Answers A, B, and D do not contain as much calcium, so they are incorrect choices.

71. **Answer C is correct.** The client receiving magnesium sulfate should have an indwelling catheter in place, and hourly intake and output should be checked. Answers A, B, and D are incorrect because they do not indicate understanding of $MgSO_4$ toxicity.

72. **Answer D is correct.** The best size cathlon to use in a child receiving blood is a 20 gauge. Answers A, B, and C are incorrect because the size is either too large or too small.

73. **Answer B is correct.** The nurse should be most concerned with laryngeal edema because of the location of the burn. Answers A, C, and D do not take priority over airway, so they are incorrect.

74. **Answer D is correct.** The nurse should tell the client to report numbness and tingling of her feet and toes because this indicates diabetic neuropathy. Answers A, B, and C do not apply to the client with diabetes mellitus, so they are incorrect.

75. **Answer D is correct.** Paresthesia of the fingers should be reported because it is associated with compartment syndrome. Answer A is incorrect because pain beneath the cast is expected at this time. Answers B and C are incorrect choices because warmth in the fingers and the presence of pulses are expected.

76. **Answer B is correct.** The client should be taught to avoid the use of herbals because they may interfere with the effectiveness of antiviral medication. Answers A, C, and D are not related to the use of the medication, so they are incorrect.

77. **Answer D is correct.** It is not necessary to wear gloves to check the IV infusion rate. The healthcare workers in Answers A, B, and C indicate knowledge by their actions.

78. **Answer D is correct.** A blood pressure cuff is applied to the client's arm prior to the initiation of ECT. Answers A, B, and C are incorrect choices because they are not done prior to ECT.

79. Answer A is correct. Pinworms cause rectal itching. Answers B, C, and D are incorrect because they are not symptoms of pinworms.

80. Answer B is correct. Bed linen should be washed in hot water. Answer A is incorrect because special shampoos can be used by children under age 10. Answers C and D are incorrect statements; therefore, they are wrong.

81. Answer A is correct. The nurse who is pregnant should be assigned to care for the client with HIV being treated with Pentam (pentamidine). The clients in Answers B, C, and D pose a risk to the fetus; therefore, these answers are incorrect.

82. Answer A is correct. The client with MRSA should be assigned to a private room because contact transmission-based precautions will be used. The clients in Answers B, C, and D may room with other clients.

83. Answer D is correct. Answers A, B, and C are incorrect because they apply to other wrongful acts. Negligence is failing to perform care for the client, a tort is a wrongful act committed on the client or their belongings, and assault is a violent physical or verbal attack.

84. Answer D is correct. Prior to administering oral potassium, the nurse should check the creatinine level to determine renal function. Answers A, B, and C do not apply to the administration of potassium; therefore, they are incorrect.

85. Answer B is correct. The mother is most likely describing a newborn rash known as erythema toxicum. About 50% of all newborns have a rash on the face and forehead that dissipates in approximately one month. Answers A, C, and D are incorrect actions.

86. Answer B is correct. Isotonic solutions such as 0.9% sodium chloride and Lactated Ringer's solution are usually ordered for the client with kidney disease. Answers A, C, and D are not suitable for the client with renal disease, so they are incorrect.

87. Answer B is correct. A discrepancy in narcotic count is reportable to the state board of nursing. The Joint Commission on Accreditation of Hospitals will probably be interested in the problems in Answers A, C, and D.

88. Answer B is correct. The nurse would expect an order for a hypertonic solution (3% sodium chloride) to correct the severe hyponatremia associated with SIADH. Answers A, C, and D are incorrect treatments for managing severe hyponatremia.

89. Answer D is correct. The client who should be seen first is the client with relapsing-remitting multiple sclerosis who is being treated with intravenous corticosteroids. Answers A, B, and C are more stable and can be seen later.

90. Answer B is correct. The client who is pregnant and the client with a fractured arm are the best choices for placing in the same room. The clients in Answers A, C, and D need to be placed in separate rooms due to the serious natures of their injuries.

91. Answer A is correct. Before instilling the eardrops, the nurse should consider the age of the child because the ear of the toddler should be pulled down and out to best deliver the drops in the ear canal. Answers B, C, and D are not considerations when administering eardrops to a small child.

92. **Answer C is correct.** Answer C is correct because the size and shape of the hotdog poses a risk of aspiration. Answers A, B, and D are incorrect because white grape juice, a grilled cheese sandwich, and ice cream pose less of a risk of aspiration for a child.

93. **Answer C is correct.** A viral load of 200 copies per mL is extremely low. This indicates that the client has a low risk for opportunistic illnesses. Answers A, B, and D are not true statements.

94. **Answer B is correct.** Lantus (glargine) insulin should not be mixed with other insulins. Answers A, C, and D are not correct methods of administering Lantus insulin.

95. **Answer C is correct.** A priority diagnosis for the child following a tonsillectomy is risk for injury/aspiration. Answers A, B, and D are incorrect since they do not take priority over airway.

96. **Answer A is correct.** Hypertension is a classic manifestation of glomerulonephritis. Answers B, C, and D are not classic manifestations of glomerulonephritis; therefore, they are wrong.

97. **Answer B is correct.** A child with epiglottitis has the possibility of complete obstruction of the airway. For this reason, the nurse should not evaluate the airway using a tongue blade. Answers A, C, and D are part of the nursing care and are therefore incorrect.

98. **Answer C is correct.** The client should take the medication in the morning with water. Answers A, B, and D are incorrect statements regarding the administration of synthetic thyroid hormone.

99. **Answer D is correct.** The child with celiac disease should be on a gluten-free diet. Answers A, B, and C all contain gluten, while Answer D gives the only choice of foods that do not contain gluten.

100. **Answer C is correct.** The first action by the nurse should be to apply oxygen by mask. Answers A, B, and D do not take priority over administering oxygen.

101. **Answer B is correct.** An amniotomy is an artificial rupture of membranes and normal amniotic fluid is clear, straw-colored and odorless. Answers A, C, and D are abnormal findings.

102. **Answer D is correct.** Diabeta (glyburide) is an antidiabetic medication that can result in hypoglycemia. Answers A, B, and C are incorrect because they are not related to Diabeta (glyburide).

103. **Answer B is correct.** The first action the nurse should take is to turn the client to the left side and apply oxygen. The normal fetal heart rate is 120–160bpm; 100–110bpm is bradycardia. Answer A is not indicated at this time. Answer C is not the best action for clients experiencing bradycardia. There is no data to indicate the need to move the client to the delivery room at this time; therefore answer D is incorrect.

104. **Answer D is correct.** Arterial ulcers are painful to touch. Answers A, B, and C are incorrect because they do not describe arterial ulcers.

105. **Answer B is correct.** Applying a fetal heart monitor is the correct action at this time. There is no need to prepare for a Caesarean section or to place the client in genupectoral position (knee-chest), so Answers A and C are incorrect. Answer D is incorrect because there is no need for an ultrasound based on the finding.

106. **Answer B is correct.** The nurse decides to apply an external monitor because the membranes are intact. Answers A, C, and D are incorrect statements.

107. **Answer D is correct.** Ice chips may be allowed during labor, but the amount of fluid might not be sufficient to prevent fluid volume deficit. Answer A, impaired gas exchange related to hyperventilation, would be indicated during the transition phase. Answers B and C are not correct choices in relation to the stem.

108. **Answer D is correct.** This information indicates a late deceleration. This type of deceleration is caused by uteroplacental insufficiency. Answers A, B, and C are not associated with late decelerations.

109. **Answer C is correct.** The initial action by the nurse observing a variable deceleration should be to turn the client to the side—preferably, the left side. Administering oxygen is also indicated. Answer A might be necessary, but not before turning the client to her side. Answer B is not necessary at this time. Answer D is incorrect because there is no data to indicate that the monitor has been applied incorrectly.

110. **Answer D is correct.** A deceleration to 90–100bpm at the end of contractions are late decelerations. This finding is ominous and should be reported to the physician. Answers A, B, and C are normal findings and are therefore incorrect choices.

111. **Answer C is correct.** Epidural anesthesia decreases the urge to void and sensation of a full bladder. A full bladder will decrease the progression of labor. Answers A, B, and D are incorrect for the stem.

112. **Answer B is correct.** Lutenizing hormone released by the pituitary is responsible for ovulation. Answers A, C, and D are incorrect because estrogen levels are high at the beginning of ovulation, the endometrial lining is thick, not thin, and the progesterone levels are high, not low.

113. **Answer C is correct.** The success of the rhythm method of birth control is dependent on the client's menses being regular. It is not dependent on the age of the client, frequency of intercourse, or range of the client's temperature; therefore, Answers A, B, and D are incorrect choices.

114. **Answer C is correct.** The best method of birth control for the client with diabetes is the diaphragm. A permanent intrauterine device can cause a continuing inflammatory response in diabetics that should be avoided, oral contraceptives tend to elevate blood glucose levels, and contraceptive sponges are not good at preventing pregnancy. Therefore, Answers A, B, and D are incorrect.

115. **Answer D is correct.** The signs of an ectopic pregnancy are vague until the Fallopian tube ruptures. The client will complain of sudden, stabbing pain in the lower quadrant that radiates down the leg or up into the chest. Painless vaginal bleeding is a sign of

placenta previa, abdominal cramping is a sign of labor, and throbbing pain in the upper quadrant is not a sign of an ectopic pregnancy, making Answers A, B, and C incorrect.

116. **Answer C is correct.** All of the choices are tasty, but the pregnant client needs a diet that is balanced and has increased amounts of calcium. Answer A is lacking in fruits and milk. Answer B contains the potato chips, which contain a large amount of sodium. Answer C contains meat, fruit, potato salad, and yogurt, which has about 360mg of calcium. Answer D is not the best diet because it lacks vegetables and milk products.

117. **Answer B is correct.** The client with hyperemesis gravidarum is at risk for developing metabolic acidosis due to vomiting and dehydration. Answers A, C, and D are not associated with hyperemesis gravidarum.

118. **Answer B is correct.** The most definitive sign of pregnancy is the presence of fetal heart tones. The signs in Answers A, C, and D are subjective and might be related to other medical conditions.

119. **Answer C is correct.** The infant of a diabetic mother is usually large for gestational age. After birth, glucose levels fall rapidly due to the absence of glucose from the mother. Answer A is incorrect because the infant will not be small for gestational age. Answer B is incorrect because the infant will not be hyperglycemic. Answer D is incorrect because the infant will be large, not small, and will be hypoglycemic, not hyperglycemic.

120. **Answer B is correct.** When the client is taking oral contraceptives and begins antibiotics, another method of birth control should be used. Antibiotics decrease the effectiveness of oral contraceptives. Answers A, C, and D are not true statements so they are incorrect choices.

121. **Answer B is correct.** Clients with HIV should not breastfeed because the virus can be transmitted to the baby through breast milk. Answers A, C, and D are incorrect because the clients can breastfeed.

122. **Answer A is correct.** The nurse's first action should be to assess the fetal heart tones because the client's symptoms are consistent with placenta previa. Answer B is incorrect because cervical checks for dilation are contraindicated because they can increase bleeding. Answers C and D are incorrect choices because they are not the first actions to be taken.

123. **Answer D is correct.** The client should be advised to come to the hospital when the contractions are five minutes apart and consistent. She should also be told to report to the hospital if she experiences rupture of membranes or extreme bleeding. She should not wait until the contractions are every two minutes or until she has bloody discharge, so Answers A and B are incorrect. Answer C is a vague answer and can be related to a urinary tract infection so it is incorrect.

124. **Answer A is correct.** Infants of mothers who smoke are often low birth weight. Infants who are large for gestational age are associated with diabetic mothers, so Answer B is incorrect. Preterm births are associated with smoking, but not with appropriate size

for gestation, making Answer C incorrect. Growth retardation is associated with smoking, but this does not affect the infant's length; therefore, Answer D is incorrect.

125. **Answer A is correct.** To provide protection against antibody production, RhoGAM should be given within 72 hours of delivery. Answers B, C, and D are incorrect because the administration times are too late to provide antibody protection.

126. **Answer B is correct.** After amniotomy, the nurse's first action should be to check fetal heart tones. When the membranes rupture, there is often a transient drop in the fetal heart tones. The heart tones should return to baseline quickly. Any alteration in fetal heart tones, such as bradycardia or tachycardia, should be reported. After the fetal heart tones are assessed, the nurse should evaluate the cervical dilation, vital signs, and level of discomfort, making Answers A, C, and D incorrect.

127. **Answer A is correct.** The active phase of labor occurs when the client is dilated 4cm–7cm. The latent or early phase of labor is from 1cm to 3cm in dilation, so Answers B and D are incorrect. The transition phase of labor is 8cm –10cm in dilation, making Answer C incorrect.

128. **Answer B is correct.** The newborn of an addicted mother will undergo withdrawal. Snugly wrapping the newborn in a blanket will help reduce muscle irritability. Answers A, C, and D are not appropriate interventions for the newborn experiencing withdrawal.

129. **Answer C is correct.** Following epidural anesthesia, the client should be checked for hypotension and signs of shock. The client can be checked for cervical dilation later after she is stable. The client should not be positioned supine because the anesthesia can move above the diaphragm and interfere with breathing. Fetal heart tones should be assessed after the blood pressure is checked; therefore, Answers A, B, and D are incorrect.

130. **Answer B is correct.** The best way to prevent post-operative wound infection is hand washing. Use of prescribed antibiotics will treat infection, not prevent infections, making Answer A is incorrect. Wearing a mask and asking the client to cover her mouth are good practices, but will not prevent wound infections; therefore, Answers C and D are incorrect.

131. **Answer B is correct.** The client with a hip fracture will most likely exhibit disalignment. Answer A is incorrect because other types of fractures cause pain. Answers C and D are incorrect choices because they are associated with compromised circulation.

132. **Answer B is correct.** Hormonal changes after menopause affect the ability to absorb and utilize calcium. Answers A, C, and D are not the most common causes of osteoporosis in women, so they are incorrect.

133. **Answer B is correct.** The buttocks should be off the bed approximately 15° in Bryant's traction. Answers A and C are incorrect because they do not indicate that the traction is working properly. Answer D is incorrect because Bryant's traction is a skin traction, not a skeletal traction.

134. Answer A is correct. Balanced skeletal traction uses pins and screws. A Steinman pin is used to stabilize large bones such as the femur. Answer B is incorrect because only the affected leg is in traction. Kirschner wires are used to stabilize small bones such as fingers and toes, as in Answer C. Answer D is incorrect because this type of traction is not used for fractured hips.

135. Answer A is correct. Bleeding is a common complication following orthopedic surgery. The blood-collection device should be checked frequently to ensure that the client is not hemorrhaging. The client's pain should be assessed, but this is not life-threatening. When the client is in less danger, the nutritional status should be assessed, and an immobilizer is not used; thus, Answers B, C, and D are incorrect.

136. Answer A is correct. The client's family member should be taught to flush and clamp the tube after each feeding. Answer B is incorrect because tube placement should be checked before feedings. Answer C is incorrect because indigestion may occur with the PEG tube feeding. Answer D is simply an incorrect statement.

137. Answer C is correct. The client with a total knee replacement should be assessed for blood loss. An Hgb of 7gm/dL is low and a blood transfusion might be required. Answers A, B, and D do not require notification of the doctor, so they are incorrect.

138. Answer B is correct. Exposure to lead used in making stained glass products increases the risk of plumbism in children. Answers A, C, and D are incorrect because they are not associated with plumbism.

139. Answer A is correct. A raised commode seat will help the client with a hip replacement with activities of daily living. Answers B, C, and D are assistive aids for clients with rheumatoid arthritis or stroke.

140. Answer B is correct. Complaints of tight burning pain in the leg following cast application raises the possibility of compartment syndrome. Answers A, C, and D are associated with fracture, not compartment syndrome.

141. Answer B is correct. Placement with a 12-year-old with a fractured humerus is best because of his gender, age, and diagnosis. Answers A, C, and D offer less suitable roommates.

142. Answer B is correct. Celebrex (celecoxib), a cox II inhibitor, has been associated with heart attacks and strokes. Any changes in cardiac status or signs of a stroke should be reported immediately. Answers A, C, D are not associated with the medication, so they are incorrect choices.

143. Answer D is correct. Fiberglass casts dry very quickly, allowing the client to weight bear in 30 minutes. Answers A, B, and C are incorrect actions.

144. Answer A is correct. There is no reason that the client's friends should not be allowed to autograph the cast; it will not harm the cast in any way, so Answers B, C, and D are incorrect.

145. **Answer A is correct.** The RN should assist by opening sterile packages and peroxide. The LPN is performing the pin care correctly when she uses sterile gloves and cotton-tipped applicators. Answers B, C, and D are incorrect statements.

146. **Answer A is correct.** Auscultating bowel sounds are specific to the care of the client in a body cast. Answers B, C, and D are not specific to the care of a client with a body cast; therefore, they are incorrect.

147. **Answer C is correct.** To be effective, the weights must hang freely. Answers A, B, and D are not true statements regarding care of the patient with skeletal traction.

148. **Answer B is correct.** The controller for the continuous passive-motion device should be placed out of the client's reach to prevent the client tampering with it. Answer A is incorrect because the client is in the bed when the CPM device is in place. Answer C is incorrect because the client may have pain when the device is in place. Answer D is incorrect because the CPM device does not eliminate the need for physical therapy.

149. **Answer A is correct.** The client's palms should rest lightly on the handles. Answers B, C, and D are incorrect actions when using a walker, so they are wrong choices.

150. **Answer C is correct.** The client with a prolapsed cord should be treated by elevating the hips and covering the cord with a moist, sterile saline gauze. Answers A, B, and D are incorrect. The nurse should not attempt to replace the cord, turn the client on the side, or cover with a dry gauze.

151. **Answer B is correct.** Chest tubes serve as a method of draining blood and serous fluid as well as reinflating the lungs. Answers A, C, and D are incorrect choices because they are not primary rationales for the insertion of chest tubes.

152. **Answer D is correct.** Success with breastfeeding depends on many factors, but the most dependable reason for success is desire and willingness to continue the breast-feeding until the infant and mother have time to adapt. The educational level, the infant's birth weight, and the size of the mother's breast have nothing to do with success, so Answers A, B, and C are incorrect.

153. **Answer C is correct.** Green-tinged amniotic fluid is indicative of meconium staining. This finding indicates fetal distress. The presence of scant bloody discharge is normal, as are frequent urination and moderate uterine contractions, making Answers A, B, and D incorrect.

154. **Answer C is correct.** Duration is measured from the beginning of one contraction to the end of the same contraction. Answer A refers to frequency. Answers B and D are incorrect statements.

155. **Answer B is correct.** The client receiving Pitocin (oxytocin) should be monitored for decelerations. There is no association with Pitocin (oxytocin) use and hypoglycemia, maternal hyperreflexia, or fetal movement; therefore, Answers A, C, and D are incorrect.

156. **Answer D is correct.** Fetal development depends on adequate nutrition and insulin regulation. Insulin needs increase during the second and third trimesters, insulin requirements do not moderate as the pregnancy progresses, and elevated human

chorionic gonadotropin elevates insulin needs, not decreases them; therefore, Answers A, B, and C are incorrect.

157. **Answer A is correct.** A calm environment is needed to prevent seizure activity. Any stimulation can precipitate seizures. Obtaining a diet history should be done later, and administering an analgesic is not indicated because there is no data in the stem to indicate pain. Therefore, Answers B and C are incorrect. Assessing the fetal heart tones is important, but this is not the highest priority in this situation as stated in Answer D.

158. **Answer A is correct.** The client who is age 42 is at increased risk for fetal anomalies such as Down syndrome. Answers B, C, and D are incorrect because the client's infant is not at increased risk for respiratory distress syndrome, pathological jaundice, or Turner syndrome.

159. **Answer C is correct.** The client with a missed abortion will most likely be treated with Prostin E (dinoprostone) to soften the cervix. Magnesium sulfate is used for preterm labor and preeclampsia, calcium gluconate is the antidote for magnesium sulfate toxicity, and Parlodel (bromocriptine) is a dopamine receptor stimulant used to treat Parkinson's disease; therefore, Answers A, B, and D are incorrect. Parlodel is an older medication that was once used to dry up breast milk.

160. **Answer A is correct.** The deep tendon reflexes and urinary output are normal findings, so the nurse should continue the magnesium sulfate and monitor the client's blood pressure. Answers B, C, and D are incorrect actions based on the DTRs and urine output.

161. **Answer C is correct.** Affected parents have a one-in-four chance of passing on a defective gene. Autosomal recessive disorders include sickle cell anemia and cystic fibrosis. Answers A, B, and D do not describe autosomal recessive patterns of inheritance.

162. **Answer D is correct.** Alpha fetoprotein is a screening test done to detect neural tube defects such as spina bifida. The test is not mandatory, as stated in Answer A. It does not detect cardiovascular defects, and the mother's age has no bearing on the need for the test, so Answers B and C are incorrect.

163. **Answer B is correct.** During pregnancy, the thyroid gland might enlarge. This makes it more difficult to regulate thyroid medication. Answer A is incorrect because there could be a need for thyroid medication during pregnancy. Answer C is incorrect because the thyroid function does not slow. Fetal growth is not arrested if thyroid medication is continued, so Answer D is incorrect.

164. **Answer C is correct.** Cyanosis of the feet and hands of the neonate is known as acrocyanosis. This is a normal finding one minute after birth. Answers A, B, and D are not expected findings in the neonate; therefore, they are incorrect choices.

165. **Answer A is correct.** The laboring client with sickle cell anemia may experience hypoxia and signs of sickle cell crisis; therefore, the nurse should anticipate a need for supplemental oxygen. Answers B, C, and D are not specific to the care of the client with sickle cell anemia who is in labor.

166. **Answer A is correct.** Before ultrasonography, the client should be taught to drink plenty of fluids and not void. The client may ambulate, an enema is not needed, and there is no need to withhold food for eight hours. Therefore, Answers B, C, and D are incorrect.

167. **Answer D is correct.** By six months of age, the infant is expected to double his birth weight. Answers A, B, and C are incorrect weights based on the birth weight.

168. **Answer B is correct.** A nonstress test is done to evaluate periodic movement of the fetus. It is not done to evaluate lung maturity as in Answer A. An oxytocin challenge test shows the effect of contractions on fetal heart rate and neurological well-being of the fetus, so Answers C and D are incorrect.

169. **Answer D is correct.** Prior to beginning the medication, the physician will most likely order a TB skin test. Answers A, B, and C are not likely to be ordered because there is no indication before beginning the medication.

170. **Answer A is correct.** Transition is the time during labor when the client loses concentration due to intense contractions. Potential for injury related to precipitate delivery has nothing to do with the dilation of the cervix, so Answer B is incorrect. There is no data to indicate that the client has had anesthesia or fluid volume deficit, making Answers C and D incorrect.

171. **Answer C is correct.** Antiviral agents such as acyclovir or valacyclovir are usually ordered for children who are at high risk because of immunosuppressive medication or generalized malignancies such as leukemia. Answers A, B, and D are not indicated for the treatment of varicella. Aspirin is avoided because of the increased risk of Reyes syndrome.

172. **Answer B is correct.** Atropine is not indicated in the care of clients with chest pain. Clients with chest pain may be treated with nitroglycerin, Inderal (propranolol), or Calan (verapamil); therefore, answers A, C, and D are incorrect.

173. **Answer B is correct.** Anti-inflammatory drugs should be taken with meals to avoid stomach upset. Answers A, C, and D are incorrect statements.

174. **Answer D is correct.** Morphine should be avoided by the client with acute pancreatitis because the medication causes spasms of the sphincter of Oddi. Answers A, B, and C may be used by the client with acute pancreatitis; therefore, they are incorrect.

175. **Answer B is correct.** Hallucinogenic drugs induce a state of altered perceptions. Answers A, C, and D are not true statements regarding hallucinogenic drugs.

176. **Answer B is correct.** Signs of mild barbiturate intoxication include nystagmus, diplopia, strabismus, slowness of speech, and positive Romberg sign. Answers A, C, and D are not signs of barbiturate intoxication, so they are incorrect.

177. **Answer A is correct.** If the fetal heart tones are heard loudest in the upper right quadrant, the infant is in a breech presentation. If the infant is positioned in the right occipital anterior presentation, the FHTs will be loudest in the right lower quadrant, so answer B is incorrect. If the fetus is in the sacral position, the FHTs will be loudest in the center of the abdomen, so answer C is incorrect. If the FHTs are loudest in the left

lower abdomen, the infant is most likely in the left occipital transverse position, making answer D incorrect.

178. **Answer D is correct.** Physical and psychological stresses are considered factors in the development of intrinsic asthma. Answers A, B, and C are incorrect because they are factors in the development of extrinsic asthma.

179. **Answer A is correct.** The client with mania should be served high-calorie foods that she can carry with her. Answers B, C, and D do not meet the client's nutritional needs and are not appropriate interventions for the client with mania.

180. **Answer B is correct.** To maintain Bryant's traction, the hips should be slightly elevated above the bed with the legs suspended at a right angle to the bed. Answer A is incorrect because the hips should not be resting on the bed. Answer C is incorrect because the hips should not be above the level of the body. Answer D is incorrect because the hips and legs should not be flat on the bed.

181. **Answer B is correct.** Wearing gloves during care will help prevent transmission of the virus. Answer A is incorrect because covering the lesions with a sterile gauze is not necessary. Answer C is incorrect because acetaminophen, not aspirin, is given for discomfort. Answer D is incorrect because Zovirax (acyclovir) should be administered within 24 to 48 hours of the outbreak.

182. **Answer B is correct.** The trough level should be drawn prior to the fourth infusion. Answers A, C, and D are incorrect times for drawing trough levels.

183. **Answer B is correct.** The client using a diaphragm should store the diaphragm in a cool place. Answers A, C, and D are incorrect statements. She should refrain from leaving the diaphragm in longer than eight hours, not four hours. She should have the diaphragm resized when she gains or loses 10 pounds or has abdominal surgery.

184. **Answer C is correct.** Mothers who plan to breastfeed should drink plenty of liquids. Four glasses is not enough in a 24-hour period for breast feeding. Wearing a support bra is a good practice for the mother who is breastfeeding as well as the mother who plans to bottle-feed, so Answer A is incorrect. Expressing milk from the breast will stimulate milk production, making Answer B incorrect. Allowing the water to run over the breast will also facilitate "letdown" when the milk begins to be produced; therefore, Answer D is incorrect.

185. **Answer A is correct.** If damage occurs to the facial nerve (CN VII), facial pain will occur. Answers B, C, and D are incorrect because they are not associated with damage to the facial nerve.

186. **Answer B is correct.** Clients taking Pyridium should be taught that the medication will turn the urine orange or red in color. The medication is not associated with diarrhea, mental confusion, or changes in taste; therefore, Answers A, C, and D are incorrect.

187. **Answer B is correct.** A pregnancy test should be done before beginning therapy with Accutane (isotretinoin), a pregnancy category X drug. It is not necessary to check the calcium, potassium, or creatinine levels before beginning therapy; therefore, Answers A, C, and D are incorrect.

188. **Answer D is correct.** The nurse should encourage the client to drink at least eight glasses of water a day to reduce the risk of renal toxicity. Limiting activity is not necessary. Supplementing the diet with high-carbohydrate food sources is not necessary. Use of an incentive spirometer is not specific to clients taking acyclovir; therefore, Answers A, B, and C are incorrect.

189. **Answer A is correct.** CAT scans are x-rays passed through the body at many angles, allowing varying degrees of penetration. Contraindications include allergy to shellfish or iodine, pregnancy, unstable vital signs, morbid obesity, and claustrophobia. Clients with a titanium hip replacement can have a CAT scan, so Answer B is incorrect. No egg-containing products are used with a CAT scan, so Answer C is incorrect. The client should remain still only when instructed, so Answer D is incorrect.

190. **Answer D is correct.** Changes in skin color may indicate liver toxicity in the client taking Abelcet (amphotericin B). Answers A, B, and C are not associated with toxicity to the medication; therefore, they are incorrect.

191. **Answer C is correct.** The client with chest pain and a history of angina should be seen first because his symptoms may indicate a myocardial infarction. Answers A, B, and D have conditions that do not take priority over the client with chest pain, so they are incorrect.

192. **Answer B is correct.** Pancreatic enzymes should be given with meals and snacks to promote digestion and absorption. Answers A, C, and D are incorrect times for administering pancreatic enzymes.

193. **Answer C is correct.** The lens allows light to pass through the pupil and focus light on the retina. The lens does not stimulate the retina, assist with eye movement, or magnify small objects, so Answers A, B, and D are incorrect.

194. **Answer C is correct.** Miotic eye drops constrict the pupil and allow aqueous humor to flow out of the Canal of Schlemm, thereby reducing intraocular pressure. They do not anesthetize the cornea, dilate the pupil, or paralyze the muscles of accommodation, making Answers A, B, and D incorrect.

195. **Answer A is correct.** The nurse should allow five minutes between the two medications. Answers B, C, and D are incorrect times for administering multiple eye medications.

196. **Answer B is correct.** Clients with color blindness have problems distinguishing violets, blues, and green. The colors in Answers A, C, and D are not associated with color blindness.

197. **Answer D is correct.** The client with a pacemaker should be taught to count and record his pulse rate. Answers A, B, and C are incorrect. Ankle edema is a sign of right-sided heart failure. Although this is not normal, it is often present in clients with heart disease. If the edema is present in the hands and face, it should be reported. Checking the blood pressure daily is not necessary for these clients. The client with a pacemaker can use a microwave oven, but he should stand about five feet from the oven while it is operating.

198. **Answer A is correct.** Clients who are being retrained for bladder control should be taught to withhold fluids after about 7 p.m., or 1900. The times in Answers B, C, and D are too early in the day.

199. **Answer D is correct.** Cranberry juice and prune juice acidify the urine and inhibit bacterial growth in the urine. Answers A, B, and C do not help reduce the risk of recurrent urinary tract infections, so they are incorrect choices.

200. **Answer C is correct.** NPH insulin peaks in 8–12 hours, so a snack should be eaten at that time. NPH insulin onsets in 90–120 minutes, so Answer A is incorrect. Answer B is untrue because NPH insulin is time released and does not cause sudden hypoglycemia. Answer D is incorrect, but the client should eat a bedtime snack.

201. **Answer D is correct.** The client taking Zyvox (linezolid) should avoid foods high in tyramine in order to prevent serotonin syndrome. Answers A, B, and C are suitable foods for the client taking the medication, so they are incorrect.

202. **Answer B is correct.** The nurse should not administer the medication if the client is allergic to neomycin. Answers A, C, and D are not contraindicated when administering the medication.

203. **Answer B is correct.** Zantac (ranitidine), a histamine blocker, should be given 30 to 60 minutes before eating for optimal effect. Answers A, C, and D are incorrect dosing times.

204. **Answer C is correct.** The proximal end of the double-barrel colostomy opens on the right side of the abdomen. Answers A, B, and D are not correct statements, so they are incorrect choices.

205. **Answer A is correct.** Displacement of the fundus to the right or to the left indicates a full bladder. Answers B, C, and D are not associated with fundal displacement, so they are incorrect.

206. **Answer C is correct.** Clients with an internal defibrillator or a pacemaker should not have an MRI because it may cause the pacemaker to work improperly. If the client has a need for oxygen, is claustrophobic, or is deaf, he can have an MRI, but provisions such as extension tubes for the oxygen, sedatives, or a signal system should be made to accommodate the client's needs; therefore, Answers A, B, and D are incorrect.

207. **Answer C is correct.** A soft book is the best toy for the developmental level of a one-year-old. Answers A, B, and D are suited to the skills of a toddler, so they are incorrect.

208. **Answer C is correct.** Encouraging rest periods throughout the day will conserve the client's energy and prevent fatigue, a major factor in the exacerbations of multiple sclerosis. Answers A, B, and D are not part of the management of the client with multiple sclerosis, so they are incorrect choices.

209. **Answer B is correct.** The client with a proctoepisiotomy will need stool softeners such as (Colace) docusate sodium. Answer A is incorrect because suppositories are usually not given to a client with a proctoepisiotomy. Answers C and D are incorrect answers because they are used to treat post-partal bleeding and to treat the client with Parkinson's.

210. **Answer C is correct.** TPN is a high-glucose solution that may elevate the blood glucose, leading to a need for insulin. Answers A, B, and D are incorrect statements regarding TPN.

211. **Answer B is correct.** The client who is 10 weeks pregnant should be assessed to determine how she feels about the pregnancy. It's too early to discuss preterm labor, and it's too late to discuss whether she was using a method of birth control and what her plans are for continuing school; therefore, Answers A, C, and D are incorrect.

212. **Answer A is correct.** The best IV fluid for correction of moderate dehydration is Lactated Ringer's. Answers B, C, and D are not suitable solutions for correcting moderate dehydration.

213. **Answer A is correct.** A thyroid scan uses an iodine dye, so the client should be assessed for allergies to iodine. The client will not have a bolus of fluid, will not be given an anxiolytic, and will not have a urinary catheter inserted, so Answers B, C, and D are incorrect.

214. **Answer B is correct.** RhoGAM is used to prevent formation of Rh antibodies. It does not provide immunity to Rh isoenzymes, eliminate circulating Rh antibodies, or convert the Rh factor from negative to positive; therefore, Answers A, C, and D are incorrect.

215. **Answer B is correct.** A client with a fractured foot often has a short leg cast applied to stabilize the fracture. Answer A is incorrect because a walking boot is used after the fracture is healed. Answers C and D are incorrect choices because they are not used for foot fractures.

216. **Answer A is correct.** Iridium seeds can be expelled during urination, so the client should be taught to strain his urine and report to the doctor if any of the seeds are expelled. Increasing fluids, reporting urinary frequency, and avoiding prolonged sitting are not necessary; therefore, Answers B, C, and D are incorrect.

217. **Answer C is correct.** To increase the effects of the antitubercular therapy, the client may also be given Benemid (probenecid). Answers A, B, and D have no effect on increasing the effect of the medication, so they are incorrect choices.

218. **Answer A is correct.** Mydriatic drops will be used to dilate the pupil, making cataract removal easier. Answers B, C, and D do not apply to the client having cataract surgery, so they are incorrect.

219. **Answer C is correct.** Placing simple signs that indicate the location of rooms where the client sleeps, eats, and bathes will help the client be more independent. Providing mirrors and pictures is not recommended with the client who has Alzheimer's disease because mirrors and pictures tend to cause agitation, and alternating healthcare workers confuses the client; therefore, Answers A, B, and D are incorrect.

220. **Answer C is correct.** A Jackson-Pratt drain is a serum-collection device commonly used in abdominal surgery. A Jackson-Pratt drain will not prevent the need for dressing changes, reduce edema of the incision, or keep the common bile duct open, so Answers A, B, and D are incorrect.

221. **Answer C is correct.** The newborn who is at 32 weeks gestation will not be able to control his head, so head lag will be present. Answers A, B, and D are incorrect because they are expected findings in the term newborn.

222. **Answer A is correct.** Hematuria in a client with a pelvic fracture can indicate trauma to the bladder or impending hemorrhage. It is not unusual for the client to complain of muscles spasms with multiple fractures, so Answer B is incorrect. Dizziness can be associated with blood loss and is nonspecific, making Answer C incorrect. Nausea, as stated in Answer D, is also common in the client with multiple traumas.

223. **Answer C is correct.** The client's symptom is known as formication. Answers A, B, and D are incorrect.

224. **Answer B is correct.** Because the nurse is unaware of when the bottle was opened or whether the saline is sterile, it is safest to obtain a new bottle. Answers A, C, and D are not safe practices.

225. **Answer C is correct.** The newborn with an Apgar score of 9 at five minutes is most likely due to the presence of acrocyanosis. It is not related to the newborn being hypothermic, experiencing bradycardia, or being lethargic; therefore, Answers A, B, and D are incorrect.

226. **Answer A is correct.** Rapid continuous rewarming of a frostbite primarily lessens cellular damage. It does not prevent formation of blisters. It does promote movement, but this is not the primary reason for rapid rewarming. It might increase pain for a short period of time as the feeling comes back into the extremity; therefore, Answers B, C, and D are incorrect.

227. **Answer D is correct.** Hemodialysis works by using a dialyzing membrane to filter waste that has accumulated in the blood. It does not pass water through a dialyzing membrane nor does it eliminate plasma proteins or lower the pH, so Answers A, B, and C are incorrect.

228. **Answer B is correct.** The nurse should contact the physician regarding an order for immune globulin. Answer A is incorrect because antibiotics are not indicated unless the client develops a bacterial infection. Answer C is incorrect because the client is already on antiviral medication. Answer D is incorrect because airborne isolation is indicated for the client with measles, not the client who has been exposed.

229. **Answer D is correct.** Precautions used for infections spread by contact include the use of gloves, a gown, and a mask. Answers A, B, and C are incorrect statements regarding contact precautions.

230. **Answer B is correct.** Phantom limb pain is due to interruption in the peripheral nervous system. Answer A is incorrect because phantom limb pain can last several months or indefinitely. Answer C is incorrect because it is not psychological. It is also not due to infections, as stated in Answer D.

231. **Answer A is correct.** A Whipple procedure involves the removal of the head of the pancreas. Answers B, C, and D are not correct regarding a Whipple procedure.

232. **Answer C is correct.** Pepper is unprocessed and may contain bacteria; therefore, it should be avoided by the client on a low-bacteria diet. Answers A, B, and D are incorrect because mustard, salt, and ketchup are allowed on a low-bacteria diet.

233. **Answer A is correct.** The client taking Coumadin should avoid using antihistamines containing diphenhydramine because it can increase the bleeding time. Answers B, C, and D are not associated with the use of Coumadin.

234. **Answer A is correct.** The nurse should instruct the client who is having a central venous catheter removed to take a deep breath, hold it, and bear down as the catheter is removed. This helps to prevent air from entering the line. Answers B, C, and D are not proper instructions associated with the removal of a central line.

235. **Answer B is correct.** Before streptokinase is administered, the client should be assessed for a history of strep infections because the client may have developed antibodies that render the streptokinase ineffective. There is no reason to assess the client for allergies to pineapples or bananas, there is no correlation to the use of phenytoin and streptokinase, and a history of alcohol abuse is also not a factor in the order for streptokinase; therefore, Answers A, C, and D are incorrect.

236. **Answer B is correct.** The client with leukemia should not floss between the teeth because this may result in bleeding due to low platelet counts. Using oils and cream-based soaps is allowed, as is using salt and an electric razor; therefore, Answers A, C, and D are incorrect.

237. **Answer A is correct.** The safest method for changing tracheostomy ties is to apply the new ones before removing the old ones. Answers B, C, and D are not the safest methods for changing tracheostomy ties; therefore, they are incorrect.

238. **Answer D is correct.** An hourly output of 300mL from a mediastinal tube is indicative of hemorrhage and should be reported to the physician immediately. Answers A, B, and C are not interventions for the client who is bleeding excessively from a mediastinal tube; therefore, they are incorrect.

239. **Answer A is correct.** Symptoms of fluid overload in the infant include bulging fontanels. Answers B, C, and D are not symptoms of fluid overload in the infant, so they are wrong.

240. **The correct answer is marked by an X in the diagram.** The Tail of Spence is located in the upper outer quadrant of the breast.

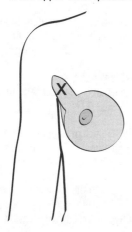

241. **Answer A is correct.** The toddler with a ventricular septal defect will tire more easily. Answers B, C, and D are not true statements regarding the child with a VSD.

242. **Answer B is correct.** A nonstress test determines periodic movement of the fetus. It does not determine lung maturity, show contractions, or measure neurological well-being, making Answers A, C, and D incorrect.

243. **Answer C is correct.** The monitor indicates variable decelerations caused by cord compression. If Pitocin is infusing, the nurse should turn off the Pitocin. Instructing the client to push is incorrect because pushing could increase the decelerations and because the client is 8cm dilated, making Answer A incorrect. Performing a vaginal exam should be done after turning off the Pitocin, and placing the client in a semi-Fowler's position is not appropriate for this situation; therefore, Answers B and D are incorrect.

244. **Answer C is correct.** The graph indicates ventricular tachycardia. The answers in A, B, and D are not noted on the ECG strip.

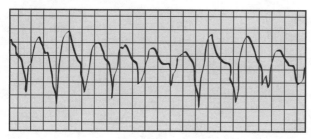

245. **Answer B is correct.** Lovenox (enoxaparin) injections should be given in the abdomen, not in the deltoid muscle. The client should not aspirate before administering the injection or clear the air from the syringe before injection; therefore, Answers A, C, and D are incorrect.

246. **Answer B is correct.** The medications should be administered separately. Answers A, C, and D are not true statements; therefore, they are incorrect choices.

247. **Answer B is correct.** The nurse should tell the client to void every three hours to prevent urine from collecting in the bladder where bacteria can collect. Answers A, C, and D do not reduce the risk of urinary tract infections, so they are incorrect choices.

248. **Answer C is correct.** Feeding the client with depression is within the scope of practice of the nursing assistant. Answers A, B, and D require the skill of the licensed nurse; therefore, they are incorrect.

249. **Answer A is correct.** A two-inch circle of blood behind the neck of the client who has had a parathyroidectomy indicates excessive bleeding. Answers B, C, and D are not complications associated with parathyroidectomy, so they are incorrect choices.

250. **Answer D is correct.** To reduce the risk of nephrotoxicity from the medication, the nurse should hydrate the client with IV fluids before and after the medication is administered. Answers A, B, and C do not reduce the risk of nephrotoxicity; therefore, they are incorrect.

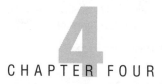

CHAPTER FOUR

Practice Exam 4 and Rationales

1. A client is admitted to the emergency room with a gunshot wound to the right arm. After dressing the wound and administering the prescribed antibiotic, the nurse should:

   ○ **A.** Ask the client if he has any medication allergies.

   ○ **B.** Check the client's immunization record.

   ○ **C.** Apply a splint to immobilize the arm.

   ○ **D.** Administer medication for pain.

Quick Answer: **302**
Detailed Answer: **304**

2. The nurse is caring for a client with suspected endometrial cancer. Which symptom is associated with endometrial cancer?

   ○ **A.** Frothy vaginal discharge

   ○ **B.** Thick, white vaginal discharge

   ○ **C.** Purulent vaginal discharge

   ○ **D.** Watery vaginal discharge

Quick Answer: **302**
Detailed Answer: **304**

3. A client with Parkinson's disease is scheduled for stereotactic surgery. Which finding indicates that the surgery had its intended effect?

   ○ **A.** The client no longer has intractable tremors.

   ○ **B.** The client has sufficient production of dopamine.

   ○ **C.** The client no longer requires any medication.

   ○ **D.** The client will have increased production of serotonin.

Quick Answer: **302**
Detailed Answer: **304**

4. A client with AIDS asks the nurse why he cannot have a pitcher of water left at his bedside. The nurse should tell the client that:

   ○ **A.** It would be best for him to drink ice water.

   ○ **B.** He should drink several glasses of juice instead.

   ○ **C.** It makes it easier to keep a record of his intake.

   ○ **D.** He should not drink water that has been sitting for a period of time.

Quick Answer: **302**
Detailed Answer: **304**

5. An elderly client is diagnosed with interstitial cystitis. Which finding differentiates interstitial cystitis from other forms of cystitis?

Quick Answer: **302**
Detailed Answer: **304**

- ○ **A.** The client is asymptomatic.
- ○ **B.** The urine is free of bacteria.
- ○ **C.** The urine contains blood.
- ○ **D.** Males are affected more often.

6. The mother of a male child with cystic fibrosis tells the nurse that she hopes her son's children won't have the disease. The nurse is aware that:

Quick Answer: **302**
Detailed Answer: **304**

- ○ **A.** There is a 25% chance that his children will have cystic fibrosis.
- ○ **B.** Most of the males with cystic fibrosis are sterile.
- ○ **C.** There is a 50% chance that his children will be carriers.
- ○ **D.** Most males with cystic fibrosis are capable of having children, so genetic counseling is advised.

7. A six-month-old is hospitalized with symptoms of botulism. What aspect of the infant's history is associated with *Clostridium botulinum* infection?

Quick Answer: **302**
Detailed Answer: **304**

- ○ **A.** The infant sucks on his fingers and toes.
- ○ **B.** The mother sweetens the infant's cereal with honey.
- ○ **C.** The infant was switched to soy-based formula.
- ○ **D.** The father recently purchased an aquarium.

8. The mother of a six-year-old with autistic disorder tells the nurse that her son has been much more difficult to care for since the birth of his sister. The best explanation for changes in the child's behavior is:

Quick Answer: **302**
Detailed Answer: **304**

- ○ **A.** The child did not want a sibling.
- ○ **B.** The child was not adequately prepared for the baby's arrival.
- ○ **C.** The child's daily routine has been upset by the birth of his sister.
- ○ **D.** The child is just trying to get the parent's attention.

9. The parents of a child with cystic fibrosis ask what determines the prognosis of the disease. The nurse knows that the greatest determinant of the prognosis is:

- ○ **A.** The degree of pulmonary involvement
- ○ **B.** The ability to maintain an ideal weight
- ○ **C.** The secretion of lipase by the pancreas
- ○ **D.** The regulation of sodium and chloride excretion

Quick Answer: **302**
Detailed Answer: **304**

10. The nurse is assessing a client hospitalized with a duodenal ulcer. Which finding should be reported to the doctor immediately?

- ○ **A.** BP 82/60, pulse 120
- ○ **B.** Pulse 68, respirations 24
- ○ **C.** BP 110/88, pulse 56
- ○ **D.** Pulse 82, respirations 16

Quick Answer: **302**
Detailed Answer: **305**

11. While caring for a client in the second stage of labor, the nurse notices a pattern of early decelerations. The nurse should:

- ○ **A.** Notify the physician immediately.
- ○ **B.** Turn the client on her left side.
- ○ **C.** Apply oxygen via a tight face mask.
- ○ **D.** Document the finding on the flow sheet.

Quick Answer: **302**
Detailed Answer: **305**

12. The nurse is teaching the client with AIDS regarding needed changes in food preparation. Which statement indicates that the client understands the nurse's teaching?

- ○ **A.** "Adding fresh ground pepper to my food will improve the flavor."
- ○ **B.** "Meat should be thoroughly cooked to the proper temperature."
- ○ **C.** "Eating cheese and yogurt will prevent AIDS-related diarrhea."
- ○ **D.** "It is important to eat four to five servings of fresh fruits and vegetables a day."

Quick Answer: **302**
Detailed Answer: **305**

13. The sputum of a client remains positive for the tubercle bacillus even though the client has been taking Laniazid (isoniazid) in combination with other antituberculars. The nurse recognizes that the client taking isoniazid should have a negative sputum culture within:

Quick Answer: **302**
Detailed Answer: **305**

- ○ **A.** Two weeks
- ○ **B.** Six weeks
- ○ **C.** Two months
- ○ **D.** Three months

14. Which person is at greatest risk for developing Lyme disease?

Quick Answer: **302**
Detailed Answer: **305**

- ○ **A.** Computer programmer
- ○ **B.** Elementary teacher
- ○ **C.** Veterinarian
- ○ **D.** Landscaper

15. The mother of a one-year-old wants to know when she should begin toilet-training her child. The nurse's response is based on the knowledge that sufficient sphincter control for toilet training is present by:

Quick Answer: **302**
Detailed Answer: **305**

- ○ **A.** 12–15 months of age
- ○ **B.** 18–24 months of age
- ○ **C.** 26–30 months of age
- ○ **D.** 32–36 months of age

16. The nurse is developing a plan of care for a client with a newly created ileostomy. The priority nursing diagnosis for this client is:

Quick Answer: **302**
Detailed Answer: **305**

- ○ **A.** Risk for deficient fluid volume related to excessive fluid loss from ostomy
- ○ **B.** Disturbed body image related to presence of ostomy
- ○ **C.** Risk for impaired skin integrity related to irritation from ostomy appliance
- ○ **D.** Deficient knowledge of ostomy care related to unfamiliarity with information resources

17. The physician has prescribed Cobex (cyanocobalamin) for a client following a gastric resection. Which lab result indicates that the medication is having its intended effect?

Quick Answer: **302**
Detailed Answer: **305**

- ○ **A.** Neutrophil count of 4500cu mm
- ○ **B.** Hgb of 14.2g/dL
- ○ **C.** Platelet count of 250,000cu mm
- ○ **D.** Eosinophil count of 200cu mm

18. A behavior-modification program has been started for an adolescent with oppositional defiant disorder. Which statement describes the use of behavior modification?

    ○ **A.** Distractors are used to interrupt repetitive or unpleasant thoughts.

    ○ **B.** Techniques using stressors and exercise are used to increase awareness of body defenses.

    ○ **C.** A system of tokens and rewards is used as positive reinforcement.

    ○ **D.** Appropriate behavior is learned through observing the action of models.

Quick Answer: **302**
Detailed Answer: **305**

19. Following eruption of the primary teeth, the mother can promote chewing by giving the toddler:

    ○ **A.** Pieces of hot dog

    ○ **B.** Carrot sticks

    ○ **C.** Pieces of cereal

    ○ **D.** Raisins

Quick Answer: **302**
Detailed Answer: **306**

20. The nurse is infusing total parenteral nutrition (TPN). The primary purpose for closely monitoring the client's intake and output is:

    ○ **A.** To determine how quickly the client is metabolizing the solution

    ○ **B.** To determine whether the client's oral intake is sufficient

    ○ **C.** To detect the development of hypovolemia

    ○ **D.** To decrease the risk of fluid overload

Quick Answer: **302**
Detailed Answer: **306**

21. An obstetrical client with diabetes has an amniocentesis at 28 weeks gestation. Which test indicates the degree of fetal lung maturity?

    ○ **A.** Alpha-fetoprotein

    ○ **B.** Estriol level

    ○ **C.** Indirect Coombs

    ○ **D.** Lecithin sphingomyelin ratio

Quick Answer: **302**
Detailed Answer: **306**

22. Which nursing assessment indicates that involutional changes have occurred in a client who is three days postpartum?

Quick Answer: **302**
Detailed Answer: **306**

  ○ **A.** The fundus is firm and three finger widths below the umbilicus.

  ○ **B.** The client has a moderate amount of lochia serosa.

  ○ **C.** The fundus is firm and even with the umbilicus.

  ○ **D.** The uterus is approximately the size of a small grapefruit.

23. When administering total parenteral nutrition, the nurse should assess the client for signs of rebound hypoglycemia. The nurse knows that rebound hypoglycemia occurs when:

Quick Answer: **302**
Detailed Answer: **306**

  ○ **A.** The infusion rate is too rapid.

  ○ **B.** The infusion is discontinued without tapering.

  ○ **C.** The solution is infused through a peripheral line.

  ○ **D.** The infusion is administered without a filter.

24. A client scheduled for disc surgery tells the nurse that she frequently uses the herbal supplement kava-kava (piper methysticum). The nurse should notify the doctor because kava-kava:

Quick Answer: **302**
Detailed Answer: **306**

  ○ **A.** Increases the effects of anesthesia and post-operative analgesia

  ○ **B.** Eliminates the need for antimicrobial therapy following surgery

  ○ **C.** Increases urinary output, so a urinary catheter will be needed post-operatively

  ○ **D.** Depresses the immune system, so infection is more of a problem

25. The physician has ordered 50mEq of potassium chloride for a client with a potassium level of 2.5mEq/L. The nurse should administer the medication:

Quick Answer: **302**
Detailed Answer: **306**

  ○ **A.** Slow, continuous IV push over 10 minutes

  ○ **B.** Continuous infusion over 30 minutes

  ○ **C.** Controlled infusion over five hours

  ○ **D.** Continuous infusion over 24 hours

26. The nurse reviewing the lab results of a client receiving Cytoxan (cyclophasphamide) for Hodgkin's lymphoma finds the following: WBC 4,200, RBC 3,800,000, platelets 25,000, and serum creatinine 1.0mg. The nurse recognizes that the greatest risk for the client at this time is:

   ○ **A.** Overwhelming infection
   ○ **B.** Bleeding
   ○ **C.** Anemia
   ○ **D.** Renal failure

Quick Answer: **302**
Detailed Answer: **306**

27. Which of the following is an adverse effect associated with the use of Adriamycin (doxorubicin)?

   ○ **A.** Ventricular arrhythmias
   ○ **B.** Alopecia
   ○ **C.** Leukopenia
   ○ **D.** Stomatitis

Quick Answer: **302**
Detailed Answer: **306**

28. A client with cervical cancer has a radioactive implant. Which statement indicates that the client understands the nurse's teaching regarding radioactive implants?

   ○ **A.** "I won't be able to have visitors while getting radiation therapy."
   ○ **B.** "I will have a urinary catheter while the implant is in place."
   ○ **C.** "I can be up to the bedside commode while the implant is in place."
   ○ **D.** "I won't have any side effects from this type of therapy."

Quick Answer: **302**
Detailed Answer: **306**

29. The nurse is teaching circumcision care to the mother of a newborn. Which statement indicates that the mother needs further teaching?

   ○ **A.** "I will apply a petroleum gauze to the area with each diaper change."
   ○ **B.** "I will clean the area carefully with each diaper change."
   ○ **C.** "I can place a heat lamp to the area to speed up the healing process."
   ○ **D.** "I should carefully observe the area for signs of infection."

Quick Answer: **302**
Detailed Answer: **307**

30. A client admitted for treatment of bacterial pneumonia has an order for intravenous ampicillin. Which specimen should be obtained prior to administering the medication?

- ○ **A.** Routine urinalysis
- ○ **B.** Complete blood count
- ○ **C.** Serum electrolytes
- ○ **D.** Sputum for culture and sensitivity

Quick Answer: **302**
Detailed Answer: **307**

31. While obtaining information about the client's current medication use, the nurse learns that the client takes ginkgo to improve mental alertness. The nurse should tell the client to:

- ○ **A.** Report signs of bruising or bleeding to the doctor.
- ○ **B.** Avoid sun exposure while using the herbal supplement.
- ○ **C.** Purchase only those brands with FDA approval.
- ○ **D.** Increase daily intake of vitamin E.

Quick Answer: **302**
Detailed Answer: **307**

32. A client with Hodgkin's lymphoma is receiving Platinol (cisplatin). To help prevent nephrotoxicity, the nurse should:

- ○ **A.** Slow the infusion rate.
- ○ **B.** Make sure the client is well hydrated.
- ○ **C.** Record the intake and output every shift.
- ○ **D.** Tell the client to report ringing in the ears.

Quick Answer: **302**
Detailed Answer: **307**

33. The chart of a client hospitalized for a total hip repair reveals that the client is colonized with MRSA. The nurse understands that the client:

- ○ **A.** Will not display symptoms of infection
- ○ **B.** Is less likely to have an infection
- ○ **C.** Can be placed in the room with others
- ○ **D.** Cannot colonize others with MRSA

Quick Answer: **302**
Detailed Answer: **307**

34. A client receiving Vancocin (vancomycin) has a serum level of 20mcg/mL. The nurse knows that the therapeutic range for vancomycin is:

- ○ **A.** 5–10mcg/mL
- ○ **B.** 10–25mcg/mL
- ○ **C.** 25–40mcg/mL
- ○ **D.** 40–60mcg/mL

Quick Answer: **302**
Detailed Answer: **307**

35. A client is admitted with symptoms of pseudomembranous colitis. Which finding is associated with *Clostridium difficile*?

    ○ **A.** Diarrhea containing blood and mucus

    ○ **B.** Cough, fever, and shortness of breath

    ○ **C.** Anorexia, weight loss, and fever

    ○ **D.** Development of ulcers on the lower extremities

Quick Answer: **302**
Detailed Answer: **307**

36. Which vitamin should be administered with INH (isoniazid) in order to prevent possible nervous system side effects?

    ○ **A.** Thiamine

    ○ **B.** Niacin

    ○ **C.** Pyridoxine

    ○ **D.** Riboflavin

Quick Answer: **302**
Detailed Answer: **307**

37. A client is admitted with suspected Legionnaires' disease. Which factor increases the risk of developing Legionnaires' disease?

    ○ **A.** Treatment of arthritis with steroids

    ○ **B.** Foreign travel

    ○ **C.** Eating fresh shellfish twice a week

    ○ **D.** Doing volunteer work at the local hospital

Quick Answer: **302**
Detailed Answer: **307**

38. A client who uses a respiratory inhaler asks the nurse to explain how he can know when half his medication is empty so that he can refill his prescription. The nurse should tell the client to:

    ○ **A.** Shake the inhaler and listen for the contents.

    ○ **B.** Drop the inhaler in water to see if it floats.

    ○ **C.** Check for a hissing sound as the inhaler is used.

    ○ **D.** Press the inhaler and watch for the mist.

Quick Answer: **302**
Detailed Answer: **308**

39. The nurse is caring for a client following a right nephrolithotomy. Post-operatively, the client should be positioned:

    ○ **A.** On the right side

    ○ **B.** Supine

    ○ **C.** On the left side

    ○ **D.** Prone

Quick Answer: **302**
Detailed Answer: **308**

40. A client is admitted with sickle cell crises and sequestration. Upon assessing the client, the nurse would expect to find:

- ○ **A.** Decreased blood pressure
- ○ **B.** Moist mucus membranes
- ○ **C.** Decreased respirations
- ○ **D.** Increased blood pressure

Quick Answer: **302**
Detailed Answer: **308**

41. A healthcare worker is referred to the nursing office with a suspected latex allergy. The first symptom of latex allergy is usually:

- ○ **A.** Oral itching after eating bananas
- ○ **B.** Swelling of the eyes and mouth
- ○ **C.** Difficulty in breathing
- ○ **D.** Swelling and itching of the hands

Quick Answer: **302**
Detailed Answer: **308**

42. A client is admitted with disseminated herpes zoster (shingles). According to the Centers for Disease Control Guidelines for Infection Control:

- ○ **A.** Airborne precautions will be needed.
- ○ **B.** No special precautions will be needed.
- ○ **C.** Only contact precautions will be needed.
- ○ **D.** Droplet precautions will be needed.

Quick Answer: **302**
Detailed Answer: **308**

43. Acticoat (silver nitrate) dressings are applied to the legs of a client with deep partial thickness burns. The nurse should:

- ○ **A.** Change the dressings once per shift.
- ○ **B.** Moisten the dressing with sterile water.
- ○ **C.** Change the dressings only when they become soiled.
- ○ **D.** Moisten the dressing with normal saline.

Quick Answer: **302**
Detailed Answer: **308**

44. The nurse is preparing to administer an injection to a six-month-old when she notices a white dot in the infant's right pupil. The nurse should:

- ○ **A.** Report the finding to the physician immediately.
- ○ **B.** Record the finding and give the infant's injection.
- ○ **C.** Recognize that the finding is a variation of normal.
- ○ **D.** Check both eyes for the presence of the red reflex.

Quick Answer: **302**
Detailed Answer: **308**

45. A client is diagnosed with stage II Hodgkin's lymphoma. The nurse recognizes that the client has involvement:

  ○ **A.** In a single lymph node or single site

  ○ **B.** In more than one node or single organ on the same side of the diaphragm

  ○ **C.** In lymph nodes on both sides of the diaphragm

  ○ **D.** In disseminated organs and tissues

Quick Answer: **302**
Detailed Answer: **308**

46. A client has been receiving Rheumatrex (methotrexate) for severe rheumatoid arthritis. The nurse should tell the client to avoid taking:

  ○ **A.** Aspirin

  ○ **B.** Multivitamins

  ○ **C.** Omega 3 fish oils

  ○ **D.** Acetaminophen

Quick Answer: **302**
Detailed Answer: **308**

47. The physician has ordered a low-residue diet for a client with Crohn's disease. Which food is not permitted in a low-residue diet?

  ○ **A.** Mashed potatoes

  ○ **B.** Smooth peanut butter

  ○ **C.** Fried fish

  ○ **D.** Rice

Quick Answer: **302**
Detailed Answer: **308**

48. A client hospitalized with cirrhosis has developed abdominal ascites. The nurse should provide the client with snacks that provide additional:

  ○ **A.** Sodium

  ○ **B.** Potassium

  ○ **C.** Protein

  ○ **D.** Fat

Quick Answer: **302**
Detailed Answer: **309**

49. A diagnosis of multiple sclerosis is often delayed because of the varied symptoms experienced by those affected with the disease. Which symptom is most common in those with multiple sclerosis?

  ○ **A.** Resting tremors

  ○ **B.** Double vision

  ○ **C.** Flaccid paralysis

  ○ **D.** "Pill-rolling" tremors

Quick Answer: **302**
Detailed Answer: **309**

50. After attending a company picnic, several clients are admitted to the emergency room with *E. coli* food poisoning. The most likely source of infection is:

    ○ **A.** Hamburger

    ○ **B.** Hot dog

    ○ **C.** Potato salad

    ○ **D.** Baked beans

Quick Answer: **302**
Detailed Answer: **309**

51. A client tells the nurse that she takes St. John's wort (hypericum perforatum) three times a day for mild depression. The nurse should tell the client that:

    ○ **A.** St. John's wort seldom relieves depression.

    ○ **B.** She should avoid eating aged cheese.

    ○ **C.** Skin reactions increase with the use of sunscreen.

    ○ **D.** The herbal is safe to use with other antidepressants.

Quick Answer: **302**
Detailed Answer: **309**

52. The physician has ordered a low-purine diet for a client with gout. Which protein source is high in purine?

    ○ **A.** Dried beans

    ○ **B.** Nuts

    ○ **C.** Cheese

    ○ **D.** Eggs

Quick Answer: **302**
Detailed Answer: **309**

53. The nurse is observing the ambulation of a client recently fitted for crutches. Which observation requires nursing intervention?

    ○ **A.** Two finger widths are noted between the axilla and the top of the crutch.

    ○ **B.** The client bears weight on his hands when ambulating.

    ○ **C.** The crutches and the client's feet move alternately.

    ○ **D.** The client bears weight on his axilla when standing.

Quick Answer: **302**
Detailed Answer: **309**

54. During the change of shift report, a nurse writes in her notes that she suspects illegal drug use by a client assigned to her care. During the shift, the notes are found by the client's daughter. The nurse could be sued for:

    ○ **A.** Libel

    ○ **B.** Slander

    ○ **C.** Malpractice

    ○ **D.** Negligence

Quick Answer: **302**
Detailed Answer: **309**

55. The nurse is caring for an adolescent with a five-year history of bulimia. A common clinical finding in the client with bulimia is:

   ○ **A.** Extreme weight loss

   ○ **B.** Dental caries

   ○ **C.** Hair loss

   ○ **D.** Decreased temperature

Quick Answer: **302**
Detailed Answer: **309**

56. A client hospitalized for treatment of congestive heart failure is to be discharged with a prescription for Digitek (digoxin) 0.25mg daily. Which of the following statements indicates that the client needs further teaching?

   ○ **A.** "I will need to take the medication at the same time each day."

   ○ **B.** "I can prevent stomach upset by taking the medication with an antacid."

   ○ **C.** "I can help prevent drug toxicity by eating foods containing fiber."

   ○ **D.** "I will need to report visual changes to my doctor."

Quick Answer: **302**
Detailed Answer: **309**

57. A client with paranoid schizophrenia has an order for Thorazine (chlorpromazine) 400mg orally twice daily. Which of the following symptoms should be reported to the physician immediately?

   ○ **A.** Fever, sore throat, weakness

   ○ **B.** Dry mouth, constipation, blurred vision

   ○ **C.** Lethargy, slurred speech, thirst

   ○ **D.** Fatigue, drowsiness, photosensitivity

Quick Answer: **302**
Detailed Answer: **310**

58. When caring for a client with an anterior cervical discectomy, the nurse should give priority to assessing for post-operative bleeding. The nurse should pay particular attention to:

   ○ **A.** Drainage on the surgical dressing

   ○ **B.** Complaints of neck pain

   ○ **C.** Bleeding from the mouth

   ○ **D.** Swelling in the posterior neck

Quick Answer: **302**
Detailed Answer: **310**

59. The initial assessment of a newborn reveals a chest circumference of 34cm and an abdominal circumference of 31cm. The chest is asymmetrical and breath sounds are diminished on the left side. The nurse should give priority to:

   ○ **A.** Providing supplemental oxygen by a ventilated mask

   ○ **B.** Performing auscultation of the abdomen for the presence of active bowel sounds

   ○ **C.** Inserting a nasogastric tube to check for esophageal patency

   ○ **D.** Positioning on the left side with head and chest elevated

60. The physician has ordered Eskalith (lithium carbonate) 500mg three times a day and Risperdal (risperidone) 2mg twice daily for a client admitted with bipolar disorder, acute manic episodes. The best explanation for the client's medication regimen is:

   ○ **A.** The client's symptoms of acute mania are typical of undiagnosed schizophrenia.

   ○ **B.** Antipsychotic medication is used to manage behavioral excitement until mood stabilization occurs.

   ○ **C.** The client will be more compliant with a medication that allows some feelings of hypomania.

   ○ **D.** Antipsychotic medication prevents psychotic symptoms commonly associated with the use of mood stabilizers.

61. During a unit card game, a client with acute mania begins to sing loudly as she starts to undress. The nurse should:

   ○ **A.** Ignore the client's behavior.

   ○ **B.** Exchange the cards for a checker board.

   ○ **C.** Send the other clients to their rooms.

   ○ **D.** Cover the client and walk her to her room.

62. A child with Down syndrome has a developmental age of four years. According to the Denver Developmental Assessment, the four-year-old should be able to:

   ○ **A.** Draw a man in six parts

   ○ **B.** Give his first and last name

   ○ **C.** Dress without supervision

   ○ **D.** Define a list of words

63. A client with paranoid schizophrenia is brought to the hospital by her elderly parents. During the assessment, the client's mother states, "Sometimes she is more than we can manage." Based on the mother's statement, the most appropriate nursing diagnosis is:

- ○ **A.** Ineffective family coping related to parental role conflict
- ○ **B.** Care-giver role strain related to chronic situational stress
- ○ **C.** Altered family process related to impaired social interaction
- ○ **D.** Altered parenting related to impaired growth and development

64. An adolescent client hospitalized with anorexia nervosa is described by her parents as "the perfect child." When planning care for the client, the nurse should:

- ○ **A.** Allow her to choose what foods she will eat
- ○ **B.** Provide activities to foster her self-identity
- ○ **C.** Encourage her to participate in morning exercise
- ○ **D.** Provide a private room near the nurse's station

65. The nurse is assigning staff to care for a number of clients with emotional disorders. Which facet of care is suitable to the skills of the nursing assistant?

- ○ **A.** Obtaining the vital signs of a client admitted for alcohol withdrawal
- ○ **B.** Helping a client with depression with bathing and grooming
- ○ **C.** Monitoring a client who is receiving electroconvulsive therapy
- ○ **D.** Sitting with a client with mania who is in seclusion

66. A client with angina is being discharged with a prescription for Transderm Nitro (nitroglycerin) patches. The nurse should tell the client to:

- ○ **A.** Shave the area before applying the patch
- ○ **B.** Remove the old patch and clean the skin with alcohol
- ○ **C.** Cover the patch with plastic wrap and tape it in place
- ○ **D.** Avoid cutting the patch because it will alter the dose

67. A client with myasthenia gravis is admitted in a cholinergic crisis. Signs of of cholinergic crisis include:

    ○ **A.** Decreased blood pressure and constricted pupils

    ○ **B.** Increased heart rate and increased respirations

    ○ **C.** Increased respirations and increased blood pressure

    ○ **D.** Anoxia and absence of the cough reflex

Quick Answer: **302**
Detailed Answer: **311**

68. The nurse is providing dietary teaching for a client with hypertension. Which food should be avoided by the client on a sodium-restricted diet?

    ○ **A.** Dried beans

    ○ **B.** Swiss cheese

    ○ **C.** Peanut butter

    ○ **D.** Colby cheese

Quick Answer: **302**
Detailed Answer: **311**

69. A client is admitted to the emergency room with partial-thickness burns to his right arm and full-thickness burns to his trunk. According to the Rule of Nines, the nurse calculates that the total body surface area (TBSA) involved is:

    ○ **A.** 20%

    ○ **B.** 35%

    ○ **C.** 45%

    ○ **D.** 60%

Quick Answer: **302**
Detailed Answer: **311**

70. The physician has ordered a paracentesis for a client with severe abdominal ascites. Before the procedure, the nurse should:

    ○ **A.** Provide the client with a urinal

    ○ **B.** Prep the area by shaving the abdomen

    ○ **C.** Encourage the client to drink extra fluids

    ○ **D.** Request an ultrasound of the abdomen

Quick Answer: **302**
Detailed Answer: **311**

71. Which of the following combinations of foods is appropriate for an eight-month-old infant?

    ○ **A.** Cocoa-flavored cereal, orange juice, and strained meat

    ○ **B.** Graham crackers, strained prunes, and pudding

    ○ **C.** Rice cereal, bananas, and strained carrots

    ○ **D.** Mashed potatoes, strained beets, and whole milk

Quick Answer: **302**
Detailed Answer: **311**

72. The mother of a nine-year-old with asthma has brought an electric CD player for her son to listen to while he is receiving oxygen therapy. The nurse should:

    ○ **A.** Explain that he does not need the added stimulation.

    ○ **B.** Allow the CD player, but ask him to wear earphones.

    ○ **C.** Tell the mother that he cannot have items from home.

    ○ **D.** Ask the mother to bring a battery-operated CD instead.

    Quick Answer: **302**
    Detailed Answer: **311**

73. Which one of the following situations represents a maturational crisis for the family?

    ○ **A.** A four-year-old entering nursery school

    ○ **B.** Development of preeclampsia during pregnancy

    ○ **C.** Loss of employment and health benefits

    ○ **D.** Hospitalization of a grandfather with a stroke

    Quick Answer: **302**
    Detailed Answer: **312**

74. A client with a history of phenylketonuria is seen at the local family planning clinic. After completing the client's intake history, the nurse provides literature for a healthy pregnancy. Which statement indicates that the client needs further teaching?

    ○ **A.** "I can help control my weight by switching from sugar to Nutrasweet."

    ○ **B.** "I need to resume my old diet before becoming pregnant."

    ○ **C.** "Fresh fruits and raw vegetables will make excellent between-meal snacks."

    ○ **D.** "I need to eliminate most sources of phenylalanine from my diet."

    Quick Answer: **302**
    Detailed Answer: **312**

75. Parents of a toddler are dismayed when they learn that their child has Duchenne's muscular dystrophy. Which statement describes the inheritance pattern of the disorder?

    ○ **A.** An affected gene is located on one of the 21 pairs of autosomes.

    ○ **B.** The disorder is caused by an over-replication of the X chromosome in males.

    ○ **C.** The affected gene is located on the Y chromosome of the father.

    ○ **D.** The affected gene is located on the X chromosome of the mother.

    Quick Answer: **302**
    Detailed Answer: **312**

76. A client with obsessive compulsive personality disorder annoys his co-workers with his rigid-perfectionistic attitude and his preoccupation with trivial details. An important nursing intervention for this client would be:

    ○ A. Helping the client develop a plan for changing his behavior

    ○ B. Contracting with him for the time he spends on a task

    ○ C. Avoiding a discussion of his annoying behavior because it will only make him worse

    ○ D. Encouraging him to set a time schedule and deadlines for himself

Quick Answer: **302**
Detailed Answer: **312**

77. The mother of a child with chickenpox wants to know if there is a medication that will shorten the course of the illness. Which medication is sometimes used to speed healing of the lesions and shorten the duration of fever and itching?

    ○ A. Zovirax (acyclovir)

    ○ B. Varivax (varicella vaccine)

    ○ C. VZIG (varicella-zoster immune globulin)

    ○ D. Periactin (cyproheptadine)

Quick Answer: **302**
Detailed Answer: **312**

78. One of the most important criteria for the diagnosis of physical abuse is inconsistency between the appearance of the injury and the history of how the injury occurred. Which one of the following situations should alert the nurse to the possibility of abuse?

    ○ A. An 18-month-old with sock and mitten burns from a fall into the bathtub

    ○ B. A six-year-old with a fractured clavicle following a fall from her bike

    ○ C. An eight-year-old with a concussion from a skateboarding accident

    ○ D. A two-year-old with burns to the scalp and face from a grease spill

Quick Answer: **302**
Detailed Answer: **312**

79. A patient refuses to take his dose of oral medication. The nurse tells the patient that if he does not take the medication that she will administer it by injection. The nurse's comments can result in a charge of:

    ○ A. Malpractice

    ○ B. Assault

    ○ C. Negligence

    ○ D. Battery

Quick Answer: **302**
Detailed Answer: **312**

80. During morning assessments, the nurse finds that a client's nephrostomy tube has been clamped. The nurse's first action should be to:

Quick Answer: 302
Detailed Answer: 312

   ○ **A.** Assess the drainage bag.

   ○ **B.** Check for bladder distention.

   ○ **C.** Unclamp the tubing.

   ○ **D.** Irrigate the tubing.

81. The nurse caring for a client with closed chest drainage notes that the collection chamber is full.

Quick Answer: 302
Detailed Answer: 313

   ○ **A.** Add more water to the suction-control chamber.

   ○ **B.** Remove the drainage using a 60mL syringe.

   ○ **C.** Milk the tubing to facilitate drainage.

   ○ **D.** Prepare a new unit for continuing collection.

82. A client with severe anemia is to receive a unit of packed red blood cells. In the event of a transfusion reaction, the first action by the nurse should be to:

Quick Answer: 302
Detailed Answer: 313

   ○ **A.** Notify the physician and the nursing supervisor.

   ○ **B.** Stop the transfusion and maintain an IV of normal saline.

   ○ **C.** Call the lab for verification of type and cross match.

   ○ **D.** Prepare an injection of Benadryl (diphenhydramine).

83. A new mother tells the nurse that she is getting a new microwave so that her husband can help prepare the baby's feedings. The nurse should:

Quick Answer: 302
Detailed Answer: 313

   ○ **A.** Explain that a microwave should never be used to warm the baby's bottles.

   ○ **B.** Tell the mother that microwaving is the best way to prevent bacteria in the formula.

   ○ **C.** Tell the mother to shake the bottle vigorously for one minute after warming in the microwave.

   ○ **D.** Instruct the parents to always leave the top of the bottle open while microwaving so heat can escape.

84. A client with HELLP syndrome is admitted to the labor and delivery unit for observation. The nurse knows that the client will have elevated:

    ○ **A.** Serum glucose levels

    ○ **B.** Liver enzymes

    ○ **C.** Pancreatic enzymes

    ○ **D.** Plasma protein levels

Quick Answer: **302**
Detailed Answer: **313**

85. To reduce the possibility of having a baby with a neural tube defect, the client should be told to increase her intake of folic acid. Dietary sources of folic acid include:

    ○ **A.** Meat, liver, eggs

    ○ **B.** Pork, fish, chicken

    ○ **C.** Spinach, beets, cantaloupe

    ○ **D.** Dried beans, sweet potatoes, Brussels sprouts

Quick Answer: **302**
Detailed Answer: **313**

86. The nurse is making room assignments for four obstetrical clients. If only one private room is available, it should be assigned to:

    ○ **A.** A multigravida with diabetes mellitus

    ○ **B.** A primigravida with preeclampsia

    ○ **C.** A multigravida with preterm labor

    ○ **D.** A primigravida with hyperemesis gravidarum

Quick Answer: **302**
Detailed Answer: **313**

87. A client has a tentative diagnosis of myasthenia gravis. The nurse recognizes that myasthenia gravis involves:

    ○ **A.** Loss of the myelin sheath in portions of the brain and spinal cord

    ○ **B.** An interruption in the transmission of impulses from nerve endings to muscles

    ○ **C.** Progressive weakness and loss of sensation that begins in the lower extremities

    ○ **D.** Loss of coordination and stiff "cogwheel" rigidity

Quick Answer: **302**
Detailed Answer: **313**

88. The physician has ordered an infusion of Osmitrol (mannitol) for a client with increased intracranial pressure. Which finding indicates the direct effectiveness of the drug?

    ○ **A.** Increased pulse rate

    ○ **B.** Increased urinary output

    ○ **C.** Decreased diastolic blood pressure

    ○ **D.** Increased pupil size

Quick Answer: **302**
Detailed Answer: **313**

89. The nurse has just received the change of shift report. Which client should the nurse assess first?

Quick Answer: 302
Detailed Answer: 313

   ○ **A.** A client with a supratentorial tumor awaiting surgery

   ○ **B.** A client admitted with a suspected subdural hematoma

   ○ **C.** A client recently diagnosed with akinetic seizures

   ○ **D.** A client transferring to the neuro rehabilitation unit

90. The physician has ordered an IV bolus of Solu-Medrol (methyl-prednisolone sodium succinate) in normal saline for a client admitted with a spinal cord injury. Solu-Medrol has been shown to be effective in:

Quick Answer: 302
Detailed Answer: 313

   ○ **A.** Preventing spasticity associated with cord injury

   ○ **B.** Decreasing the need for mechanical ventilation

   ○ **C.** Improving motor and sensory functioning

   ○ **D.** Treating post injury urinary tract infections

91. The physician has ordered a lumbar puncture for a client with suspected Guillain-Barre syndrome. The spinal fluid of a client with Guillain-Barre syndrome typically shows:

Quick Answer: 302
Detailed Answer: 314

   ○ **A.** Decreased protein concentration with a normal cell count

   ○ **B.** Increased protein concentration with a normal cell count

   ○ **C.** Increased protein concentration with an abnormal cell count

   ○ **D.** Decreased protein concentration with an abnormal cell count

92. An 18-month-old is admitted to the hospital with acute laryngotracheobronchitis. When assessing the respiratory status, the nurse should expect to find:

Quick Answer: 302
Detailed Answer: 314

   ○ **A.** Inspiratory stridor and harsh cough

   ○ **B.** Strident cough and drooling

   ○ **C.** Wheezing and intercostal retractions

   ○ **D.** Expiratory wheezing and nonproductive cough

93. The school nurse is assessing an elementary student with hemophilia who fell during recess. Which symptoms indicate hemarthrosis?

Quick Answer: **302**
Detailed Answer: **314**

- ○ **A.** Pain, coolness, and blue discoloration in the affected joint
- ○ **B.** Tingling and pain without loss of movement in the affected joint
- ○ **C.** Warmth, redness, and decreased movement in the affected joint
- ○ **D.** Stiffness, aching, and decreased movement in the affected joint

94. The physician has ordered aerosol treatments, chest percussion, and postural drainage for a client with cystic fibrosis. The nurse recognizes that the combination of therapies is to:

Quick Answer: **302**
Detailed Answer: **314**

- ○ **A.** Decrease respiratory effort and mucous production
- ○ **B.** Increase efficiency of the diaphragm and gas exchange
- ○ **C.** Dilate the bronchioles and help remove secretions
- ○ **D.** Stimulate coughing and oxygen consumption

95. The nurse is assessing a six-year-old following a tonsillectomy. Which one of the following signs is an early indication of hemorrhage?

Quick Answer: **302**
Detailed Answer: **314**

- ○ **A.** Drooling of bright red secretions
- ○ **B.** Pulse rate of 90
- ○ **C.** Vomiting of dark brown liquid
- ○ **D.** Infrequent swallowing while sleeping

96. A client is admitted for suspected bladder cancer. Which one of the following factors is most significant in the client's diagnosis?

Quick Answer: **302**
Detailed Answer: **314**

- ○ **A.** Smoking a pack of cigarettes a day for 30 years
- ○ **B.** Use of nonsteroidal anti-inflammatories
- ○ **C.** Eating foods with preservatives
- ○ **D.** Past employment involving asbestos

Quick Check

97. The nurse is teaching a client with peritoneal dialysis how to manage exchanges at home. The nurse should tell the client to notify the doctor immediately if:

   ○ **A.** The dialysate returns become cloudy in appearance.

   ○ **B.** The return of the dialysate is slower than usual.

   ○ **C.** A "tugging" sensation is noted as the dialysate drains.

   ○ **D.** A feeling of fullness is felt when the dialysate is instilled.

Quick Answer: **302**
Detailed Answer: **314**

98. The physician has prescribed nitroglycerin sublingual tablets as needed for a client with angina. The nurse should tell the client to take the medication:

   ○ **A.** After engaging in strenuous activity

   ○ **B.** Every four hours to prevent chest pain

   ○ **C.** As soon as he notices signs of chest pain

   ○ **D.** At bedtime to prevent nocturnal angina

Quick Answer: **302**
Detailed Answer: **314**

99. The nurse is caring for a client following a myocardial infarction. Which of the following enzymes are specific to cardiac damage?

   ○ **A.** SGOT and LDH

   ○ **B.** SGOT and CK BB

   ○ **C.** LDH and CK MB

   ○ **D.** LDH and CK BB

Quick Answer: **302**
Detailed Answer: **314**

100. Which of the following characterizes peer group relationships in eight- and nine-year-olds?

   ○ **A.** Activities organized around competitive games

   ○ **B.** Loyalty and strong same-sex friendships

   ○ **C.** Informal socialization between boys and girls

   ○ **D.** Shared activities with one best friend

Quick Answer: **302**
Detailed Answer: **314**

101. If the school-age child is not given the opportunity to engage in tasks and activities he can carry through to completion, he is likely to develop feelings of:

   ○ **A.** Guilt

   ○ **B.** Shame

   ○ **C.** Stagnation

   ○ **D.** Inferiority

Quick Answer: **302**
Detailed Answer: **314**

102. The physician has ordered two units of whole blood for a client following surgery. To provide for client safety, the nurse should:

    ○ **A.** Obtain a signed permit for each unit of blood.

    ○ **B.** Use a new administration set for each unit transfused.

    ○ **C.** Administer the blood using a Y connector.

    ○ **D.** Check the blood type and Rh factor three times before initiating the transfusion.

Quick Answer: **302**
Detailed Answer: **315**

103. A client with B positive blood is scheduled for a transfusion of whole blood. Which finding requires nursing intervention?

    ○ **A.** The available blood has been banked for two weeks.

    ○ **B.** The blood available for transfusion is Rh negative.

    ○ **C.** The client has a peripheral IV of D5 ½ normal saline.

    ○ **D.** The blood available for transfusion is type O positive.

Quick Answer: **302**
Detailed Answer: **315**

104. The nurse is reviewing the lab results of a client's arterial blood gases. The $PaCO_2$ indicates effective functioning of the:

    ○ **A.** Kidneys

    ○ **B.** Pancreas

    ○ **C.** Lungs

    ○ **D.** Liver

Quick Answer: **302**
Detailed Answer: **315**

105. The autopsy results in SIDS-related death will show the following consistent findings:

    ○ **A.** Abnormal central nervous system development

    ○ **B.** Abnormal cardiovascular development

    ○ **C.** Intraventricular hemorrhage and cerebral edema

    ○ **D.** Pulmonary edema and intrathoracic hemorrhages

Quick Answer: **302**
Detailed Answer: **315**

106. The nurse is caring for a newborn who is on strict intake and output. The used diaper weighs 73.5gm. The diaper's dry weight was 62gm. The newborn's urine output is:

    ○ **A.** 10mL

    ○ **B.** 11.5mL

    ○ **C.** 10gm

    ○ **D.** 12gm

Quick Answer: **302**
Detailed Answer: **315**

107. The nurse is teaching the parents of an infant with osteogenesis imperfecta. The nurse should explain the need for:

   ○ **A.** Additional calcium in the infant's diet

   ○ **B.** Careful handling to prevent fractures

   ○ **C.** Providing extra sensorimotor stimulation

   ○ **D.** Frequent testing of visual function

108. A newborn is diagnosed with respiratory distress syndrome (RDS). Which position is best for maintaining an open airway?

   ○ **A.** Prone, with his head turned to one side

   ○ **B.** Side-lying, with a towel beneath his shoulders

   ○ **C.** Supine, with his neck slightly flexed

   ○ **D.** Supine, with his neck slightly extended

109. A client with bipolar disorder is discharged with a prescription for Depakote (divalproex sodium). The nurse should remind the client of the need for:

   ○ **A.** Frequent dental visits

   ○ **B.** Frequent lab work

   ○ **C.** Additional fluids

   ○ **D.** Additional sodium

110. The physician's notes state that a client with cocaine addiction has formication. The nurse recognizes that the client has:

   ○ **A.** Tactile hallucinations

   ○ **B.** Irregular heart rate

   ○ **C.** Paranoid delusions

   ○ **D.** Methadone tolerance

111. The nurse is preparing a client with gastroesophageal reflux disease (GERD) for discharge. The nurse should tell the client to:

   ○ **A.** Eat a small snack before bedtime

   ○ **B.** Sleep on his right side

   ○ **C.** Avoid carbonated beverages

   ○ **D.** Increase his intake of citrus fruits

112. A client with a C3 spinal cord injury experiences autonomic hyper-reflexia. After placing the client in high Fowler's position, the nurse's next action should be to:

Quick Answer: 302
Detailed Answer: 316

   ○ **A.** Notify the physician

   ○ **B.** Make sure the catheter is patent

   ○ **C.** Administer an antihypertensive

   ○ **D.** Provide supplemental oxygen

113. A client is to receive Dilantin (phenytoin) via a nasogastric (NG) tube. When giving the medication, the nurse should:

Quick Answer: 302
Detailed Answer: 316

   ○ **A.** Flush the NG tube with 2–4mL of water before giving the medication

   ○ **B.** Administer the medication, flush with 5mL of water, and clamp the NG tube

   ○ **C.** Flush the NG tube with 5mL of normal saline and administer the medication

   ○ **D.** Flush the NG tube with 2–4oz of water before and after giving the medication

114. When assessing the client with acute arterial occlusion, the nurse would expect to find:

Quick Answer: 302
Detailed Answer: 316

   ○ **A.** Peripheral edema in the affected extremity

   ○ **B.** Minute blackened areas on the toes

   ○ **C.** Pain above the level of occlusion

   ○ **D.** Redness and warmth over the affected area

115. The nurse is assessing a client following the removal of a pituitary tumor. The nurse notes that the urinary output has increased and that the urine is very dilute. The nurse should give priority to:

Quick Answer: 302
Detailed Answer: 316

   ○ **A.** Notifying the doctor immediately

   ○ **B.** Documenting the finding in the chart

   ○ **C.** Decreasing the rate of IV fluids

   ○ **D.** Administering vasopressive medication

116. The physician has ordered Coumadin (sodium warfarin) for a client with a history of clots. The nurse should tell the client to avoid which of the following vegetables?

Quick Answer: 302
Detailed Answer: 316

   ○ **A.** Lettuce

   ○ **B.** Cauliflower

   ○ **C.** Beets

   ○ **D.** Carrots

117. The nurse is caring for a child in a plaster-of-Paris hip spica cast. To facilitate drying, the nurse should:

Quick Answer: **302**
Detailed Answer: **316**

- ○ **A.** Use a small hand-held hair dryer set on medium heat.
- ○ **B.** Place a small heater near the child's bed.
- ○ **C.** Turn the child at least every two hours.
- ○ **D.** Allow one side to dry before changing positions.

118. The local health clinic recommends vaccination against influenza for all its employees. The influenza vaccine is usually given annually in:

Quick Answer: **302**
Detailed Answer: **316**

- ○ **A.** November
- ○ **B.** December
- ○ **C.** January
- ○ **D.** February

119. A client is admitted with suspected Hodgkin's lymphoma. The diagnosis is confirmed by the:

Quick Answer: **302**
Detailed Answer: **316**

- ○ **A.** Overproliferation of immature white cells
- ○ **B.** Presence of Reed-Sternberg cells
- ○ **C.** Increased incidence of microcytosis
- ○ **D.** Reduction in the number of platelets

120. The nurse is caring for a client following a laryngectomy. The nurse can best help the client with communication by:

Quick Answer: **302**
Detailed Answer: **316**

- ○ **A.** Providing a pad and pencil
- ○ **B.** Checking on him every 30 minutes
- ○ **C.** Telling him to use the call light
- ○ **D.** Teaching the client simple sign language

121. A client has recently been diagnosed with primary open-angle glaucoma. The nurse should tell the client to avoid taking:

Quick Answer: **302**
Detailed Answer: **316**

- ○ **A.** Aleve (naprosyn)
- ○ **B.** Benadryl (diphenhydramine)
- ○ **C.** Tylenol (acetaminophen)
- ○ **D.** Robitussin (guaifenesin)

122. The nurse is caring for a client with an endemic goiter. The nurse recognizes that the client's condition is related to:

Quick Answer: **302**
Detailed Answer: **317**

   ○ **A.** Living in an area where the soil is depleted of iodine

   ○ **B.** Eating foods that decrease the thyroxine level

   ○ **C.** Using aluminum cookware to prepare the family's meals

   ○ **D.** Taking medications that decrease the thyroxine level

123. A client with a history of schizophrenia is seen in the local health clinic for medication follow-up. To maintain a therapeutic level of medication, the nurse should tell the client to avoid:

Quick Answer: **302**
Detailed Answer: **317**

   ○ **A.** Taking over-the-counter allergy medication

   ○ **B.** Eating cheese and pickled foods

   ○ **C.** Eating salty foods

   ○ **D.** Taking over-the-counter pain relievers

124. The nurse is formulating a plan of care for a client with a goiter. The priority nursing diagnosis for the client with a goiter is:

Quick Answer: **302**
Detailed Answer: **317**

   ○ **A.** Body image disturbance related to enlargement of the neck

   ○ **B.** Activity intolerance related to fatigue

   ○ **C.** Nutrition imbalance, less than body requirements, related to increased metabolism

   ○ **D.** Risk for ineffective airway clearance related to pressure of goiter on the trachea

125. Upon arrival to the nursery, Ilotycin (erythromycin) eyedrops are instilled in the newborn's eyes. The nurse understands that the medication will:

Quick Answer: **303**
Detailed Answer: **317**

   ○ **A.** Make the eyes less sensitive to light

   ○ **B.** Help prevent neonatal blindness

   ○ **C.** Strengthen the muscles of the eyes

   ○ **D.** Improve accommodation to near objects

126. A client has a diagnosis of discoid lupus erythematosus (DLE). The nurse recognizes that discoid lupus differs from systemic lupus erythematosus because it:

Quick Answer: **303**
Detailed Answer: **317**

   ○ **A.** Produces changes in the kidneys

   ○ **B.** Is confined to changes in the skin

   ○ **C.** Results in damage to the heart and lungs

   ○ **D.** Affects both joints and muscles

127. A client sustained a severe head injury to the occipital lobe. The nurse should carefully assess the client for:

Quick Answer: **303**
Detailed Answer: **317**

- ○ **A.** Changes in vision
- ○ **B.** Difficulty in speaking
- ○ **C.** Impaired judgment
- ○ **D.** Hearing impairment

128. The nurse observes a group of toddlers at daycare. Which of the following play situations exhibits the characteristics of parallel play?

Quick Answer: **303**
Detailed Answer: **317**

- ○ **A.** Lindie and Laura sharing clay to make cookies
- ○ **B.** Nick and Matt playing beside each other with trucks
- ○ **C.** Adrienne working a puzzle with Meredith and Ryan
- ○ **D.** Ashley playing with a busy box while sitting in her crib

129. Which of the following statements is true regarding language development of young children?

Quick Answer: **303**
Detailed Answer: **317**

- ○ **A.** Infants can discriminate speech from other patterns of sound.
- ○ **B.** Boys are more advanced in language development than girls of the same age.
- ○ **C.** Second-born children develop language earlier than first-born or only children.
- ○ **D.** Using single words for an entire sentence suggests delayed speech development.

130. A mother tells the nurse that her daughter has become quite a collector, filling her room with Beanie babies, dolls, and stuffed animals. The nurse recognizes that the child is developing:

Quick Answer: **303**
Detailed Answer: **317**

- ○ **A.** Object permanence
- ○ **B.** Post-conventional thinking
- ○ **C.** Concrete operational thinking
- ○ **D.** Pre-operational thinking

131. According to Erikson, the developmental task of the infant is to establish trust. Parents and caregivers foster a sense of trust by:

Quick Answer: **303**
Detailed Answer: **317**

- ○ **A.** Holding the infant during feedings
- ○ **B.** Speaking quietly to the infant
- ○ **C.** Providing sensory stimulation
- ○ **D.** Consistently responding to needs

132. The nurse is preparing to walk the postpartum client for the first time since delivery. Before walking the client, the nurse should:

Quick Answer: **303**
Detailed Answer: **317**

- O **A.** Give the client pain medication.
- O **B.** Assist the client in dangling her legs.
- O **C.** Have the client breathe deeply.
- O **D.** Provide the client additional fluids.

133. To minimize confusion in the elderly hospitalized client, the nurse should:

Quick Answer: **303**
Detailed Answer: **318**

- O **A.** Provide sensory stimulation by varying the daily routine.
- O **B.** Keep the room brightly lit and the television on to provide orientation to time.
- O **C.** Encourage visitors to limit visitation to phone calls to avoid overstimulation.
- O **D.** Provide explanations in a calm, caring manner to minimize anxiety.

134. A client diagnosed with tuberculosis asks the nurse when he can return to work. The nurse should tell the client that:

Quick Answer: **303**
Detailed Answer: **318**

- O **A.** He can return to work when he has three negative sputum cultures.
- O **B.** He can return to work as soon as he feels well enough.
- O **C.** He can return to work after a week of being on the medication.
- O **D.** He should think about applying for disability because he will no longer be able to work.

135. The physician has ordered lab work for a client with suspected disseminated intravascular coagulation (DIC). Which lab finding would provide a definitive diagnosis of DIC?

Quick Answer: **303**
Detailed Answer: **318**

- O **A.** Elevated erythrocyte sedimentation rate
- O **B.** Prolonged clotting time
- O **C.** Presence of fibrin split compound
- O **D.** Elevated white cell count

136. The nurse is caring for a client with rheumatoid arthritis. The nurse knows that the client's early morning symptoms will be most improved by:

Quick Answer: **303**
Detailed Answer: **318**

- ○ **A.** Taking a warm shower upon awakening
- ○ **B.** Applying ice packs to the joints
- ○ **C.** Taking two aspirin before going to bed
- ○ **D.** Going for an early morning walk

137. A client with schizophrenia has been taking Clozaril (clozapine) for the past six months. This morning the client's temperature was elevated to 102°F. The nurse should give priority to:

Quick Answer: **303**
Detailed Answer: **318**

- ○ **A.** Placing a note in the chart for the doctor
- ○ **B.** Rechecking the temperature in four hours
- ○ **C.** Notifying the physician immediately
- ○ **D.** Asking the client if he has been feeling sick

138. Which one of the following clients is most likely to develop acute respiratory distress syndrome?

Quick Answer: **303**
Detailed Answer: **318**

- ○ **A.** A 20-year-old with fractures of the tibia
- ○ **B.** A 36-year-old who is HIV positive
- ○ **C.** A 40-year-old with duodenal ulcers
- ○ **D.** A 32-year-old with barbiturate overdose

139. The complete blood count of a client admitted with anemia reveals that the red blood cells are hypochromic and microcytic. The nurse recognizes that the client has:

Quick Answer: **303**
Detailed Answer: **318**

- ○ **A.** Aplastic anemia
- ○ **B.** Iron-deficiency anemia
- ○ **C.** Pernicious anemia
- ○ **D.** Hemolytic anemia

140. While performing a neurological assessment on a client with a closed head injury, the nurse notes a positive Babinski reflex. The nurse should:

Quick Answer: **303**
Detailed Answer: **318**

- ○ **A.** Recognize that the client's condition is improving.
- ○ **B.** Reposition the client and check reflexes again.
- ○ **C.** Do nothing because the finding is an expected one.
- ○ **D.** Notify the physician of the finding.

141. The doctor has ordered neurological checks every 30 minutes for a client injured in a biking accident. Which finding indicates that the client's condition is satisfactory?

   ○ **A.** A score of 13 on the Glascow coma scale

   ○ **B.** The presence of doll's eye movement

   ○ **C.** The absence of deep tendon reflexes

   ○ **D.** Decerebrate posturing

Quick Answer: **303**
Detailed Answer: **318**

142. The nurse is developing a plan for bowel and bladder retraining for a client with paraplegia. The primary goal of a bowel and bladder retraining program is:

   ○ **A.** Optimal restoration of the client's elimination pattern

   ○ **B.** Restoration of the client's neurosensory function

   ○ **C.** Prevention of complications from impaired elimination

   ○ **D.** Promotion of a positive body image

Quick Answer: **303**
Detailed Answer: **319**

143. When checking patellar reflexes, the nurse is unable to elicit a knee-jerk response. To facilitate checking the patellar reflex, the nurse should tell the client to:

   ○ **A.** Pull against her interlocked fingers

   ○ **B.** Shrug her shoulders and hold for a count of five

   ○ **C.** Close her eyes tightly and resist opening

   ○ **D.** Cross her legs at the ankles

Quick Answer: **303**
Detailed Answer: **319**

144. The nurse is performing a physical assessment on a newly admitted client. The last step in the physical assessment is:

   ○ **A.** Inspection

   ○ **B.** Auscultation

   ○ **C.** Percussion

   ○ **D.** Palpation

Quick Answer: **303**
Detailed Answer: **319**

145. A client with schizophrenia spends much of his time pacing the floor, rocking back and forth, and moving from one foot to another. The client's behaviors are an example of:

   ○ **A.** Dystonia

   ○ **B.** Tardive dyskinesia

   ○ **C.** Akathisia

   ○ **D.** Oculogyric crisis

Quick Answer: **303**
Detailed Answer: **319**

146. The nurse is assessing a recently admitted newborn. Which finding should be reported to the physician?

Quick Answer: **303**
Detailed Answer: **319**

- ○ **A.** The umbilical cord contains three vessels.
- ○ **B.** The newborn has a temperature of 98°F.
- ○ **C.** The feet and hands are bluish in color.
- ○ **D.** A large, soft swelling crosses the suture line.

147. Which statement is true regarding the infant's susceptibility to pertussis?

Quick Answer: **303**
Detailed Answer: **319**

- ○ **A.** If the mother had pertussis, the infant will have passive immunity.
- ○ **B.** Most infants and children are highly susceptible from birth.
- ○ **C.** The newborn will be immune to pertussis for the first few months of life.
- ○ **D.** Infants under one year of age seldom get pertussis.

148. A client in labor has been given epidural anesthesia with Marcaine (bupivacaine). To reverse the hypotension associated with epidural anesthesia, the nurse should have which medication available?

Quick Answer: **303**
Detailed Answer: **319**

- ○ **A.** Narcan (naloxone)
- ○ **B.** Dobutrex (dobutamine)
- ○ **C.** Romazicon (flumazenil)
- ○ **D.** Adrenalin (epinephrine)

149. The physician has prescribed Gantrisin (sulfasoxazole) 1gm in divided doses for a client with a urinary tract infection. The nurse should administer the medication:

Quick Answer: **303**
Detailed Answer: **319**

- ○ **A.** With meals or a snack
- ○ **B.** 30 minutes before meals
- ○ **C.** 30 minutes after meals
- ○ **D.** At bedtime

150. A client with a history of depression is treated with Parnate (tranylcypromine), an MAO inhibitor. Ingestion of foods containing tyramine while taking an MAO inhibitor can result in:

Quick Answer: **303**
Detailed Answer: **319**

- ○ **A.** Extreme elevations in blood pressure
- ○ **B.** Rapidly rising temperature
- ○ **C.** Abnormal movement and muscle spasms
- ○ **D.** Damage to the eighth cranial nerve

151. A client is admitted to the emergency room after falling down a flight of stairs. Initial assessment reveals a large bump on the front of the head and a two-inch laceration above the right eye. Which finding is consistent with injury to the frontal lobe?

- ○ **A.** Complaints of blindness
- ○ **B.** Decreased respiratory rate and depth
- ○ **C.** Failure to recognize touch
- ○ **D.** Inability to identify sweet taste

Quick Answer: **303**
Detailed Answer: **319**

152. The nurse is evaluating the intake and output of a client for the first 12 hours following an abdominal cholecystectomy. Which finding should be reported to the physician?

- ○ **A.** Output of 10mL from the Jackson-Pratt drain
- ○ **B.** Foley catheter output of 285mL
- ○ **C.** Nasogastric tube output of 150mL
- ○ **D.** Absence of stool

Quick Answer: **303**
Detailed Answer: **320**

153. A community health nurse is teaching healthful lifestyles to a group of senior citizens. The nurse knows that the leading cause of death in persons 65 and older is:

- ○ **A.** Chronic pulmonary disease
- ○ **B.** Diabetes mellitus
- ○ **C.** Pneumonia
- ○ **D.** Heart disease

Quick Answer: **303**
Detailed Answer: **320**

154. A client suspected of having Alzheimer's dementia is evaluated using the Mini-Mental State Examination. At the beginning of the evaluation, the examiner names three objects. Later in the evaluation, he asks the client to name the same three objects. The examiner is testing the client's:

- ○ **A.** Attention
- ○ **B.** Orientation
- ○ **C.** Recall
- ○ **D.** Registration

Quick Answer: **303**
Detailed Answer: **320**

155. A client with end stage renal disease is being managed with peritoneal dialysis. If the dialysate return is slowed the nurse should tell the client to:

Quick Answer: **303**
Detailed Answer: **320**

- ○ **A.** Irrigate the dialyzing catheter with saline.
- ○ **B.** Skip the next scheduled infusion.
- ○ **C.** Gently retract the dialyzing catheter.
- ○ **D.** Change position or turn side to side.

156. The nurse is the first person to arrive at the scene of a motor vehicle accident. When rendering aid to the victim, the nurse should give priority to:

Quick Answer: **303**
Detailed Answer: **320**

- ○ **A.** Establishing a patent airway
- ○ **B.** Checking the quality of respirations
- ○ **C.** Observing for signs of active bleeding
- ○ **D.** Determining the level of consciousness

157. A client hospitalized with renal calculi complains of severe pain in the right flank. In addition to complaints of pain, the nurse can expect to see changes in the client's vital signs that include:

Quick Answer: **303**
Detailed Answer: **320**

- ○ **A.** Decreased pulse rate
- ○ **B.** Increased blood pressure
- ○ **C.** Decreased respiratory rate
- ○ **D.** Increased temperature

158. The nurse is using the Glascow coma scale to assess the client's motor response. The nurse places pressure at the base of the client's fingernail for 20 seconds. The client's only response is withdrawal of his hand. The nurse interprets the client's response as:

Quick Answer: **303**
Detailed Answer: **320**

- ○ **A.** A score of 6 because he follows commands
- ○ **B.** A score of 5 because he localizes pain
- ○ **C.** A score of 4 because he uses flexion
- ○ **D.** A score of 3 because he uses extension

159. A four-year-old is admitted to the hospital for treatment of Kawasaki's disease. The medication commonly prescribed for the treatment of Kawasaki's disease is:

Quick Answer: **303**
Detailed Answer: **320**

- ○ **A.** Aspirin (acetylsalicylic acid)
- ○ **B.** Benadryl (diphenhydramine)
- ○ **C.** Polycillin (ampicillin)
- ○ **D.** Betaseron (interferon beta)

160. The nurse is caring for a client with bulimia nervosa. The nurse recognizes that the major difference in the client with anorexia nervosa and the client with bulimia nervosa is the client with bulimia:

   ○ **A.** Is usually grossly overweight.

   ○ **B.** Has a distorted body image.

   ○ **C.** Recognizes that she has an eating disorder.

   ○ **D.** Struggles with issues of dependence versus independence.

Quick Answer: **303**
Detailed Answer: **320**

161. The Mantoux text is used to determine whether a person has been exposed to tuberculosis. If the test is positive, the nurse will find a:

   ○ **A.** Fluid-filled vesicle

   ○ **B.** Sharply demarcated erythema

   ○ **C.** Central area of induration

   ○ **D.** Circular blanched area

Quick Answer: **303**
Detailed Answer: **320**

162. The physician has ordered continuous bladder irrigation for a client following a prostatectomy. The nurse should:

   ○ **A.** Hang the solution 2–3 feet above the client's abdomen.

   ○ **B.** Allow air from the solution tubing to flow into the catheter.

   ○ **C.** Use a clean technique when attaching the solution tubing to the catheter.

   ○ **D.** Clamp the solution tubing periodically to prevent bladder distention.

Quick Answer: **303**
Detailed Answer: **321**

163. A pediatric client is admitted to the hospital for treatment of diarrhea caused by an infection with salmonella. Which of the following most likely contributed to the child's illness?

   ○ **A.** Brushing the family dog

   ○ **B.** Playing with a turtle

   ○ **C.** Taking a pony ride

   ○ **D.** Feeding the family cat

Quick Answer: **303**
Detailed Answer: **321**

164. Which one of the following infants needs a further assessment of growth?

Quick Answer: **303**
Detailed Answer: **321**

- ○ **A.** Four-month-old: birth weight 7lb, 6oz; current weight 14lb, 4oz
- ○ **B.** Two-week-old: birth weight 6lb, 10oz; current weight 6lb, 12oz
- ○ **C.** Six-month-old: birth weight 8lb, 8oz; current weight 15lb
- ○ **D.** Two-month-old: birth weight 7lb, 2oz; current weight 9lb, 6oz

165. The physician has ordered Pyridium (phenazopyridine) for a client with urinary urgency. The nurse should tell the client that:

Quick Answer: **303**
Detailed Answer: **321**

- ○ **A.** The urine will have a strong odor of ammonia.
- ○ **B.** The urinary output will increase in amount.
- ○ **C.** The urine will have a red-orange color.
- ○ **D.** The urinary output will decrease in amount.

166. The nurse is teaching the mother of a six-month-old with eczema. Which instruction should be included in the nurse's teaching?

Quick Answer: **303**
Detailed Answer: **321**

- ○ **A.** Dress the infant warmly to prevent undue chilling.
- ○ **B.** Cut the infant's fingernails and toenails regularly.
- ○ **C.** Use bubble bath instead of soap for bathing the infant.
- ○ **D.** Wash the infant's clothes with mild detergent and fabric softener.

167. Skeletal traction is applied to the right femur of a client injured in a fall. The primary purpose of the skeletal traction is to:

Quick Answer: **303**
Detailed Answer: **321**

- ○ **A.** Realign the tibia and fibula.
- ○ **B.** Provide traction on the muscles.
- ○ **C.** Provide traction on the ligaments.
- ○ **D.** Realign femoral bone fragments.

168. The home health nurse is visiting a client with an exacerbation of rheumatoid arthritis. To prevent deformities of the knee joints, the nurse should:

Quick Answer: **303**
Detailed Answer: **321**

- ○ **A.** Tell the client to walk without bending the knees.
- ○ **B.** Encourage movement within the limits of pain.
- ○ **C.** Instruct the client to sit only in a recliner.
- ○ **D.** Tell the client to remain in bed as long as the joints are painful.

169. The physician has ordered Dextrose 5% in normal saline for an infant admitted with gastroenteritis. The advantage of administering the infant's IV through a scalp vein is:

Quick Answer: **303**
Detailed Answer: **321**

- ○ **A.** The infant can be held and comforted more easily.
- ○ **B.** Dextrose is best absorbed from the scalp veins.
- ○ **C.** Scalp veins do not infiltrate like peripheral veins.
- ○ **D.** There are few pain receptors in the infant's scalp.

170. A newborn diagnosed with bilateral choanal atresia is scheduled for surgery soon after delivery. The nurse recognizes the immediate need for surgery because the newborn:

Quick Answer: **303**
Detailed Answer: **321**

- ○ **A.** Will have difficulty swallowing
- ○ **B.** Will be unable to pass meconium
- ○ **C.** Will regurgitate his feedings
- ○ **D.** Will be unable to breathe through his nose

171. The most appropriate means of rehydration of a seven-month-old with diarrhea and mild dehydration is:

Quick Answer: **303**
Detailed Answer: **321**

- ○ **A.** Oral rehydration therapy with an electrolyte solution
- ○ **B.** Replacing milk-based formula with a lactose-free formula
- ○ **C.** Administering intraveneous Dextrose 5% ¼ normal saline
- ○ **D.** Offering bananas, rice, and applesauce along with oral fluids

172. The nurse is caring for an infant receiving intravenous fluid. Signs of fluid overload in an infant include:

Quick Answer: **303**
Detailed Answer: **322**

- ○ **A.** Swelling of the hands and increased temperature
- ○ **B.** Increased heart rate and increased blood pressure
- ○ **C.** Swelling of the feet and increased temperature
- ○ **D.** Decreased heart rate and decreased blood pressure

173. The nurse is providing care for a 10-month-old diagnosed with Wilms tumor. Most parents of infants with Wilms tumor report finding the mass when:

Quick Answer: **303**
Detailed Answer: **322**

- ○ **A.** The infant is diapered or bathed.
- ○ **B.** The infant is unable to use his arms.
- ○ **C.** The infant is unable to follow a moving object.
- ○ **D.** The infant is unable to vocalize sounds.

174. An obstetrical client has just been diagnosed with cardiac disease. The nurse should give priority to:

Quick Answer: **303**
Detailed Answer: **322**

- ○ **A.** Instructing the client to remain on strict bed rest
- ○ **B.** Telling the client to monitor her pulse and respirations
- ○ **C.** Instructing the client to check her temperature in the evening
- ○ **D.** Telling the client to weigh herself monthly

175. The nurse is caring for a client receiving supplemental oxygen. The effectiveness of the oxygen therapy is best determined by:

Quick Answer: **303**
Detailed Answer: **322**

- ○ **A.** The rate of respirations
- ○ **B.** The absence of cyanosis
- ○ **C.** Arterial blood gases
- ○ **D.** The level of consciousness

176. A client having a colonoscopy is medicated with Versed (midazolam). The nurse recognizes that the client:

Quick Answer: **303**
Detailed Answer: **322**

- ○ **A.** Will be able to remember the procedure within 2–3 hours
- ○ **B.** Will not be able to remember having the procedure done
- ○ **C.** Will be able to remember the procedure within 2–3 days
- ○ **D.** Will not be able to remember what occurred before the procedure

177. The nurse is assessing a client with an altered level of consciousness. One of the first signs of altered level of consciousness is:

Quick Answer: **303**
Detailed Answer: **322**

- ○ **A.** Inability to perform motor activities
- ○ **B.** Complaints of double vision
- ○ **C.** Restlessness
- ○ **D.** Unequal pupil size

178. Four clients are to receive medication. Which client should receive medication first?

Quick Answer: **303**
Detailed Answer: **322**

- ○ **A.** A client with an apical pulse of 72 receiving Lanoxin (digoxin) PO daily
- ○ **B.** A client with abdominal surgery receiving Phenergan (promethazine) IM every four hours PRN for nausea and vomiting
- ○ **C.** A client with labored respirations receiving a stat dose of IV Lasix (furosemide)
- ○ **D.** A client with pneumonia receiving Polycillin (ampicillin) IVPB every six hours

179. The nurse is caring for a cognitively impaired client who begins to pull at the tape securing his IV site. To lessen the likelihood of the client dislodging the IV, the nurse should:

Quick Answer: **303**
Detailed Answer: **322**

- ○ **A.** Place tape completely around the extremity, with taped ends out of the client's vision.
- ○ **B.** Tell him that if he pulls out the IV, it will have to be restarted.
- ○ **C.** Apply clove hitch restraints to the client's hands.
- ○ **D.** Wrap the IV site loosely with Kerlix to remove it from his site.

180. A client is admitted to the emergency room with complaints of substernal chest pain radiating to the left jaw. Which ECG finding is suggestive of acute myocardial infarction?

Quick Answer: **303**
Detailed Answer: **322**

- ○ **A.** Peaked P wave
- ○ **B.** Changes in ST segment
- ○ **C.** Minimal QRS wave
- ○ **D.** Prominent U wave

181. The nurse is assessing a client with a closed reduction of a fractured femur. Which finding should the nurse report to the physician?

Quick Answer: **303**
Detailed Answer: **322**

- ○ **A.** Chest pain and shortness of breath
- ○ **B.** Ecchymosis on the side of the injured leg
- ○ **C.** Oral temperature of 99.2°F
- ○ **D.** Complaints of level two pain on a scale of five

182. The physician has ordered a guaiac test for a client with a history of intestinal polyps. Which instruction should be given to the client regarding his diet prior to the test?

- ○ **A.** Increase the intake of whole grains and cereals.
- ○ **B.** Limit the intake of dairy products.
- ○ **C.** Avoid citrus juices and vitamin C.
- ○ **D.** Increase foods containing omega 3 oils.

Quick Answer: **303**
Detailed Answer: **323**

183. A client is admitted with a diagnosis of renal calculi. The nurse should give priority to:

- ○ **A.** Initiating an intravenous infusion
- ○ **B.** Encouraging oral fluids
- ○ **C.** Administering pain medication
- ○ **D.** Straining the urine

Quick Answer: **303**
Detailed Answer: **323**

184. The Joint Commission for Accreditation of Hospital Organizations (JCAHO) specifies that two client identifiers are to be used before administering medication. Which method is best for identifying patients using two patient identifiers?

- ○ **A.** Take the medication administration record (MAR) to the room and compare it with the name and medical number recorded on the armband.
- ○ **B.** Compare the medication administration record (MAR) with the client's room number and name on the armband.
- ○ **C.** Request that a family member identify the client and then ask the client to state his name.
- ○ **D.** Ask the client to state his full name and then to write his full name.

Quick Answer: **303**
Detailed Answer: **323**

185. A client complains of sharp, stabbing pain in the right lower quadrant that is graded as level 8 on a scale of 10. The nurse knows that pain of this severity can best be managed using:

- ○ **A.** Aleve (naproxen sodium)
- ○ **B.** Tylenol with codeine (acetaminophen with codeine)
- ○ **C.** Toradol (ketorolac)
- ○ **D.** Morphine sulfate (morphine sulfate)

Quick Answer: **303**
Detailed Answer: **323**

186. A client has had diarrhea for the past three days. Which acid/base imbalance would the nurse expect the client to have?

    ○ **A.** Respiratory alkalosis

    ○ **B.** Metabolic acidosis

    ○ **C.** Metabolic alkalosis

    ○ **D.** Respiratory acidosis

Quick Answer: **303**
Detailed Answer: **323**

187. The nurse is planning the diet of a client who is recovering from acute pancreatitis. The nurse should select foods that are

    ○ **A.** High in carbohydrate and protein

    ○ **B.** Low in sodium but high fat

    ○ **C.** High in protein and sodium

    ○ **D.** Low in fat and low protein

Quick Answer: **303**
Detailed Answer: **323**

188. The nurse is reviewing the lab reports of a client who is HIV positive. Which lab report provides information regarding the effectiveness of the client's medication regimen?

    ○ **A.** ELISA

    ○ **B.** Western Blot

    ○ **C.** Viral load

    ○ **D.** CD4 count

Quick Answer: **303**
Detailed Answer: **323**

189. A client taking antiretroviral drugs reports his last blood work showed a drop of 3 units in the viral load. The nurse understands that:

    ○ **A.** The virus is no longer detectable.

    ○ **B.** 90% of the viral load has been eliminated.

    ○ **C.** 95% of the viral load has been eliminated.

    ○ **D.** 99% of the viral load has been eliminated.

Quick Answer: **303**
Detailed Answer: **323**

190. The nurse is caring for a client with suspected AIDS dementia complex. The first sign of dementia in the client with AIDS is:

    ○ **A.** Changes in gait

    ○ **B.** Loss of concentration

    ○ **C.** Problems with speech

    ○ **D.** Seizures

Quick Answer: **303**
Detailed Answer: **324**

191. The physician has ordered Activase (alteplase) for a client admitted with a myocardial infarction. The desired effect of Activase is:

    ○ **A.** Prevention of congestive heart failure

    ○ **B.** Stabilization of the clot

    ○ **C.** Increased tissue oxygenation

    ○ **D.** Destruction of the clot

Quick Answer: **303**
Detailed Answer: **324**

192. The mother of a two-year-old asks the nurse when she should schedule her son's first dental visit. The nurse's response is based on the knowledge that most children have all their deciduous teeth by:

    ○ **A.** 15 months

    ○ **B.** 18 months

    ○ **C.** 24 months

    ○ **D.** 30 months

Quick Answer: **303**
Detailed Answer: **324**

193. The nurse is caring for a child with Down syndrome. Which characteristics are commonly found in the child with Down syndrome?

    ○ **A.** Fragile bones, blue sclera, and brittle teeth

    ○ **B.** Epicanthal folds, broad hands, and transpalmar creases

    ○ **C.** Low posterior hairline, webbed neck, and short stature

    ○ **D.** Developmental regression and cherry-red macula

Quick Answer: **303**
Detailed Answer: **324**

194. After several hospitalizations for respiratory ailments, a six-month-old has been diagnosed as having HIV. The infant's respiratory ailments were most likely due to:

    ○ **A.** Pneumocystis jiroveci

    ○ **B.** Cytomegalovirus

    ○ **C.** Cryptosporidiosis

    ○ **D.** Herpes simplex

Quick Answer: **303**
Detailed Answer: **324**

195. A client has returned from having a bronchoscopy. Before offering the client sips of water, the nurse should assess the client's:

    ○ **A.** Blood pressure

    ○ **B.** Pupilary response

    ○ **C.** Gag reflex

    ○ **D.** Pulse rate

Quick Answer: **303**
Detailed Answer: **324**

196. The physician has ordered injections of Neumega (oprelvekin) for a client receiving chemotherapy for prostate cancer. Which finding suggests that the medication is having its desired effect?

- ○ **A.** Hct 12.8g
- ○ **B.** Platelets 250,000mm^3
- ○ **C.** Neutrophils 4,000mm^3
- ○ **D.** RBC 4.7 million

197. A child suspected of having cystic fibrosis is scheduled for a quantitative sweat test. The nurse knows that the quantitative sweat test will be analyzed using:

- ○ **A.** Pilocarpine iontophoresis
- ○ **B.** Choloride iontophoresis
- ○ **C.** Sodium iontophoresis
- ○ **D.** Potassium iontophoresis

198. The nurse is caring for a client with a Brown-Sequard spinal cord injury. The nurse should expect the client to have:

- ○ **A.** Total loss of motor, sensory, and reflex activity
- ○ **B.** Incomplete loss of motor function
- ○ **C.** Loss of sensory function with potential for recovery
- ○ **D.** Loss of sensation on the side opposite the injury

199. A client with cirrhosis has developed signs of heptorenal syndrome. Which diet is most appropriate for the client at this time?

- ○ **A.** High protein, moderate sodium
- ○ **B.** High carbohydrate, moderate sodium
- ○ **C.** Low protein, low sodium
- ○ **D.** Low carbohydrate, high protein

200. The nurse is caring for a client with a basal cell epithelioma. The primary cause of basal cell epithelioma is:

- ○ **A.** Sun exposure
- ○ **B.** Smoking
- ○ **C.** Ingestion of alcohol
- ○ **D.** Food preservatives

201. A client with in situ bladder cancer is receiving intravesical therapy using BCG. During treatment, the nurse should

Quick Answer: **303**
Detailed Answer: **325**

- ○ **A.** Ask the client to remain still after the medication is instilled.
- ○ **B.** Offer the client additional oral fluids.
- ○ **C.** Ask the client to change positions every fifteen minutes.
- ○ **D.** Ask the client to void every hour.

202. A client is receiving a blood transfusion following surgery. In the event of a transfusion reaction, any unused blood should be:

Quick Answer: **303**
Detailed Answer: **325**

- ○ **A.** Sealed and discarded in a red bag
- ○ **B.** Flushed down the client's commode
- ○ **C.** Sealed and discarded in the sharp's container
- ○ **D.** Returned to the blood bank

203. The physician has ordered a trivalent botulism antitoxin for a client with botulism poisoning. Before administering the medication, the nurse should assess the client for a history of allergies to:

Quick Answer: **303**
Detailed Answer: **325**

- ○ **A.** Eggs
- ○ **B.** Horses
- ○ **C.** Shellfish
- ○ **D.** Pork

204. The physician has ordered increased oral hydration for a client with renal calculi. Unless contraindicated, the recommended oral intake for helping with the removal of renal calculi is:

Quick Answer: **303**
Detailed Answer: **325**

- ○ **A.** 75mL per hour
- ○ **B.** 100mL per hour
- ○ **C.** 150mL per hour
- ○ **D.** 200mL per hour

205. The nurse is caring for a client with acquired immunodeficiency syndrome who has oral candidiasis. The nurse should clean the client's mouth using:

Quick Answer: **303**
Detailed Answer: **325**

- ○ **A.** A toothbrush
- ○ **B.** A soft gauze pad
- ○ **C.** Antiseptic mouthwash
- ○ **D.** Lemon and glycerin swabs

206. A client taking anticoagulant medication has developed a cardiac tamponade. Which finding is associated with cardiac tamponade?

Quick Answer: **303**
Detailed Answer: **325**

- ○ **A.** A decrease in systolic blood pressure during inspiration
- ○ **B.** An increase in diastolic blood pressure during expiration
- ○ **C.** An increase in systolic blood pressure during inspiration
- ○ **D.** A decrease in diastolic blood pressure during expiration

207. The nurse is preparing a client for discharge following the removal of a cataract. The nurse should tell the client to:

Quick Answer: **303**
Detailed Answer: **325**

- ○ **A.** Take aspirin for discomfort
- ○ **B.** Avoid bending over to put on his shoes
- ○ **C.** Remove the eye shield before going to sleep
- ○ **D.** Continue showering as usual

208. The physician has ordered Pentam (pentamidine) IV for a client with pneumocystis jirovecki. While receiving the medication, the nurse should carefully monitor the client's:

Quick Answer: **303**
Detailed Answer: **325**

- ○ **A.** Blood pressure
- ○ **B.** Temperature
- ○ **C.** Heart rate
- ○ **D.** Respirations

209. Intra-arterial chemotherapy primarily benefits the client by applying greater concentrations of medication directly to the malignant tumor. An additional benefit of intra-arterial chemotherapy is:

Quick Answer: **303**
Detailed Answer: **325**

- ○ **A.** Prevention of nausea and vomiting
- ○ **B.** Treatment of micro-metastasis
- ○ **C.** Eradication of bone pain
- ○ **D.** Prevention of therapy-induced anemia

210. A client with rheumatoid arthritis is receiving injections of Myochrysine (gold sodium thiomalate). Before administering the client's medication, the nurse should:

Quick Answer: **303**
Detailed Answer: **325**

- ○ **A.** Check the lab work.
- ○ **B.** Administer an antiemetic.
- ○ **C.** Obtain the blood pressure.
- ○ **D.** Administer a sedative.

211. The nurse is caring for a client following a Whipple procedure. The nurse notes that the drainage from the nasogastric tube is bile tinged in appearance and has increased in the past hour. The nurse should:

- ○ **A.** Document the finding and continue to monitor the client.
- ○ **B.** Irrigate the drainage tube with 10mL of normal saline.
- ○ **C.** Decrease the amount of intermittent suction.
- ○ **D.** Notify the physician of the findings.

212. A client with AIDS tells the nurse that he regularly takes echinacea to boost his immune system. The nurse should tell the client that:

- ○ **A.** Herbals can interfere with the action of antiviral medication.
- ○ **B.** Supplements have proven effective in prolonging life.
- ○ **C.** Herbals have been shown to decrease the viral load.
- ○ **D.** Supplements appear to prevent replication of the virus.

213. A client with rheumatoid arthritis has Sjogren's syndrome. The nurse can help relieve the symptoms of Sjogren's syndrome by:

- ○ **A.** Providing heat to the joints
- ○ **B.** Instilling eyedrops
- ○ **C.** Administering pain medication
- ○ **D.** Providing small, frequent meals

214. Which one of the following symptoms is common in the client with duodenal ulcers?

- ○ **A.** Vomiting shortly after eating
- ○ **B.** Epigastric pain following meals
- ○ **C.** Frequent bouts of diarrhea
- ○ **D.** Presence of blood in the stools

215. A client with end-stage renal failure receives hemodialysis via an arteriovenous fistula (AV) placed in the right arm. When caring for the client, the nurse should:

- ○ **A.** Take the blood pressure in the right arm above the AV fistula.
- ○ **B.** Flush the AV fistula with IV normal saline to keep it patent.
- ○ **C.** Auscultate the AV fistula for the presence of a bruit.
- ○ **D.** Perform needed venopunctures distal to the AV fistula.

216. The nurse is reviewing the lab results of four clients. Which finding should be reported to the physician?

Quick Answer: **303**
Detailed Answer: **326**

- ○ **A.** A client with chronic renal failure with a serum creatinine of 5.6mg/dL
- ○ **B.** A client with rheumatic fever with a positive C reactive protein
- ○ **C.** A client with gastroenteritis with a hematocrit of 52%
- ○ **D.** A client with epilepsy with a white cell count of 3,800mm^3

217. The physician has prescribed a Becloforte (beclomethasone) inhaler two puffs twice a day for a client with asthma. The nurse should tell the client to report:

Quick Answer: **303**
Detailed Answer: **326**

- ○ **A.** Increased weight
- ○ **B.** A sore throat
- ○ **C.** Difficulty in sleeping
- ○ **D.** Changes in mood

218. A client treated for depression has developed symptoms of serotonin syndrome. The nurse recognizes that serotonin syndrome might result when the client takes both a prescribed antidepressant and

Quick Answer: **303**
Detailed Answer: **326**

- ○ **A.** St. John's wort
- ○ **B.** Ginko biloba
- ○ **C.** Black cohosh
- ○ **D.** Saw palmetto

219. The nurse is caring for a client following a transphenoidal hypophysectomy. Post-operatively, the nurse should:

Quick Answer: **303**
Detailed Answer: **327**

- ○ **A.** Provide the client a toothbrush for mouth care.
- ○ **B.** Check the nasal dressing for the "halo sign."
- ○ **C.** Tell the client to cough forcibly every two hours.
- ○ **D.** Ambulate the client when he is fully awake.

220. The physician has inserted an esophageal balloon tamponade in a client with bleeding esophageal varices. The nurse should maintain the esophageal balloon at a pressure of:

Quick Answer: **303**
Detailed Answer: **327**

- ○ **A.** 5–10mmHg
- ○ **B.** 10–15mmHg
- ○ **C.** 15–20mmHg
- ○ **D.** 20–25mmHg

221. The nurse is caring for a client with Lyme disease. The nurse should carefully monitor the client for signs of neurological complications, which include:

- ○ **A.** Complaints of a "drawing" sensation and paralysis on one side of the face
- ○ **B.** Presence of an unsteady gait, intention tremor, and facial weakness
- ○ **C.** Complaints of excruciating facial pain brought on by talking, smiling, or eating
- ○ **D.** Presence of fatigue when talking, dysphagia, and involuntary facial twitching

222. When caring for the child with autistic disorder, the nurse should:

- ○ **A.** Take the child to the playroom to be with peers.
- ○ **B.** Assign a consistent caregiver.
- ○ **C.** Place the child in a ward with other children.
- ○ **D.** Assign several staff members to provide care.

223. A client is admitted with suspected pernicious anemia. Which findings support the diagnosis of pernicious anemia?

- ○ **A.** The client complains of feeling tired and listless.
- ○ **B.** The client has waxy, pale skin.
- ○ **C.** The client exhibits loss of coordination and position sense.
- ○ **D.** The client has a rapid pulse rate and a detectable heart murmur.

224. The physician has prescribed Cyclogel (cyclopentolate hydrochloride) drops for a client following a scleral buckling. The nurse knows that the purpose of the medication is to:

- ○ **A.** Rest the muscles of accommodation
- ○ **B.** Prevent post-operative infection
- ○ **C.** Constrict the pupils
- ○ **D.** Reduce the production of aqueous humor

225. Which finding is associated with secondary syphilis?

- ○ **A.** Painless, papular lesions on the perineum, fingers, and eyelids
- ○ **B.** Absence of lesions
- ○ **C.** Deep asymmetrical granulomatous lesions
- ○ **D.** Well-defined generalized lesions on the palms, soles, and perineum

226. A client is transferred to the intensive care unit following a coronary artery bypass graft. Which one of the post-surgical assessments should be reported to the physician?

   - **A.** Urine output of 50ml in the past hour
   - **B.** Temperature of 99°F
   - **C.** Strong pedal pulses bilaterally
   - **D.** Central venous pressure 15mmH$_2$O

227. Which symptom is not associated with glaucoma?

   - **A.** Veil-like loss of vision
   - **B.** Foggy loss of vision
   - **C.** Seeing halos around lights
   - **D.** Complaints of eye pain

228. When caring for a ventilator-dependent client who is receiving tube feedings, the nurse can help prevent aspiration of gastric secretions by:

   - **A.** Keeping the head of the bed flat
   - **B.** Elevating the head of the bed 30–45°
   - **C.** Placing the client on his left side
   - **D.** Raising the foot of the bed 10–20°

229. When gathering evidence from a victim of rape, the nurse should place the victim's clothing in a:

   - **A.** Plastic zip-lock bag
   - **B.** Rubber tote
   - **C.** Paper bag
   - **D.** Padded manila envelope

230. The nurse on an orthopedic unit is assigned to care for four clients with displaced bone fractures. Which client will not be treated with the use of traction?

   - **A.** A client with fractures of the femur
   - **B.** A client with fractures of the cervical spine
   - **C.** A client with fractures of the humerus
   - **D.** A client with fractures of the ankle

231. A client is hospitalized with an acute myocardial infarction. Which nursing diagnosis reflects an understanding of the cause of acute myocardial infarction?

Quick Answer: **303**
Detailed Answer: **328**

   ○ **A.** Decreased cardiac output related to damage to the myocardium

   ○ **B.** Impaired tissue perfusion related to an occlusion in the coronary vessels

   ○ **C.** Acute pain related to cardiac ischemia

   ○ **D.** Ineffective breathing patterns related to decreased oxygen to the tissues

232. The nurse in the emergency department is responsible for the triage of four recently admitted clients. Which client should the nurse send directly to the treatment room?

Quick Answer: **303**
Detailed Answer: **328**

   ○ **A.** A 23-year-old female complaining of headache and nausea

   ○ **B.** A 76-year-old male complaining of dysuria

   ○ **C.** A 56-year-old male complaining of exertional short-ness of breath

   ○ **D.** A 42-year-old female complaining of recent sexual assault

233. The physician has ordered an injection of morphine for a client with post-operative pain. Before administering the medication, it is essential that the nurse assess the client's:

Quick Answer: **303**
Detailed Answer: **328**

   ○ **A.** Heart rate

   ○ **B.** Respirations

   ○ **C.** Temperature

   ○ **D.** Blood pressure

234. The nurse is caring for a client with a closed head injury. A late sign of increased intracranial pressure is:

Quick Answer: **303**
Detailed Answer: **328**

   ○ **A.** Changes in pupil equality and reactivity

   ○ **B.** Restlessness and irritability

   ○ **C.** Complaints of headache

   ○ **D.** Nausea and vomiting

235. The newly licensed nurse has been asked to perform a procedure that he feels unqualified to perform. The nurse's best response at this time is to:

- ○ **A.** Attempt to perform the procedure.
- ○ **B.** Refuse to perform the procedure and give a reason for the refusal.
- ○ **C.** Request to observe a similar procedure and then attempt to complete the procedure.
- ○ **D.** Agree to perform the procedure if the client is willing.

Quick Answer: **303**
Detailed Answer: **328**

236. A client is admitted to the emergency department with complaints of crushing chest pain that radiates to the left jaw. After obtaining a stat electrocardiogram the nurse should:

- ○ **A.** Obtain a history of prior cardiac problems
- ○ **B.** Begin an IV using a large-bore catheter
- ○ **C.** Administer oxygen at 2L per minute via nasal cannula
- ○ **D.** Perform pupil checks for size and reaction to light

Quick Answer: **303**
Detailed Answer: **328**

237. Which of the following techniques is recommended for removing a tick from the skin?

- ○ **A.** Grasping the tick with a tissue and quickly jerking it away from the skin
- ○ **B.** Placing a burning match close the tick and watching for it to release
- ○ **C.** Using tweezers, grasp the tick close to the skin and pull the tick free using a steady, firm motion
- ○ **D.** Covering the tick with petroleum jelly and gently rubbing the area until the tick releases

Quick Answer: **303**
Detailed Answer: **328**

238. A nurse is observing a local softball game when one of the players is hit in the nose with a ball. The player's nose is visibly deformed and bleeding. The best way for the nurse to control the bleeding is to:

- ○ **A.** Tilt the head back and pinch the nostrils.
- ○ **B.** Apply a wrapped ice compress to the nose.
- ○ **C.** Pack the nose with soft, clean tissue.
- ○ **D.** Tilt the head forward and pinch the nostrils.

Quick Answer: **303**
Detailed Answer: **329**

239. What is the responsibility of the nurse in obtaining an informed consent for surgery?

  ○ **A.** Describing in a clear and simply stated manner what the surgery will involve

  ○ **B.** Explaining the benefits, alternatives, and possible risks and complications of surgery

  ○ **C.** Using the nurse/client relationship to persuade the client to sign the operative permit

  ○ **D.** Providing the informed consent for surgery and witnessing the client's signature

Quick Answer: **303**
Detailed Answer: **329**

240. During the change of shift report, the nurse states that the client's last pulse strength was a 1+. The oncoming nurse recognizes that the client's pulse was:

  ○ **A.** Bounding

  ○ **B.** Full

  ○ **C.** Normal

  ○ **D.** Weak

Quick Answer: **303**
Detailed Answer: **329**

241. The RN is making assignments for the day. Which one of the following duties can be assigned to the unlicensed assistive personnel?

  ○ **A.** Notifying the physician of an abnormal lab value

  ○ **B.** Providing routine catheter care with soap and water

  ○ **C.** Administering two aspirin to a client with a headache

  ○ **D.** Setting the rate of an infusion of normal saline

Quick Answer: **303**
Detailed Answer: **329**

242. The nurse is observing the respirations of a client when she notes that the respiratory cycle is marked by periods of apnea lasting from 10 seconds to one minute. The apnea is followed by respirations that gradually increase in depth and frequency. The nurse should document that the client is experiencing:

  ○ **A.** Cheyne-Stokes respirations

  ○ **B.** Kussmaul respirations

  ○ **C.** Biot respirations

  ○ **D.** Diaphragmatic respirations

Quick Answer: **303**
Detailed Answer: **329**

243. A client seen in the doctor's office for complaints of nausea and vomiting is sent home with directions to follow a clear-liquid diet for the next 24–48 hours. Which of the following is not permitted on a clear-liquid diet?

- ○ **A.** Sweetened tea
- ○ **B.** Chicken broth
- ○ **C.** Ice cream
- ○ **D.** Orange gelatin

244. When administering a tuberculin skin test, the nurse should insert the needle at a:

- ○ **A.** 15° angle
- ○ **B.** 30° angle
- ○ **C.** 45° angle
- ○ **D.** 90° angle

245. The nurse is preparing to discharge a client following a trabeculo-plasty for the treatment of glaucoma. The nurse should instruct the client to:

- ○ **A.** Wash her eyes with baby shampoo and water twice a day
- ○ **B.** Take only tub baths for the first month following surgery
- ○ **C.** Begin using her eye makeup again one week after surgery
- ○ **D.** Wear eye protection for several months after surgery

246. Which type of endotracheal tube is recommended by the Centers for Disease Control (CDC) for reducing the risk of ventilator-associated pneumonia?

- ○ **A.** Uncuffed
- ○ **B.** CASS
- ○ **C.** Fenestrated
- ○ **D.** Nasotracheal

247. Which client is at greatest risk for complications following abdominal surgery?

Quick Answer: **303**
Detailed Answer: **330**

- ○ **A.** A 68-year-old obese client with non-insulin-dependent diabetes
- ○ **B.** A 27-year-old client with a recent history of urinary tract infections
- ○ **C.** A 16-year-old client who smokes a half-pack of cigarettes per day
- ○ **D.** A 40-year-old client who exercises regularly, with no history of medical conditions

248. The nurse is preparing a client for surgery. Which lab finding should be reported to the physician?

Quick Answer: **303**
Detailed Answer: **330**

- ○ **A.** Potassium 2.5mEq/L
- ○ **B.** Hemoglobin 14.5g/dL
- ○ **C.** Blood glucose 75mg/dL
- ○ **D.** White cell count 8,000mm^3

249. A client is diagnosed with bleeding from the upper gastrointestinal system. The nurse would expect the client's stools to be:

Quick Answer: **303**
Detailed Answer: **330**

- ○ **A.** Brown
- ○ **B.** Black
- ○ **C.** Clay colored
- ○ **D.** Green

250. In order to reduce the risk of hypotension and "red man syndrome" infusions of Vancocin (vancomycin) should be administered:

Quick Answer: **303**
Detailed Answer: **330**

- ○ **A.** Within 15 minutes
- ○ **B.** Only after giving Benadryl (diphenhydramine)
- ○ **C.** Over one hour
- ○ **D.** With Zantac (ranitidine) or other histamine blocker

Quick Answers

1. B	32. B	63. B	94. C
2. D	33. A	64. B	95. A
3. A	34. B	65. B	96. A
4. D	35. A	66. D	97. A
5. B	36. C	67. A	98. C
6. B	37. A	68. D	99. C
7. B	38. B	69. C	100. A
8. C	39. C	70. A	101. D
9. A	40. A	71. C	102. D
10. A	41. D	72. D	103. C
11. D	42. A	73. A	104. C
12. B	43. B	74. A	105. D
13. D	44. A	75. D	106. B
14. D	45. B	76. B	107. B
15. B	46. B	77. A	108. D
16. A	47. C	78. A	109. B
17. B	48. C	79. B	110. A
18. C	49. B	80. C	111. C
19. C	50. A	81. D	112. B
20. C	51. B	82. B	113. D
21. D	52. A	83. A	114. B
22. A	53. D	84. B	115. A
23. B	54. A	85. C	116. B
24. A	55. B	86. B	117. C
25. C	56. B	87. B	118. A
26. B	57. A	88. B	119. B
27. A	58. C	89. B	120. A
28. B	59. D	90. C	121. B
29. C	60. B	91. B	122. A
30. D	61. D	92. A	123. A
31. A	62. B	93. D	124. D

125. B	157. B	189. D	221. A
126. B	158. C	190. B	222. B
127. A	159. A	191. D	223. C
128. B	160. C	192. D	224. A
129. A	161. C	193. B	225. D
130. C	162. A	194. A	226. D
131. D	163. B	195. C	227. A
132. B	164. B	196. B	228. B
133. D	165. C	197. A	229. C
134. A	166. B	198. D	230. D
135. C	167. D	199. C	231. B
136. A	168. B	200. A	232. D
137. C	169. A	201. C	233. B
138. D	170. D	202. D	234. A
139. B	171. A	203. B	235. B
140. D	172. B	204. D	236. C
141. A	173. A	205. B	237. C
142. C	174. B	206. A	238. B
143. A	175. C	207. B	239. D
144. B	176. B	208. A	240. D
145. C	177. C	209. B	241. B
146. D	178. C	210. A	242. A
147. B	179. D	211. D	243. C
148. D	180. B	212. A	244. A
149. B	181. A	213. B	245. D
150. A	182. C	214. D	246. B
151. C	183. A	215. C	247. A
152. B	184. A	216. D	248. A
153. D	185. D	217. B	249. B
154. C	186. B	218. A	250. C
155. D	187. D	219. B	
156. A	188. C	220. D	

Answers and Rationales

1. **Answer B is correct.** The nurse should check the client's immunization record to determine the date of the last tetanus immunization. The nurse should question the client regarding allergies to medications before administering medication; therefore, answer A is incorrect. Answer C is incorrect because a sling, not a splint, should be applied to immobilize the arm and prevent dependent edema. Answer D is incorrect because pain medication would be given before cleaning and dressing the wound, not afterward.

2. **Answer D is correct.** Watery vaginal discharge and painless bleeding are associated with endometrial cancer. Frothy vaginal discharge describes trichomonas infection; thick, white vaginal discharge describes infection with candida albicans; and purulent vaginal discharge describes pelvic inflammatory disease. Therefore, answers A, B, and C are incorrect.

3. **Answer A is correct.** Stereotactic surgery destroys areas of the brain responsible for intractable tremors. The surgery does not increase production of dopamine, making answer B incorrect. Answer C is incorrect because the client will continue to need medication. Serotonin production is not associated with Parkinson's disease; therefore, answer D is incorrect.

4. **Answer D is correct.** The client with AIDS should not drink water that has been sitting longer than 15 minutes because of bacterial contamination. Answer A is incorrect because ice water is not better for the client. Answer B is incorrect because juices should not replace water intake. Answer C is not an accurate statement.

5. **Answer B is correct.** The finding that differentiates interstitial cystitis from other forms of cystitis is the absence of bacteria in the urine. Answer A is incorrect because symptoms that include burning and pain on urination characterize all forms of cystitis. Answer C is incorrect because blood in the urine is a characteristic of interstitial as well as other forms of cystitis. Answer D is an incorrect statement because females are affected more often than males.

6. **Answer B is correct.** Approximately 99% of males with cystic fibrosis are sterile due to obstruction of the vas deferens. Answers A, C, and D are incorrect because most males with cystic fibrosis are incapable of reproduction.

7. **Answer B is correct.** Infants under the age of two years should not be fed honey because of the danger of infection with *Clostridium botulinum.* Answers A, C, and D are not related to the situation; therefore, they are incorrect.

8. **Answer C is correct.** Children with autistic disorder engage in ritualistic behaviors and are easily upset by changes in daily routine. Changes in the environment are usually met with behaviors that are difficult to control. Answers A, B, and D are incorrect because they do not focus on autistic disorder.

9. **Answer A is correct.** The degree of pulmonary involvement is the greatest determinant in the prognosis of cystic fibrosis. Answers B, C, and D are affected by cystic fibrosis; however, they are not major determinants of the prognosis of the disease.

10. **Answer A is correct.** Decreased blood pressure and increased pulse rate are associated with bleeding and shock. Answers B, C, and D are within normal limits; thus, incorrect.

11. **Answer D is correct.** Early decelerations during the second stage of labor are benign and are the result of fetal head compression that occurs during normal contractions. No action is necessary other than documenting the finding on the flow sheet. Answers A, B, and C are interventions for the client with late decelerations, which reflect ureteroplacental insufficiency.

12. **Answer B is correct.** The client's statement that meat should be thoroughly cooked to the appropriate temperature indicates an understanding of the nurse's teaching regarding food preparation. Undercooked meat is a source of toxoplasmosis cysts. Toxoplasmosis is a major cause of encephalitis in clients with AIDS. Answer A is incorrect because fresh-ground pepper contains bacteria that can cause illness in the client with AIDS. Answer C is an incorrect choice because cheese contains molds and yogurt contains live cultures that the client with AIDS must avoid. Answer D is incorrect because fresh fruit and vegetables contain microscopic organisms that can cause illness in the client with AIDS.

13. **Answer D is correct.** The client taking isoniazid should have a negative sputum culture within three months. Continued positive cultures reflect noncompliance with therapy or the development of strains resistant to the medication. Answers A, B, and C are incorrect because there has not been sufficient time for the medication to be effective.

14. **Answer D is correct.** Lyme disease is transmitted by ticks found on deer and mice in wooded areas. The people in answers A and B have little risk of the disease. Veterinarians are exposed to dog ticks, which carry Rocky Mountain Spotted Fever, so answer C is incorrect.

15. **Answer B is correct.** Children ages 18–24 months normally have sufficient sphincter control necessary for toilet training. Answer A is incorrect because the child is not developmentally capable of toilet training. Answers C and D are incorrect choices because toilet training should already be established.

16. **Answer A is correct.** The priority nursing diagnosis is risk for deficient fluid volume related to excessive fluid loss from the ostomy. The client with a new ileostomy might experience a high volume output of 1000–1800mL per day when peristalsis returns. The client needs to increase fluid intake to 2–3 liters a day. Fluid intake should include sports drinks to help replenish sodium and potassium lost in the ileostomy output. Answers B, C, and D apply to clients with an ileostomy, but they do not take priority over the risk for deficient fluid volume; therefore, they are incorrect.

17. **Answer B is correct.** Cobex is an injectable form of cyanocobalamin or vitamin B12. Increased Hgb levels reflect the effectiveness of the medication. Answers A, C, and D do not reflect the effectiveness of the medication; therefore, they are incorrect.

18. **Answer C is correct.** Behavior modification relies on the principles of operant conditioning. Tokens or rewards are given for appropriate behavior. Answers A and B are incorrect because they refer to techniques used to reduce anxiety, such as thought stopping and bioenergetic techniques, respectively. Answer D is incorrect because it refers to modeling.

19. **Answer C is correct.** Small pieces of cereal promote chewing and are easily managed by the toddler. Pieces of hot dog, carrot sticks, and raisins are unsuitable for the toddler because of the risk of aspiration.

20. **Answer C is correct.** Complications of TPN therapy are osmotic diuresis and hypovolemia. Answer A is incorrect because the intake and output would not reflect metabolic rate. Answer B is incorrect because the client is most likely receiving no oral fluids. Answer D is incorrect because the complication of TPN therapy is hypovolemia, not hypervolemia.

21. **Answer D is correct.** L/S ratios are an indicator of fetal lung maturity. Answer A is incorrect because it is the diagnostic test for neural tube defects. Answer B is incorrect because it measures fetal well-being. Answer C is incorrect because it detects circulating antibodies against red blood cells.

22. **Answer A is correct.** By the third postpartum day, the fundus should be located three finger widths below the umbilicus. Answer B is incorrect because the discharge would be light in amount. Answer C is incorrect because the fundus is not even with the umbilicus at three days. Answer D is incorrect because the uterus is not enlarged.

23. **Answer B is correct.** Rapid discontinuation of TPN can result in hypoglycemia. Answer A is incorrect because rapid infusion of TPN results in hyperglycemia. Answer C is incorrect because TPN is administered through a central line. Answer D is incorrect because the infusion is administered with a filter.

24. **Answer A is correct.** Kava-kava can increase the effects of anesthesia and postoperative analgesia. Answers B, C, and D are not related to the use of kava-kava; therefore, they are incorrect.

25. **Answer C is correct.** The maximum recommended rate of an intravenous infusion of potassium chloride is 5–10mEq per hour, never to exceed 20mEq per hour. An intravenous infusion controller is always used to regulate the flow. Answer A is incorrect because potassium chloride is not given IV push. Answer B is incorrect because the infusion time is too brief. Answer D is incorrect because the infusion time is excessive.

26. **Answer B is correct.** The normal platelet count is 150,000–400,000; therefore, the client is at high risk for spontaneous bleeding. Answer A is incorrect because the WBC is a low normal; therefore, overwhelming infection is not a risk at this time. The RBC is low, but anemia at this point is not life threatening; therefore, answer C is incorrect. Answer D is incorrect because the serum creatinine is within normal limits.

27. **Answer A is correct.** Cardiac toxicity including delayed congestive heart failure, ventricular arrhythmias, and acute left ventricular failure are adverse effects of Adriamycin. Alopecia, leukopenia, and stomatitis are side effects of the medication; therefore, Answers B, C, and D are incorrect.

28. **Answer B is correct.** The client will have a urinary catheter inserted to keep the bladder empty during radiation therapy. Answer A is incorrect because visitors are allowed to see the client for short periods of time, as long as they maintain a distance of six feet from the client. Answer C is incorrect because the client is on bed rest. Side effects from radiation therapy include pain, nausea, vomiting, and dehydration; therefore, answer D is incorrect.

29. **Answer C is correct.** The mother does not need to place an external heat source near the newborn. It will not promote healing, and there is a chance that the newborn could be burned, so the mother needs further teaching. Answers A, B, and D indicate correct understanding of the care of the newborn who has been circumcised and are incorrect choices.

30. **Answer D is correct.** A sputum specimen for culture and sensitivity should be obtained before the antibiotic is administered to determine whether the organism is sensitive to the prescribed medication. A routine urinalysis, complete blood count, and serum electrolytes can be obtained after the medication is initiated; therefore, answers A, B, and C are incorrect.

31. **Answer A is correct.** Ginkgo interacts with many medications to increase the risk of bleeding; therefore, bruising or bleeding should be reported to the doctor. Photosensitivity is not a side effect of ginkgo; therefore, answer B is incorrect. Answer C is incorrect because the FDA does not regulate herbals and natural products. The client does not need to take additional vitamin E, so answer D is incorrect.

32. **Answer B is correct.** The client should be well hydrated before and during treatment to prevent nephrotoxicity. The client should be encouraged to drink 2,000–3,000mL of fluid a day to promote excretion of uric acid. Answer A is incorrect because it does not prevent nephrotoxicity. Answer C is incorrect because the intake and output should be recorded hourly. Answer D is incorrect because it refers to ototoxicity, which is also an adverse side effect of the medication but is not accurate for this stem.

33. **Answer A is correct.** The client who is colonized with MRSA will have no symptoms associated with infection. Answer B is incorrect because the client is more likely to develop an infection with MRSA following invasive procedures. Answer C is incorrect because the client should not be placed in the room with others. Answer D is incorrect because the client can colonize others, including healthcare workers, with MRSA.

34. **Answer B is correct.** The therapeutic range for vancomycin is 10–25mcg/mL. Answer A is incorrect because the range is too low to be therapeutic. Answers C and D are incorrect because they are too high.

35. **Answer A is correct.** Pseudomembranous colitis resulting from infection with *Clostridium difficile* produces diarrhea containing blood, mucus, and white blood cells. Answers B, C, and D are incorrect because they are not specific to infection with *Clostridium difficile*.

36. **Answer C is correct.** Pyridoxine (vitamin B6) is usually administered with INH (isoniazid) in order to prevent nervous system side effects. Answers A, B, and D are not associated with the use of INH; therefore, they are incorrect choices.

37. **Answer A is correct.** Factors associated with the development of Legionnaires' disease include immunosuppression, advanced age, alcoholism, and pulmonary disease. Answer B is incorrect because it is associated with the development of SARS. Answer C is associated with food-borne illness, not Legionnaires' disease, and answer D is not related to the question.

38. **Answer B is correct.** The client can check the inhaler by dropping it into a container of water. If the inhaler is half full, it will float upside down with one-fourth of the container remaining above the water line. Answers A, C, and D do not help determine the amount of medication remaining; therefore, they are incorrect.

39. **Answer C is correct.** Following a nephrolithotomy, the client should be positioned on the unoperative side. Answers A, B, and D are incorrect positions for the client following a right nephrolithotomy.

40. **Answer A is correct.** The client with sickle cell crisis and sequestration can be expected to have signs of hypovolemia, including decreased blood pressure. Answer B is incorrect because the client would have dry mucus membranes. Answer C is incorrect because the client would have increased respirations because of pain associated with sickle cell crisis. Answer D is incorrect because the client's blood pressure would be decreased.

41. **Answer D is correct.** The first sign of latex allergy is usually contact dermatitis, which includes swelling and itching of the hands. Answers A, B, and C can also occur but are not the first signs of latex allergy.

42. **Answer A is correct.** The nurse caring for the client with disseminated herpes zoster (shingles) should use airborne precautions as outlined by the CDC. Answer B is incorrect because precautions are needed to prevent transmission of the disease. Answers C and D are incorrect because airborne precautions are used, not contact or droplet precautions.

43. **Answer B is correct.** Acticoat, a commercially prepared dressing, should be moistened with sterile water. Answers A and C are incorrect because Acticoat dressings remain in place up to five days. Answer D is incorrect because normal saline should not be used to moisten the dressing.

44. **Answer A is correct.** The presence of a white or gray dot (a cat's eye reflex) in the pupil is associated with retinoblastoma, a highly malignant tumor of the eye. The nurse should report the finding to the physician immediately so that it can be further evaluated. Simply recording the finding can delay diagnosis and treatment; therefore, answer B is incorrect. Answer C is incorrect because it is not a variation of normal. Answer D is incorrect because the presence of the red reflex is a normal finding.

45. **Answer B is correct.** Stage II indicates that multiple lymph nodes or organs are involved on the same side of the diaphragm. Answer A refers to stage I Hodgkin's lymphoma, answer C refers to stage III Hodgkin's lymphoma, and answer D refers to stage IV Hodgkin's lymphoma.

46. **Answer B is correct.** The client taking methotrexate should avoid multivitamins because multivitamins contain folic acid. Methotrexate is a folic acid antagonist. Answers A and D are incorrect because aspirin and acetaminophen are given to relieve pain and inflammation associated with rheumatoid arthritis. Answer C is incorrect because omega 3 and omega 6 fish oils have proven beneficial for the client with rheumatoid arthritis.

47. **Answer C is correct.** Fried foods are not permitted on a low-residue diet. Answers A, B, and D are all allowed on a low-residue diet and, therefore, are incorrect.

48. **Answer C is correct.** The client with cirrhosis and abdominal ascites requires additional protein and calories. (Note: if the ammonia level increases, protein intake should be restricted or eliminated.) Answer A is incorrect because the client needs a low-sodium diet. Answer B is incorrect because the client does not need to increase his intake of potassium. Answer D is incorrect because the client does not need additional fat.

49. **Answer B is correct.** The most common symptom reported by clients with multiple sclerosis is double vision. Answers A, C, and D are not symptoms commonly reported by clients with multiple sclerosis, so they are wrong.

50. **Answer A is correct.** Common sources of *E. coli* are undercooked beef and shellfish. Answers B, C, and D are incorrect because they are not sources of *E. coli*.

51. **Answer B is correct.** St. John's wort has properties similar to those of monoamine oxidase inhibitors (MAOI). Eating foods high in tryramine (example: aged cheese, chocolate, salami, liver) can result in a hypertensive crisis. Answer A is incorrect because it can relieve mild to moderate depression. Answer C is incorrect because use of a sunscreen prevents skin reactions to sun exposure. Answer D is incorrect because St. John's wort should not be used with MAOI antidepressants.

52. **Answer A is correct.** Foods high in purine include dried beans, peas, spinach, oatmeal, poultry, fish, liver, lobster, and oysters. Answers B, C, and D are incorrect because they are low in purine. Other sources low in purine include most vegetables, milk, and gelatin.

53. **Answer D is correct.** The nurse should tell the client to avoid bearing weight on the axilla when using crutches because it can result in nerve damage. Answer A is incorrect because the finger width between the axilla and the crutch is appropriate. Answer B is incorrect because the client should bear weight on his hands when ambulating with crutches. Answer C is incorrect because it describes the correct use of the four-point gait.

54. **Answer A is correct.** By writing down her suspicions, the nurse leaves herself open for a suit of libel, a defamatory tort that discloses a privileged communication and leads to a lowering of opinion of the client. Defamatory torts include libel and slander. Libel is a written statement, whereas slander is an oral statement. Thus, answer B is incorrect because it involves oral statements. Malpractice is an unreasonable lack of skill in performing professional duties that result in injury or death; therefore, answer C is incorrect. Negligence is an act of omission or commission that results in injury to a person or property, making answer D incorrect.

55. **Answer B is correct.** The client with bulimia is prone to tooth erosion and dental caries caused by frequent bouts of self-induced vomiting. Answers A, C, and D are findings associated with anorexia nervosa, not bulimia, and are incorrect.

56. **Answer B is correct.** Antacids should not be taken within two hours of taking digoxin; therefore, the nurse needs to do additional teaching regarding the client's medication. Answers A, C, and D are true statements indicating that the client understands the nurse's teaching, so they are incorrect.

57. **Answer A is correct.** Fever, sore throat, and weakness need to be reported immediately. Adverse reactions to Thorazine include agranulocytosis, which makes the client vulnerable to overwhelming infection. Answers B, C, and D are expected side effects that occur with the use of Thorazine; therefore, it is not necessary to notify the doctor immediately.

58. **Answer C is correct.** The anterior approach for cervical discectomy lends itself to covert bleeding. The nurse should pay particular attention to bleeding coming from the mouth. Answer A is incorrect because bleeding will be obvious on the surgical dressing. Answer B is incorrect because complaints of neck pain are expected and will be managed by the use of analgesics. Answer D is incorrect because swelling in the posterior neck can be expected. The nurse should observe for swelling in the anterior neck as well as changes in voice quality, which can indicate swelling of the airway.

59. **Answer D is correct.** The assessment suggests the presence of a diaphragmatic hernia. The newborn should be positioned on the left side with the head and chest elevated. This position will allow the lung on the right side to fully inflate. Supplemental oxygen for newborns is not provided by mask; therefore, answer A is incorrect. Answer B is incorrect because bowel sounds would not be heard in the abdomen since abdominal contents occupy the chest cavity in the newborn with diaphragmatic hernia. Inserting a nasogastric tube to check for esophageal patency refers to the newborn with esophageal atresia; therefore, answer C is incorrect.

60. **Answer B is correct.** It takes 1–2 weeks for mood stabilizers to achieve a therapeutic effect; therefore, antipsychotic medications can also be used during the first few days or weeks to manage behavioral excitement. Answers A and D are not true statements and, therefore, are incorrect. Answer C is incorrect because the combination of medications will not allow for hypomania.

61. **Answer D is correct.** The nurse should first provide for the client's safety, including protecting her from an embarrassing situation. Answer A is incorrect because it allows the client to continue unacceptable behavior. Answer B is incorrect because it does not stop the client's behavior. Answer C is incorrect because it focuses on the other clients, not the client with inappropriate behavior.

62. **Answer B is correct.** According to the Denver Developmental Assessment, a four-year-old should be able to state his first and last name. Answers A and C are expected abilities of a five-year-old, and answer D is an expected ability of a five- and six-year-old.

63. **Answer B is correct.** The mother's statement reflects the stress placed on her by her daughter's chronic mental illness. Answer A is incorrect because there is no indication of ineffective family coping. Answer C is incorrect because it is not the most appropriate nursing diagnosis. Answer D is incorrect because there is no indication of altered parenting.

64. **Answer B is correct.** Clients with anorexia nervosa have problems with developing self-identity. They are often described by others as "passive," "perfect," and "introverted." Poor self-identity and low self-esteem lead to feelings of personal ineffectiveness. Answer A is incorrect because she will choose only low-calorie food items. Answer C is incorrect because the client with anorexia is restricted from exercising because it promotes weight loss. Placement in a private room increases the likelihood that the client will continue activities that prevent weight gain; therefore, answer D is incorrect.

65. **Answer B is correct.** The nursing assistant has skills suited to assisting the client with activities of daily living, such as bathing and grooming. Answer A is incorrect because the nurse should monitor the client's vital signs. Answer C is incorrect because the client will have an induced generalized seizure, and the nurse should monitor the client's response before, during, and after the procedure. Answer D is incorrect because staff does not remain in the room with a client in seclusion; only the nurse should monitor clients who are in seclusion.

66. **Answer D is correct.** Transderm Nitro is a reservoir patch that releases the medication via a semipermeable membrane. Cutting the patch allows too much of the drug to be released. Answer A is incorrect because the area should not be shaved; this can cause skin irritation. Answer B is incorrect because the skin is cleaned with soap and water. Answer C is incorrect because the patch should not be covered with plastic wrap because it can cause the medication to absorb too rapidly.

67. **Answer A is correct.** Cholinergic crisis is the result of overmedication with anti-cholinesterase inhibitors. Symptoms of cholinergic crisis are nausea, vomiting, diarrhea, blurred vision, pallor, decreased blood pressure, and constricted pupils. Answers B, C, and D are incorrect because they are symptoms of myasthenia crisis, which is the result of undermedication with cholinesterase inhibitors.

68. **Answer D is correct.** The client should avoid eating American and processed cheeses, such as Colby and Cheddar, because they are high in sodium. Dried beans, peanut butter, and Swiss cheese are low in sodium; therefore, answers A, B, and C are incorrect.

69. **Answer C is correct.** According to the Rule of Nines, the arm (9%) + the trunk (36%) = 45% TBSA burn injury. Answers A, B, and D are inaccurate calculations for the TBSA.

70. **Answer A is correct.** The client should void before the paracentesis to prevent accidental trauma to the bladder. Answer B is incorrect because the abdomen is not shaved. Answer C is incorrect because the client does not need extra fluids, which would cause bladder distention. Answer D is incorrect because the physician, not the nurse, would request an ultrasound, if needed.

71. **Answer C is correct.** Rice cereal, mashed ripe bananas, and strained carrots are appropriate foods for an eight-month-old infant. Answer A is incorrect because the cocoa-flavored cereal contains chocolate and sugar, orange juice is too acidic for the infant, and strained meat is difficult to digest. Answer B is incorrect because graham crackers contain wheat flour and sugar. Pudding contains sugar and additives unsuitable for the eight-month-old. Answer D is incorrect because whole milk is not given before the age of one year.

72. **Answer D is correct.** A battery-operated CD player is a suitable diversion for the nine-year-old who is receiving oxygen therapy for asthma. He should not have an electric player while receiving oxygen therapy because of the danger of fire. Answer A is incorrect because he does need diversional activity. Answer B is incorrect because there is no need for him to wear earphones while he is listening to music. Answer C is incorrect because he can have items from home.

73. **Answer A is correct.** Maturational crises are normal expected changes that face the family. Entering nursery school is a maturational crisis because the child begins to move away from the family and spend more time in the care of others. It is a time of adjustment for both the child and the parents. Answers B, C, and D are incorrect because they represent situational crises.

74. **Answer A is correct.** The client with a history of phenylketonuria should not use Nutrasweet or other sugar substitutes containing aspartame because aspartame is not adequately metabolized by the client with PKU. Answers B and C indicate an understanding of the nurse's teaching; therefore, they are incorrect. The client needs to resume a low-phenylalanine diet, making answer D incorrect.

75. **Answer D is correct.** Duchenne's muscular dystrophy is a sex-linked disorder, with the affected gene located on the X chromosome of the mother. Answer A is incorrect because the affected gene is not located on the autosomes. Over-replication of the X chromosomes in males is known as Klinefelter's syndrome; therefore, answer B is incorrect. Answer C is incorrect because the disorder is not located on the Y chromosome of the father.

76. **Answer B is correct.** The nurse and the client should work together to form a contract that outlines the amount of time he spends on a task. Answer A is incorrect because the client with a personality disorder will see no reason to change. The nurse should discuss his behavior and its effects on others with him, so answer C is incorrect. Answer D is incorrect because the client will not be able to set schedules and deadlines for himself.

77. **Answer A is correct.** Zovirax (acyclovir) shortens the course of chickenpox; however, the American Academy of Pediatrics does not recommend it for healthy children because of the cost. Answer B is incorrect because it is the vaccine used to prevent chickenpox. Answer C is incorrect because it is the immune globulin given to those who have been exposed to chickenpox. Answer D is incorrect because it is an antihistamine used to control itching associated with chickenpox.

78. **Answer A is correct.** Sock and mitten burns, burns confined to the hands and feet, indicate submersion in a hot liquid. Falling into the tub would not have produced sock burns; therefore, the nurse should be alert to the possibility of abuse. Answer B and C are within the realm of possibility, given the active play of the school-aged child; therefore, they are incorrect. Answer D is within the realm of possibility; therefore, it is incorrect.

79. **Answer B is correct.** Assault is the intentional threat to bring about harmful or offensive contact. The nurse's threat to give the medication by injection can be considered as assault. Answers A, C, and D do not relate to the nurse's statement; therefore, they are incorrect.

80. **Answer C is correct.** A nephrostomy tube is placed directly into the kidney and should not be clamped or irrigated because of the damage that can result to the kidney. Answers A and B are incorrect because the first action should be to relieve pressure on the affected kidney. Answer D is incorrect because the tubing should not be irrigated.

81. **Answer D is correct.** When the collection chamber is full, the nurse should prepare a new unit for continuing the collection. Answer A is incorrect because the unit is providing suction, so the amount of water does not need to be increased. Answer B is incorrect because the drainage is not to be removed using a syringe. Milking a chest tube requires a doctor's order, and because the tube is draining in this case, there is no need to milk it, so answer C is incorrect.

82. **Answer B is correct.** The first action by the nurse is to stop the transfusion and maintain an IV of normal saline. Answers A, C, and D are incorrect because they are not the first action the nurse would take.

83. **Answer A is correct.** Microwaving can cause uneven heating and "hot spots" in the formula, which can cause burns to the baby's mouth and throat. Answers B, C, and D are incorrect because the infant's formula should never be prepared using a microwave.

84. **Answer B is correct.** HELLP syndrome is characterized by hemolytic anemia, elevated liver enzymes, and low platelet counts. Answers A, C, and D have no connection to HELLP syndrome, so they are incorrect.

85. **Answer C is correct.** Dark green, leafy vegetables; members of the cabbage family; beets; kidney beans; cantaloupe; and oranges are good sources of folic acid (B9). Answers A, B, and D are incorrect because they are not sources of folic acid. Meat, liver, eggs, dried beans, sweet potatoes, and Brussels sprouts are good sources of B12; pork, fish, and chicken are good sources of B6.

86. **Answer B is correct.** The client with preeclampsia should be kept as quiet as possible, to minimize the possibility of seizures. The client should be kept in a dimly lit room with little or no stimulation. The clients in answers A, C, and D do not require a private room; therefore, they are incorrect.

87. **Answer B is correct.** Myasthenia gravis is caused by a loss of acetylcholine receptors, which results in the interruption of the transmission of nerve impulses from nerve endings to muscles. Answer A is incorrect because it refers to multiple sclerosis. Answer C is incorrect because it refers to Guillain-Barre syndrome. Answer D is incorrect because it refers to Parkinson's disease.

88. **Answer B is correct.** Osmitrol (mannitol) is an osmotic diuretic, which inhibits reabsorption of sodium and water. The first indication of its effectiveness is an increased urinary output. Answers A, C, and D do not relate to the effectiveness of the drug, so they are incorrect.

89. **Answer B is correct.** The client with a suspected subdural hematoma is more critical than the other clients and should be assessed first. Answers A, C, and D have more stable conditions; therefore, they are incorrect.

90. **Answer C is correct.** When given within eight hours of the injury, Solu-Medrol has proven effective in reducing cord swelling, thereby improving motor and sensory function. Answer A is incorrect because Solu-Medrol does not prevent spasticity. Answer B is incorrect because Solu-Medrol does not decrease the need for mechanical ventilation. Answer D is incorrect because Solu-Medrol is used to reduce inflammation, not used to treat infections.

91. **Answer B is correct.** The spinal fluid of a client with Guillain-Barre has an increased protein concentration with normal or near-normal cell counts. Answers A, C, and D are inaccurate statements; therefore, they are incorrect.

92. **Answer A is correct.** The child with laryngotracheobronchitis has inspiratory stridor and a harsh, "brassy" cough. Answer B refers to the child with epiglotttis, answer C refers to the child with bronchiolitis, and answer D refers to the child with asthma.

93. **Answer D is correct.** Hemarthrosis or bleeding into the joints is characterized by stiffness, aching, tingling, and decreased movement in the affected joint. Answers A, B, and C do not describe hemarthrosis, so they are incorrect.

94. **Answer C is correct.** The objective of therapy using aerosol treatments and chest percussion and postural drainage is to dilate the bronchioles and help loosen secretions. Answers A, B, and D are inaccurate statements, so they are incorrect.

95. **Answer A is correct.** Drooling of bright red secretions indicates active bleeding. Answer B is incorrect because the heart rate is within normal range for a six-year-old. Answer C is incorrect because it indicates old bleeding. Answer D is incorrect because the child would have frequent, not infrequent, swallowing.

96. **Answer A is correct.** Cigarette smoking is the number one cause of bladder cancer. Answer B is incorrect because it is not associated with bladder cancer. Answer C is a primary cause of gastric cancer, and answer D is a cause of certain types of lung cancer.

97. **Answer A is correct.** Cloudy or whitish dialysate returns should be reported to the doctor immediately because it indicates infection and impending peritonitis. Answers B, C, and D are expected with peritoneal dialysis and do not require the doctor's attention.

98. **Answer C is correct.** Nitroglycerin tablets should be used as soon as the client first notices chest pain or discomfort. Answer A is incorrect because the medication should be used before engaging in activity. Strenuous activity should be avoided. Answer B is incorrect because the medication should be used when pain occurs, not on a regular schedule. Answer D is incorrect because the medication will not prevent nocturnal angina.

99. **Answer C is correct.** The LDH and CK MB are specific for diagnosing cardiac damage. Answers A, B, and D are not specific to cardiac function; therefore, they are incorrect.

100. **Answer A is correct.** The school-age child (eight or nine years old) engages in cooperative play. These children enjoy competitive games in which there are rules and guidelines for winning. Answers B and D describe peer-group relationships of the preschool child, and answer C describes peer-group relationships of the preteen.

101. **Answer D is correct.** According to Erikson, the school-age child needs the opportunity to be involved in tasks that he can complete so that he can develop a sense of industry. If he is not given these opportunities, he is likely to develop feelings of inferiority. Answers A, B, and C are not associated with the psychosocial development of the school-age child; therefore, they are incorrect.

102. **Answer D is correct.** Before initiating a transfusion, the nurse should check the identifying information, including blood type and Rh, at least three times with another staff member. It is not necessary to obtain a signed permit for each unit of blood; therefore, answer A is incorrect. It is not necessary to use a new administration set for each unit transfused; therefore, answer B is incorrect. Administering the blood using a Y connector is not related to client safety; therefore, answer C is incorrect.

103. **Answer C is correct.** The client should have a peripheral IV of normal saline for initiating the transfusion. Solutions containing dextrose are unsuitable for administering blood. Blood that has been banked for two weeks is suitable for transfusion; therefore, answer A is incorrect. The client with B positive blood can receive Rh negative and type O positive blood; therefore, answers B and D are incorrect.

104. **Answer C is correct.** The $PaCO_2$ (partial pressure of alveolar carbon dioxide) indicates the effective functioning of the lungs. Adequate exchange of carbon dioxide is one of the major determinants in acid/base balance. Answers A, B, and D are incorrect because they are not represented by the $PaCO_2$.

105. **Answer D is correct.** Although the cause remains unknown, autopsy results consistently reveal the presence of pulmonary edema and intrathoracic hemorrhages in infants dying with SIDS. Answers A, B, and C have not been linked to SIDS deaths; therefore, they are incorrect.

106. **Answer B is correct.** To obtain the urine output, the weight of the dry diaper (62g) is subtracted from the weight of the used diaper (73.5g), for a urine output of 11.5mL. Answers A, C, and D contain wrong amounts; therefore, they are incorrect.

107. **Answer B is correct.** The infant with osteogenesis imperfecta (ribbon bones) should be handled with care, to prevent fractures. Adding calcium to the infant's diet will not improve the condition; therefore, answer A is incorrect. Answers C and D are not related to the disorder, so they are incorrect.

108. **Answer D is correct.** Placing the infant supine with the neck slightly extended helps to maintain an open airway. Answers A, B, and C are incorrect because they do not help to maintain an open airway.

109. **Answer B is correct.** Adverse reactions to Depakote (divalproex sodium) include thrombocytopenia, leukopenia, bleeding tendencies, and hepatotoxicity; therefore, the client will need frequent lab work. Answer A is associated with the use of Dilantin (phenytoin), and answers C and D are associated with the use of Eskalith (lithium carbonate); therefore, they are incorrect.

110. **Answer A is correct.** The client with cocaine addiction frequently reports formication, or "cocaine bugs," which are tactile hallucinations. Answers B and C occur in those addicted to cocaine but do not refer to formication; therefore, they are incorrect. Answer D is not related to the formication; therefore, it is incorrect.

111. **Answer C is correct.** Carbonated beverages increase the pressure in the stomach and increase the incidence of gastroesophageal reflux. Answer A is incorrect because the client with GERD should not eat 3–4 hours before going to bed. Answer B is incorrect because the client should sleep on his left side to prevent reflux. Answer D is incorrect because spicy, acidic foods and beverages are irritating to the gastric mucosa.

112. **Answer B is correct.** After raising the client's head to lower the blood pressure, the nurse should make sure that the catheter is patent. Answers A and C are not the first or second actions the nurse should take; therefore, they are incorrect. The client with autonomic hyperreflexia has an extreme elevation in blood pressure. The use of supplemental oxygen is not indicated; therefore, answer D is incorrect.

113. **Answer D is correct.** The nurse should flush the NG tube with 2–4oz of water before and after giving the medication. Answers A and B are incorrect because they do not use sufficient amounts of water. Answer C is incorrect because water, not normal saline, is used to flush the NG tube.

114. **Answer B is correct.** Acute arterial occlusion results in blackened or gangrenous areas on the toes. Answer A is incorrect because it describes venous occlusion. Answer C is incorrect because the pain is located below the level of occlusion. Answer D is incorrect because the area is cool, pale, and pulseless.

115. **Answer A is correct.** The client's symptoms suggest the development of diabetes insipidus, which can occur with surgery on or near the pituitary. Although the finding will be documented in the chart, it is not the main priority at this time; therefore, answer B is incorrect. Answers C and D must be ordered by the doctor, making them incorrect.

116. **Answer B is correct.** The client taking Coumadin (sodium warfarin) should limit his intake of vegetables such as cauliflower, cabbage, spinach, turnip greens, and collards because they are high in vitamin K. Answers A, C, and D do not contain large amounts of vitamin K; thus, they are incorrect.

117. **Answer C is correct.** Turning the child every two hours will help the cast to dry and help prevent complications related to immobility. Answers A and B are incorrect because the cast will transmit heat to the child, which can result in burns. External heat prevents complete drying of the cast because the outside will feel dry while the inside remains wet. Answer D is incorrect because the child should be turned at least every two hours.

118. **Answer A is correct.** The influenza vaccine is usually given in October and November. Answers B, C, and D are not usually the times for administering the influenza vaccine, so they are incorrect.

119. **Answer B is correct.** The presence of Reed-Sternberg cells, sometimes referred to as "owl's eyes," are diagnostic for Hodgkin's lymphoma. Answers A, C, and D are not associated with Hodgkin's lymphoma and are incorrect.

120. **Answer A is correct.** Providing the client a pad and pencil allows him a way to communicate with the nurse. Answers B and C are important in the client's care; however, they do not provide a means for the client to "talk" with the nurse. Answer D is not realistic and is likely to be frustrating to the client, so it is incorrect.

121. **Answer B is correct.** Antihistamines should not be used by the client with primary open-angle glaucoma because they dilate the pupil and prevent the outflow of aqueous humor, which raises pressures in the eye. Answers A, C, and D are safe for use in the client with primary open-angle glaucoma; therefore, they are incorrect.

122. **Answer A is correct.** Persons with endemic goiter live in areas where the soil is depleted of iodine. Answers B and D refer to sporadic goiter, and answer C is not related to the occurrence of goiter.

123. **Answer A is correct.** The client should avoid over-the-counter allergy medications because many of them contain Benadryl (diphenhydramine). Benadryl is used to counteract the effects of antipsychotic medications that are prescribed for schizophrenia. Answer B refers to the client taking an MAO inhibitor, and answer C refers to the client taking lithium; therefore, they are incorrect. Over-the-counter pain relievers are safe for the client taking antipsychotic medication, so answer D is incorrect.

124. **Answer D is correct.** The priority nursing diagnosis for the client with a goiter is risk for ineffective airway clearance related to pressure of the goiter on the trachea. Answers A, B, and C apply to the client with a goiter; however, they do not take priority over airway clearance and are, therefore, incorrect choices.

125. **Answer B is correct.** The purpose of instilling Ilotycin (erythromycin) eyedrops in the newborn's eyes is to prevent neonatal blindness that can result from contamination with *Neisseria gonorrhoeae*. Answers A, C, and D are inaccurate statements and, therefore, are incorrect.

126. **Answer B is correct.** Discoid lupus produces discoid or "coinlike" lesions on the skin. Answers A, C, and D refer to systemic lupus; therefore, they are incorrect.

127. **Answer A is correct.** The visual center of the brain is located in the occipital lobe, so damage to that region results in changes in vision. Answers B and D are associated with the temporal lobe, and answer C is associated with the frontal lobe.

128. **Answer B is correct.** Parallel play, the form of play used by toddlers, involves playing beside one another with like toys but without interaction. Answer A is incorrect because it describes associative play, typical of the preschooler. Answer C is incorrect because it describes cooperative play, typical play of the school-age child. Answer D is incorrect because it describes solitary play, typical play of the infant.

129. **Answer A is correct.** Infants can discriminate speech and the human voice from other patterns of sound. Answers B, C, and D are inaccurate statements; therefore, they are incorrect.

130. **Answer C is correct.** As the school-age child develops concrete operational thinking, she becomes more selective and discriminating in her collections. Answer A refers to the cognitive development of the infant; answer B refers to moral, not cognitive, development; and answer D refers to the cognitive development of the toddler and preschool child. Therefore, all are incorrect.

131. **Answer D is correct.** Consistently responding to the infant's needs fosters a sense of trust. Failure or inconsistency in meeting the infant's needs results in a sense of mistrust. Answers A, B, and C are important to the development of the infant but do not necessarily foster a sense of trust; therefore, they are incorrect.

132. **Answer B is correct.** Before walking the client for the first time after delivery, the nurse should ask the client to sit on the side of the bed and dangle her legs, to prevent postural hypotension. Pain medication should not be given before walking, making answer A incorrect. Answers C and D have no relationship to walking the client, so they are incorrect.

133. **Answer D is correct.** Hospitalized elderly clients frequently become confused. Providing simple explanations in a calm, caring manner will help minimize anxiety and confusion. Answers A and B will increase the client's confusion, and answer C is incorrect because personal visits from family and friends would benefit the client.

134. **Answer A is correct.** The client can return to work when he has three negative sputum cultures. Answers B, C, and D are inaccurate statements, so they are incorrect.

135. **Answer C is correct.** The presence of fibrin split compound provides a definitive diagnosis of DIC. An elevated erythrocyte sedimentation rate is associated with inflammatory diseases; therefore, answer A is incorrect. Answer B is incorrect because the client with DIC clots too readily, forming microscopic thrombi. Answer D is incorrect because an elevated white cell count is associated with infection.

136. **Answer A is correct.** The symptoms of rheumatoid arthritis are worse upon awakening. Taking a warm shower helps relieve the stiffness and soreness associated with the disease. Answer B is incorrect because heat is the most beneficial way of relieving the symptoms. Large doses of aspirin are given in divided doses throughout the day, making answer C incorrect. Answer D is incorrect because the client has more problems with mobility early in the morning.

137. **Answer C is correct.** Temperature elevations in the client receiving antipsychotics (sometimes referred to as neuroleptics) such as Clozaril (clozapine) should be reported to the physician immediately. Antipsychotics can produce adverse reactions that include dystonia, agranulocytosis, and neuromalignant syndrome (NMS). Answers A and B are incorrect because they jeopardize the safety of the client. Answer D is incorrect because the client with schizophrenia is often unaware of his condition; therefore, the nurse must rely on objective signs of illness.

138. **Answer D is correct.** Drug overdose is a primary cause of acute respiratory distress syndrome. Answers A, B, and C are incorrect because they are not associated with the development of acute respiratory distress syndrome.

139. **Answer B is correct.** With iron-deficiency anemia, the RBCs are described as hypochromic and microcytic. Answer A is incorrect because the RBCs would be normochromic and normocytic but would be reduced in number. Answer C is incorrect because the RBCs would be normochromic and macrocytic. Answer D refers to anemias due to an abnormal shape or shortened life span of the RBCs rather than the color or size of the RBC; therefore, it is incorrect.

140. **Answer D is correct.** A positive Babinski reflex in adults should be reported to the physician because it indicates a lesion of the corticospinal tract. Answer A is incorrect because it does not indicate that the client's condition is improving. Answer B is incorrect because changing the position will not alter the finding. Answer C is incorrect because a positive Babinski reflex is an expected finding in an infant, but not in an adult.

141. **Answer A is correct.** The Glascow coma scale, which measures verbal response, motor response, and eye opening, ranges from 0 to 15. A score of 13 indicates the client's condition is satisfactory. Answer B is incorrect because the presence of doll's eye movement indicates damage to the brainstem or oculomotor nerve. Answer C is incorrect because absent deep tendon reflexes are associated with deep coma. Answer D is incorrect because decerebrate posturing is associated with injury to the brain stem.

142. **Answer C is correct.** The primary goal of a bowel and bladder retraining program is to prevent complications that can result from impaired elimination. Answer A is incorrect because the retraining will not restore the client's preinjury elimination pattern. Answer B is incorrect because the retraining will not restore the client's neurosensory function. The client's body image will improve with retraining; however, it is not the primary goal, so answer D is incorrect.

143. **Answer A is correct.** Pulling against interlocked fingers will focus the client's attention away from the area being examined, thus making it easier to elicit a knee-jerk response. Answer B is incorrect because it is a means of checking the spinal accessory nerve. Answer C is incorrect because it is a means of checking the oculomotor nerve. Answer D is incorrect because it will not facilitate checking the patellar reflex.

144. **Answer B is correct.** Auscultation is the last step performed in a physical assessment. Answers A, C, and D are incorrect because they are performed before auscultation.

145. **Answer C is correct.** Akathesia, an extrapyramidal side effect of antipsychotic medication, results in an inability to sit still or stand still. Dystonia, in answer A, refers to a muscle spasm in any muscle of the body; answer B refers to abnormal, involuntary movements of the face, neck, and jaw; and answer D refers to an involuntary deviation and fixation of the eyes; therefore, they are incorrect.

146. **Answer D is correct.** The large soft swelling that crosses the suture line indicates that the newborn has a caput succedaneum. This finding should be reported to the physician. Answer A is incorrect because the umbilical cord normally contains three vessels (two arteries and one vein). Answer B is incorrect because the temperature is normal for the newborn. Answer C refers to acrocyanosis, which is normal in the newborn.

147. **Answer B is correct.** Infants and children are highly susceptible to infection with pertussis. Answers A, C, and D are inaccurate statements; therefore, they are incorrect.

148. **Answer D is correct.** Epidural anesthesia produces vasodilation and lowers the blood pressure; therefore, adrenalin should be available to reverse hypotension. Answer A is incorrect because it is a narcotic antagonist. Answer B is incorrect because it is an adrenergic that increases cardiac output. Answer C is incorrect because it is a benzodiazepine antagonist.

149. **Answer B is correct.** Gantrisin and other sulfa drugs should be given 30 minutes before meals, to enhance absorption. Answer A is incorrect because the medication should be given before eating. Answer C is incorrect because the medication should be given on an empty stomach. Answer D is incorrect because the medication is to be given in divided doses throughout the day.

150. **Answer A is correct.** The client taking Parnate and other MAO inhibitors should avoid ingesting foods containing tyramine, which can result in extreme elevations in blood pressure. Answers B, C, and D are not associated with the use of MAO inhibitors; therefore, they are incorrect.

151. **Answer C is correct.** The frontal lobe interprets sensation, so the client's failure to recognize touch confirms a frontal lobe injury. Answer A is incorrect because the occipital lobe is the visual center. Answer B is incorrect because the medulla is the respiratory center. Taste impulses are interpreted in the parietal lobe; therefore, answer D is incorrect.

152. **Answer B is correct.** The normal urinary output is 30–50mL per hour. The client's urinary output is below normal, indicating that additional fluids are needed. The amount of output from the Jackson-Pratt drain should be small; therefore, answer A is incorrect. The amount of drainage from the nasogastric tube is not excessive, so answer C is incorrect. Answer D is incorrect because the client would not be expected to have a stool in the first 12 hours following surgery.

153. **Answer D is correct.** According to the National Center for Health Statistics, heart disease is the number one cause of death in persons 65 and older. Chronic pulmonary disease is the fourth-leading cause of death in this age group; therefore, answer A is incorrect. Diabetes mellitus is the sixth-leading cause of death in this age group, and pneumonia is the fifth-leading cause of death in this age group; therefore, answers B and C are incorrect.

154. **Answer C is correct.** Recall is the client's ability to restate items mentioned at the beginning of the evaluation. Attention is evaluated by having the client count backward by 7 beginning at 100, so answer A is incorrect. Orientation is evaluated by having the client state the year, month, date, and day, so answer B is incorrect. Registration is evaluated by having the client immediately repeat the name of three items just named by the examiner; thus, answer D is incorrect.

155. **Answer D is correct.** The nurse should tell the client to change position or turn side to side in order to improve the dialysate return. Answers A, B, and C are incorrect ways of managing peritoneal dialysis; therefore, they are incorrect choices.

156. **Answer A is correct.** The nurse should give priority to maintaining the client's airway. The ABCDs of trauma care are airway with cervical spine immobilization, breathing, circulation, and disabilities (neurological); therefore, answers B, C, and D are incorrect.

157. **Answer B is correct.** The client in pain usually has an increased blood pressure. Answers A and C are incorrect because the client in pain will have an increased pulse rate and increased respiratory rate. Temperature is not affected by pain; therefore, answer D is incorrect.

158. **Answer C is correct.** A score of 4 indicates normal flexion. Normal flexion caused the client to withdraw his whole hand from the stimuli. Answers A, B, and D are incorrect because they do not relate to the client's response to the stimulus.

159. **Answer A is correct.** Management of Kawasaki's disease includes the use of large doses of aspirin. Answers B, C, and D are incorrect because they are not used in the treatment of Kawasaki's disease.

160. **Answer C is correct.** The client with bulimia nervosa recognizes that she has an eating disorder but feels helpless to correct it. Answer A is incorrect because the client with bulimia nervosa is usually of normal weight. Answers B and D are incorrect because they describe both the client with anorexia nervosa and the client with bulimia nervosa.

161. **Answer C is correct.** A positive Mantoux test is indicated by the presence of induration. Answers A, B, and D are incorrect because they do not describe the findings of a positive Mantoux test.

162. **Answer A is correct.** The solution bag should be hung 2–3 feet above the client's abdomen to allow a slow, steady irrigation. Answer B is incorrect because it will distend the bladder and cause trauma. Answer C is incorrect because the nurse should use sterile technique when attaching the tubing. Answer D is incorrect because it would be an intermittent irrigation rather than a continuous one.

163. **Answer B is correct.** Salmonella infection is commonly associated with turtles and reptiles. Answers A, C, and D are incorrect because they are not sources of salmonella infection.

164. **Answer B is correct.** The infant is not gaining weight as he should. Further assessment of feeding patterns as well as organic causes for growth failure should be investigated. Answers A, C, and D are incorrect because they are within the expected range for growth.

165. **Answer C is correct.** Pyridium causes the urine to become red-orange in color, so the client should be informed of this. Answers A, B, and D are not associated with the use of Pyridium; therefore, they are incorrect.

166. **Answer B is correct.** The infant's fingernails and toenails should be kept short to prevent scratching the skin. Answers A, C, and D are incorrect because keeping the infant warm will increase itching; bubble bath and perfumed soaps should not be used because they can cause skin irritations; and the infant's clothes should be washed in mild detergent and rinsed in plain water to reduce skin irritations.

167. **Answer D is correct.** Skeletal traction is used to realign bone fragments. Answer A is incorrect because it does not apply to the fractures of the femur. Answers B and C refer to skin traction, so they are incorrect.

168. **Answer B is correct.** The client with rheumatoid arthritis benefits from activity within the limits of pain because it decreases the likelihood of joints becoming nonfunctional. Answer A is incorrect because the client needs to use the knees to prevent further stiffness and disuse. Answer C is incorrect because the client can sit in chairs other than a recliner. Answer D is incorrect because it predisposes the client to further complications associated with immobility.

169. **Answer A is correct.** Use of a scalp vein for IV infusions allows the infant to be picked up and held more easily. Answers B, C, and D are inaccurate statements; therefore, they are incorrect.

170. **Answer D is correct.** The newborn with choanal atresia will not be able to breathe through his nose because of the presence of a bony obstruction that blocks the passage of air through the nares. Answers A, B, and C are not associated with choanal atresia; therefore, they are incorrect.

171. **Answer A is correct.** The most appropriate means of rehydrating the seven-month-old with diarrhea and mild dehydration is to provide oral electrolyte solutions. Answer B is incorrect because formula feedings should be delayed until symptoms improve. Answer C is incorrect because the seven-month-old has symptoms of mild dehydration, which can be managed with oral fluid replacement. Answer D is incorrect because a BRAT diet (bananas, rice, applesauce, toast) is no longer recommended by some pediatricians. In the event it is used, it would be instituted after rehydration had taken place.

172. **Answer B is correct.** Signs of fluid overload in an infant include increased heart rate and increased blood pressure. Temperature would not be increased by fluid overload; therefore, answers A and C are incorrect. Heart rate and blood pressure are not decreased by fluid overload; therefore, answer D is incorrect.

173. **Answer A is correct.** Most parents report finding Wilms tumor when the infant is being diapered or bathed. Answers B, C, and D are not associated with Wilms tumor; therefore, they are incorrect.

174. **Answer B is correct.** Monitoring her pulse and respirations will provide information on her cardiac status. Answer A is incorrect because she should not remain on strict bed rest. Answer C is incorrect because it does not provide information on her cardiac status. Answer D is incorrect because she needs to weigh more often to determine unusual gain, which could be related to her cardiac status.

175. **Answer C is correct.** The effectiveness of oxygen therapy is best determined by arterial blood gases. Answers A, B, and D are less helpful in determining the effectiveness of oxygen therapy, so they are incorrect.

176. **Answer B is correct.** Versed produces conscious sedation, so the client will not be able to remember having the procedure. Answers A, C, and D are inaccurate statements.

177. **Answer C is correct.** Early indicators of an altered level of consciousness include restlessness and irritability. Answer A is incorrect because it is a sign of impaired motor function. Answer B is incorrect because it is a sign of damage to the optic chiasm or optic nerve. Answer D is incorrect because it is a sign of increased intracranial pressure.

178. **Answer C is correct.** The client receiving a stat dose of medication should receive his medication first. Answers A, B, and D are incorrect because they are regularly scheduled medications for clients whose conditions are more stable.

179. **Answer D is correct.** Wrapping the IV site with Kerlex removes the area from the client's line of vision, allowing his attention to be directed away from the site. Answer A is incorrect because it impedes circulation at and distal to the IV site. Answer B is incorrect because reasoning is a cognitive function and the client has cognitive impairment. Answer C is incorrect because the use of restraints would require a doctor's order, and only one hand would be restrained.

180. **Answer B is correct.** Changes in the ST segment are associated with acute myocardial infarction. Peaked P waves, minimal QRS wave, and prominent U wave are not associated with acute myocardial infarction; therefore, answers A, C, and D are incorrect choices.

181. **Answer A is correct.** Chest pain and shortness of breath following a fracture of the long bones is associated with pulmonary embolus, which requires immediate intervention. Answer B is incorrect because ecchymosis is common following fractures. Answer C is incorrect because a low-grade temperature is expected because of the inflammatory response. Answer D is incorrect because level-two pain is expected in the client with a recent fracture.

182. **Answer C is correct.** The client should avoid citrus juices, vitamin C, and red meat for three days prior to the guaiac test. Answers A, B, and D are not part of the preparation of the client for a guaiac test; therefore, they are incorrect.

183. **Answer A is correct.** The nurse should give priority to beginning intravenous fluids. Increasing the client's fluid intake to 3,000mL per day will help prevent the obstruction of urine flow by increasing the frequency and volume of urinary output. Answer B is incorrect because the catheter is in the bladder and will do nothing to affect the flow of urine from the kidney. Answer C is important but has no effect on preventing or alleviating the obstruction of urine flow from the kidney; therefore, it is incorrect. Answer D is incorrect because it will help prevent the formation of some stones but will not prevent the obstruction of urine flow.

184. **Answer A is correct.** JCAHO guidelines state that at least two client identifiers should be used whenever administering medications or blood products, whenever samples or specimens are taken, and when providing treatments. Neither of the identifiers is to be the client's room number. Answer B is incorrect because the client's room number is not used as an identifier. Answer C and D are incorrect because the best identifiers according to the JCAHO are the client's armband, medical record number, and/or date of birth.

185. **Answer D is correct.** The client's level of pain is severe and requires narcotic analgesia. Morphine, an opioid, is the strongest medication listed. Answer A is incorrect because it is effective only with mild pain. Answers B and C are incorrect because they are not strong enough to relieve severe pain.

186. **Answer B is correct.** Persistent diarrhea results in the loss of bicarbonate (base) so that the client develops metabolic acidosis. Answers A and D are incorrect because the problem of diarrhea is metabolic, not respiratory, in nature. Answer C is incorrect because the client is losing bicarbonate (base); therefore, he cannot develop alkalosis, caused by excess base.

187. **Answer D is correct.** The client recovering from acute pancreatitis should be provided with foods that are low in fat and protein. Answers A, B, and C are incorrect because they include food sources that are not suitable for the client recovering from acute pancreatitis.

188. **Answer C is correct.** The viral load or viral burden test provides information on the effectiveness of the client's medication regimen as well as progression of the disease. Answers A and B are incorrect because they are screening tests to detect the presence of HIV. Answer D is incorrect because it is a measure of the number of helper cells.

189. **Answer D is correct.** A drop of 3 units indicates that the viral load has decreased by 99%. Answer A is incorrect because an undetectable viral load indicates that the amount of virus is extremely low and cannot be found in the blood using current technology; however, it does not mean that the virus is gone. Answer B is incorrect because a drop of 1 unit indicates that the viral load has decreased by 90%. Answer C is incorrect because a drop of 2 units indicates that the viral load has decreased by 95%.

190. **Answer B is correct.** Loss of memory and loss of concentration are the first signs of AIDS dementia complex. Answers A, C, and D are symptoms associated with toxoplasmosis encephalitis, so they are not correct.

191. **Answer D is correct.** Activase (alteplase) is a thrombolytic agent that destroys the clot. Answer A is incorrect because the medication does not prevent congestive heart failure. Answer B is incorrect because it does not stabilize the clot. Answer C is incorrect because Alteplase does not directly increase oxygenation.

192. **Answer D is correct.** The majority of children have all their deciduous teeth by age 30 months, which should coincide with the child's first visit with the dentist. Answers A, B, and C are incorrect because the deciduous teeth are probably not all erupted.

193. **Answer B is correct.** The child with Down syndrome has epicanthal folds, broad hands, and transpalmar creases. Answer A describes the child with osteogenesis imperfecta, answer C describes the child with Turner's syndrome, and answer D describes the child with Tay Sach's disease; therefore, they are incorrect.

194. **Answer A is correct.** The most common opportunistic infection in infants and children with HIV is *Pneumocystis jiroveci* (PCP) pneumonia. Answers B, C, and D are incorrect because they are not the most common cause of opportunistic infection in the infant with HIV.

195. **Answer C is correct.** The nurse should ensure that the client's gag reflex is intact before offering sips of water or other fluids in order to reduce the risk of aspiration. Answers A and D should be assessed because the client has returned from having a diagnostic procedure, but they are not related to the question; therefore, they are incorrect. Answer B is not related to the question, so it is incorrect.

196. **Answer B is correct.** Neumega stimulates the production of platelets, so a finding of $250,000mm^3$ suggests that the medication is working. Answers A and D are associated with the use of Epogen, and answer C is associated with the use of Neupogen; therefore, they are incorrect.

197. **Answer A is correct.** Pilocarpine, a substance that stimulates sweating, is used to diagnose cystic fibrosis. Chloride and sodium levels in the sweat are measured by the test, but they do not stimulate sweating; therefore, answers B and C are incorrect. Answer D is incorrect because it is not associated with cystic fibrosis.

198. **Answer D is correct.** The client with a Brown Sequard spinal cord injury will have a loss of sensation on the side opposite the cord injury. Answer A is incorrect because it describes a complete cord lesion. Answer B is incorrect because it describes central cord syndrome. Answer C is incorrect because it describes cauda equina syndromes.

199. **Answer C is correct.** The client with signs of heptorenal syndrome should have a diet that is low in protein and sodium, to decrease serum ammonia levels. Answer A is incorrect because the client will not benefit from a high-protein diet, and sodium will be restricted. A high-carbohydrate diet will provide the client with calories; however, sodium intake is restricted, making answer B incorrect. Answer D is incorrect because the client will not benefit from a high-protein diet, which would increase ammonia levels.

200. **Answer A is correct.** Basal cell epithelioma, or skin cancer, is related to sun exposure. Answers B, C, and D are incorrect because they are not associated with the development of basal cell epithelioma.

201. **Answer C is correct.** The nurse should tell the client to change positions every fifteen minutes to provide maximum contact of the BCG with all areas of the bladder. Answer A is incorrect because the client does not need to remain still. Answer B is incorrect because oral fluids should be encouraged after the treatment time is completed. Answer D is incorrect because the client needs to void before the BCG is instilled, not during treatment time.

202. **Answer D is correct.** Any unused blood should be returned to the blood bank. Answers A, B, and C are incorrect because they are improper ways of handling the unused blood.

203. **Answer B is correct.** Trivalent botulism antitoxin is made from horse serum; therefore, the nurse needs to assess the client for allergies to horses. Answers A, C, and D are incorrect because they are not involved in the manufacturing of trivalent botulism anti-toxin.

204. **Answer D is correct.** Unless contraindicated, the client with renal calculi should receive 200mL of fluid per hour to help flush the calculi from the kidneys. Answers A, B, and C are incorrect choices because the amounts are inadequate.

205. **Answer B is correct.** A soft gauze pad should be used to clean the oral mucosa of a client with oral candidiasis. Answer A is incorrect because it is too abrasive to the mucosa of a client with oral candidiasis. Answer C is incorrect because the mouthwash contains alcohol, which can burn the client's mouth. Answer D is incorrect because lemon and glycerin will cause burning and drying of the client's oral mucosa.

206. **Answer A is correct.** The client with a cardiac tamponade will exhibit a decrease of 10mmHg or greater in systolic blood pressure during inspirations. This phenomenon, known as pulsus paradoxus, is related to blood pooling in the pulmonary veins during inspiration. Answers B, C, and D are incorrect because they contain inaccurate statements.

207. **Answer B is correct.** Following removal of a cataract, the client should avoid bending over for several days because this increases intraocular pressure. The client should avoid aspirin because it increases the likelihood of bleeding, and the client should keep the eye shield on when sleeping, so answers A and C are incorrect. Answer D is incorrect because the client should not face into the shower stream after having cataract removal because this can cause trauma to the operative eye.

208. **Answer A is correct.** A severe toxic side effect of pentamidine is hypotension. Answers B, C, and D are not related to the administration of pentamidine; therefore, they are incorrect.

209. **Answer B is correct.** A secondary benefit of intra-arterial chemotherapy is that it helps in the treatment of micro-metastasis from cancerous tumors. Intra-arterial chemotherapy lessens systemic effects but does not prevent or eradicate them; therefore, answers A, C, and D are incorrect.

210. **Answer A is correct.** Before administering gold salts, the nurse should check the lab work for the complete blood count and urine protein level because gold salts are toxic to the kidneys and the bone marrow. Answer B is incorrect because it is not necessary to give an antiemetic before administering the medication. Changes in vital signs are not associated with the medication, and a sedative is not needed before receiving the medication; therefore, answers C and D are incorrect.

211. **Answer D is correct.** The appearance of increased drainage that is clear, colorless, or bile tinged indicates disruption or leakage at one of the anastamosis sites, requiring the immediate attention of the physician. Answer A is incorrect because the client's condition will worsen without prompt intervention. Answers B and C are incorrect choices because they cannot be performed without a physician's order.

212. **Answer A is correct.** Herbals such as echinacea can interfere with the action of antiviral medications; therefore, the client should discuss the use of herbals with his physician. Answer B is incorrect because supplements have not been shown to prolong life. Answer C is incorrect because herbals have not been shown to be effective in decreasing the viral load. Answer D is incorrect because supplements do not prevent replication of the virus.

213. **Answer B is correct.** The client with Sjogren's syndrome complains of dryness of the eyes. The nurse can help relieve the client's symptoms by instilling artificial tears. Answers A, C, and D do not relieve the symptoms of Sjogren's syndrome; therefore, they are incorrect.

214. **Answer D is correct.** Melena, or blood in the stool, is common in the client with duodenal ulcers. Answers A and B are symptoms of gastric ulcers, and diarrhea is not a symptom of duodenal ulcers; therefore, answers A, B, and C are incorrect.

215. **Answer C is correct.** The nurse should auscultate the fistula for the presence of a bruit, which indicates that the fistula is patent. Answer A is incorrect because repeated compressions such as obtaining the blood pressure can result in damage to the AV fistula. Answer B is incorrect because the AV fistula is not used for the administration of IV fluids. Answer D is incorrect because venopunctures are not done in the arm with an AV fistula.

216. **Answer D is correct.** A client with epilepsy is managed with anticonvulsant medication. An adverse side effect of anticonvulsant medication is decreased white cell count. Answer A is incorrect because elevations in serum creatinine are expected in the client with chronic renal failure. Answer B is incorrect because a positive C reactive protein is expected in the client with rheumatic fever. Elevations in hematocrit are expected in a client with gastroenteritis because of dehydration; therefore, answer C is incorrect.

217. **Answer B is correct.** Clients who use steroid medications, such as beclomethasone, can develop adverse side effects, including oral infections with candida albicans. Symptoms of candida albicans include sore throat and white patches on the oral mucosa. Increased weight, difficulty sleeping, and changes in mood are expected side effects; therefore, answers A, C, and D are incorrect.

218. **Answer A is correct.** Symptoms of serotonin syndrome can result when the client takes both a prescribed antidepressant and St. John's wort. The use of ginko biloba, black cohosh, and saw palmetto with prescribed antidepressants is not associated with an increased risk of serotoin syndrome; therefore, answers B, C, and D are incorrect.

219. Answer B is correct. The nurse should check the nasal packing for the presence of the "halo sign," or a light yellow color at the edge of clear drainage on the nasal dressing. The presence of the halo sign indicates leakage of cerebral spinal fluid. Answer A is incorrect because the nurse provides mouth care using oral washes not a toothbrush. Answer C is incorrect because coughing increases pressure in the incisional area and can lead to a cerebral spinal fluid leak. Answer D is incorrect because the client should not be ambulated for 1–3 days after surgery.

220. Answer D is correct. The esophageal balloon tamponade should be maintained at a pressure of 20–25mmHg to help decrease bleeding from the esophageal varices. Answers A, B, and C are incorrect because the pressures are too low to be effective.

221. Answer A is correct. The most common neurological complication of Lyme disease is Bell's palsy. Symptoms of Bell's palsy include complaints of a "drawing" sensation and paralysis on one side of the face. Answer B is incorrect because it describes symptoms of multiple sclerosis. Answer C is incorrect because it describes symptoms of trigeminal neuralgia. Answer D is incorrect because it describes symptoms of amyotrophic lateral sclerosis. Multiple sclerosis, trigeminal neuralgia, and amyotrophic lateral sclerosis are not associated with Lyme disease.

222. Answer B is correct. The child with autistic disorder is easily upset by changes in routine; therefore, the nurse should assign a consistent caregiver. Answers A, C, and D are incorrect because they provide too much stimulation and change in routine for the child with autistic disorder.

223. Answer C is correct. Pernicious anemia is characterized by changes in neurological function such as loss of coordination and loss of position sense. Answers A, B, and D are applicable to all types of anemia; therefore, they are incorrect.

224. Answer A is correct. Cyclogel is a cycloplegic medication that inhibits constriction of the pupil and rests the muscles of accommodation. Answer B is incorrect because the medication does not prevent post-operative infection. Answer C is incorrect because the medication keeps the pupil from constricting. Answer D is incorrect because it does not decrease the production of aqueous humor.

225. Answer D is correct. Secondary syphilis is characterized by well-defined generalized lesions on the palms, soles, and perineum. Lesions can enlarge and erode, leaving highly contagious pink or grayish-white lesions. Answer A describes the chancre associated with primary syphilis, answer B describes the latent stage of syphilis, and answer C describes late syphilis.

226. Answer D is correct. The central venous pressure of 15mm H_2O indicates fluid overload. Answers A, B, and C are incorrect because they are not a cause for concern; therefore, they do not need to be reported to the physician.

227. Answer A is correct. Veil-like loss of vision is a symptom of a detached retina, not glaucoma. Answers B, C, and D are symptoms associated with glaucoma; therefore, they are incorrect.

228. Answer B is correct. According to the Centers for Disease Control (CDC), the ventilator-dependent client who is receiving tube feedings should have the head of the bed elevated 30–45° to prevent aspiration of gastric secretions. Keeping the head of the bed flat has been shown to increase aspiration of gastric secretions; therefore, answer A is incorrect. Answer C is incorrect because placing the client on his left side has not been shown to decrease the incidence of aspiration of gastric secretions. Answer D is incorrect because it would increase the incidence of aspiration of gastric secretions.

229. Answer C is correct. A paper bag should be used for the victim's clothing because it will allow the clothes to dry without destroying evidence. Answers A and B are incorrect because plastic and rubber retain moisture that can deteriorate evidence. Answer D is incorrect because padded envelopes are plastic lined, and plastic retains moisture that can deteriorate evidence.

230. Answer D is correct. Because of the anatomic location, fractures of the ankle are not treated with traction. Answers A, B, and C are incorrect because they are treated by the use of traction.

231. Answer B is correct. The cause of acute myocardial infarction is occlusion in the coronary vessels by a clot or atherosclerotic plaque. Answers A and C are incorrect because they are the result, not the cause, of acute myocardial infarction. Answer D is incorrect because it reflects a compensatory action in which the depth and rate of respirations changes to compensate for decreased cardiac output.

232. Answer D is correct. The client complaining of sexual assault should be taken immediately to a private area rather than left sitting in the waiting room. Answers A, B, and C require intervention, but the clients can remain in the waiting room.

233. Answer B is correct. Morphine is an opiate that can severely depress the client's respirations. The word *essential* implies that this vital sign must be assessed to provide for the client's safety. Answers A, C, and D are incorrect choices because they are not necessarily associated before administering morphine.

234. Answer A is correct. Changes in pupil equality and reactivity, including sluggish pupil reaction, are late signs of increased intracranial pressure. Answers B, C, and D are incorrect because they are early signs of increased intracranial pressure.

235. Answer B is correct. If the newly licensed nurse thinks he is unqualified to perform a procedure at this time, he should refuse, give a reason for the refusal, and request training. Answers A, C, and D can result in injury to the client and bring legal charges against the nurse; therefore, they are incorrect choices.

236. Answer C is correct. The nurse should give priority to administering oxygen via nasal cannula. Answer A is incorrect because the history of prior cardiac problems can be obtained after the client's condition has stabilized. Answer B is incorrect because starting an IV is done after the client's oxygen needs are met. Answer D is incorrect because pupil checks are part of a neurological assessment, which is not indicated for the situation.

237. Answer C is correct. The recommended way of removing a tick is to use tweezers. The tick is grasped close to the skin and removed using a steady, firm motion. Quickly jerking the tick away from the skin, placing a burning match close to the tick, and covering the tick with petroleum jelly increases the likelihood that the tick will regurgitate contaminated saliva into the wound; therefore, answers A, B, and D are incorrect.

238. **Answer B is correct.** The application of a wrapped ice compress will help decrease bleeding by causing vasoconstriction. Answer A is incorrect because the client's head should be tilted forward, not back. Nothing should be placed inside the nose except by the physician; therefore, answer C is incorrect. Answer D is incorrect because the nostrils should not be pinched due to a visible deformity.

239. **Answer D is correct.** The nurse's responsibility in obtaining an informed consent for surgery is providing the client with the consent form and witnessing the client's signature. Answers A and B are the responsibility of the physician, not the nurse. Answer C is incorrect because the nurse-client relationship should never be used to persuade the client to sign a permit for surgery or other medical treatments.

240. **Answer D is correct.** A pulse strength of 1+ is a weak pulse. Answer A is incorrect because it refers to a pulse strength of 4+. Answer B is incorrect because it refers to a pulse strength of 3+. Answer C is incorrect because it refers to a pulse strength of 2+.

241. **Answer B is correct.** Unlicensed assistive personnel can perform routine catheter care with soap and water. Answers A, C, and D are incorrect because they are actions that must be performed by the licensed nurse.

242. **Answer A is correct.** The client's respiratory pattern is that of Cheyne-Stokes respirations. Answer B is incorrect because Kussmaul respirations, associated with diabetic ketoacidosis, are characterized by an increase in the rate and depth of respirations. Answer C is incorrect because Biot respirations are characterized by several short respirations followed by long, irregular periods of apnea. Answer D is incorrect because diaphragmatic respirations refer to abdominal breathing.

243. **Answer C is correct.** Milk and milk products are not permitted on a clear-liquid diet. Answers A, B, and D are permitted on a clear-liquid diet; therefore, they are incorrect.

244. **Answer A is correct.** The tuberculin skin test is given by intradermal injection. Intradermal injections are administered by inserting the needle at a 5–15° angle. Answers B, C, and D are incorrect because the angle is not used for intradermal injections.

245. **Answer D is correct.** Following a trabeculoplasty, the client is instructed to wear eye protection continuously for several months. Eye protection can be in the form of protective glasses or an eye shield that is worn during sleep. Answer A is not correct because the client is instructed to keep soap and water away from the eyes. Answer B is incorrect because showering is permitted as long as soap and water are kept away from the eyes. Answer C is incorrect because the client should avoid using eye make-up for at least a month after surgery.

246. **Answer B is correct.** The CASS (continuous aspiration of subglottic secretions) tube features an evacuation port above the cuff, making it possible to remove secretions above the cuff. Use of an uncuffed tube increases the incidence of ventilator pneumonia by allowing aspiration of secretions, making answer A incorrect. Answer C is incorrect because the fenestrated tube has openings that increase the risk of pneumonia. Answer D is incorrect because *nasotracheal* refers to one of the routes for inserting an endotracheal tube, not a type of tube.

247. **Answer A is correct.** This client has multiple risk factors for complications following abdominal surgery, including age, weight, and an endocrine disorder. Answer B is incorrect because the client has only one significant factor, the recent urinary tract infection. Answer C is incorrect because the client has only one significant factor, the use of tobacco. Answer D is incorrect because the client has no significant factors for post-operative complications.

248. **Answer A is correct.** The client's potassium level is low. The normal potassium level is 3.5–5.5mEq/L. Answers B, C, and D are within normal range and, therefore, are incorrect.

249. **Answer B is correct.** Black or tarry stools are associated with upper gastrointestinal bleeding. Normal stools are brown in color, clay-colored stools are associated with biliary obstruction, and green stools are associated with infection or large amounts of bile; therefore, answers A, C, and D are incorrect.

250. **Answer C is correct.** In order to reduce the risk of hypotension and "red man syndrome" associated with the infusion of Vancocin (vancomycin), the medication should be infused over one hour. Answer A is incorrect because the time is too brief. Answers B and D are not generally recommended ways of reducing the risk of hypotension and "red man syndrome" associated with the medication; therefore, they are incorrect.

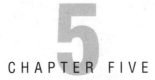

CHAPTER FIVE

Practice Exam 5 and Rationales

Quick Check

1. The nurse at a college campus is preparing to medicate several students who have been exposed to meningococcal meningitis. Which would the nurse most likely administer?

   ○ **A.** Ampicillin (Omnipen)

   ○ **B.** Ciprofoxacin (Cipro)

   ○ **C.** Vancomycin (Vancocin)

   ○ **D.** Piperacillin/Tazobactam (Zosyn)

Quick Answer: **388**
Detailed Answer: **390**

2. A 65-year-old client is admitted after a stroke. Which nursing intervention would best improve tissue perfusion to prevent skin problems?

   ○ **A.** Assessing the skin daily for breakdown

   ○ **B.** Massaging any erythematous areas on the skin

   ○ **C.** Changing incontinence pads as soon as they become soiled with urine or feces

   ○ **D.** Performing range-of-motion exercises and turning and repositioning the client

Quick Answer: **388**
Detailed Answer: **390**

3. Which diet selection by a client with a decubitus ulcer would indicate a clear understanding of the proper diet for healing of the ulcer?

   ○ **A.** Tossed salad, milk, and a slice of caramel cake

   ○ **B.** Vegetable soup and crackers, and a glass of iced tea

   ○ **C.** Baked chicken breast, broccoli, wheat roll, and an orange

   ○ **D.** Hamburger, French fries, and corn on the cob

Quick Answer: **388**
Detailed Answer: **390**

4. The nurse is assessing elderly clients at a community center. Which of the following findings would be the most cause for concern?

Quick Answer: **388**
Detailed Answer: **390**

- ○ **A.** Dry mouth
- ○ **B.** Loss of one inch of height in the last year
- ○ **C.** Stiffened joints
- ○ **D.** Rales bilaterally on chest auscultation

5. A client with chronic pain is being treated with opioid administration via epidural route. Which medication would it be most important to have available due to a possible complication of this pain relief procedure?

Quick Answer: **388**
Detailed Answer: **390**

- ○ **A.** Ketorolac (Toradol)
- ○ **B.** Naloxone (Narcan)
- ○ **C.** Diphenhydramine (Benadryl)
- ○ **D.** Promethazine (Phenergan)

6. The nurse is assessing an adult female client for hypovolemia. Which laboratory result would help the nurse in confirming a volume deficit?

Quick Answer: **388**
Detailed Answer: **390**

- ○ **A.** Hematocrit 55%
- ○ **B.** Potassium 5.0mEq/L
- ○ **C.** Urine specific gravity 1.016
- ○ **D.** BUN 18mg/dL

7. A nurse is triaging in the emergency room when a client enters complaining of muscle cramps and a feeling of exhaustion after a running competition. Which of the following would the nurse suspect?

Quick Answer: **388**
Detailed Answer: **390**

- ○ **A.** Hypernatremia
- ○ **B.** Hyponatremia
- ○ **C.** Hyperkalemia
- ○ **D.** Hypokalemia

8. A client was transferred to the hospital unit as a direct admit. While the nurse is obtaining part of the admission history information, the client suddenly becomes semiconscious. Assessment reveals a systolic BP of 70, heart rate of 130, and respiratory rate of 24. What is the nurse's best initial action?

- ○ **A.** Lower the head of the client's bed.
- ○ **B.** Initiate an IV with a large bore needle.
- ○ **C.** Notify the physician of the assessment results.
- ○ **D.** Call for the cardiopulmonary resuscitation team.

Quick Answer: **388**
Detailed Answer: **390**

9. The nurse is caring for a client post-myocardial infarction on the cardiac unit. The client is exhibiting symptoms of shock. Which clinical manifestation is the best indicator that the shock is cardiogenic rather than anaphylactic?

- ○ **A.** BP 90/60
- ○ **B.** Chest pain
- ○ **C.** Increased anxiety
- ○ **D.** Temp 98.6°F

Quick Answer: **388**
Detailed Answer: **390**

10. While reading the progress notes on a client with cancer, the nurse notes a TNM classification of T1, N1, M0. What does this classification indicate?

- ○ **A.** The tumor is in situ, no regional lymph nodes are involved, and there is no metastasis.
- ○ **B.** No evidence of primary tumor exists, lymph nodes can't be assessed, and metastasis can't be assessed.
- ○ **C.** The tumor is extended, with regional lymph node involvement and distant metastasis.
- ○ **D.** The tumor is extended and regional lymph nodes are involved, but there is no metastasis.

Quick Answer: **388**
Detailed Answer: **391**

11. The nurse is caring for a client with leukemia who has received the drug Daunorubicin (Cerubidine). Which of the following common side effects would cause the most concern?

- ○ **A.** Nausea
- ○ **B.** Vomiting
- ○ **C.** Cardiotoxicity
- ○ **D.** Alopecia

Quick Answer: **388**
Detailed Answer: **391**

12. The nurse is caring for an organ donor client with a severe head injury from an MVA. Which of the following is most important when caring for the organ donor client?

Quick Answer: **388**
Detailed Answer: **391**

  ○ **A.** Maintenance of the BP at 90mmHg or greater
  ○ **B.** Maintenance of a normal temperature
  ○ **C.** Keeping the hematocrit at less than 28%
  ○ **D.** Ensuring a urinary output of at least 300mL/hr

13. A client is being admitted with syndrome of inappropriate diuretic hormone. Which does the nurse expect to observe?
Select all that apply.

Quick Answer: **388**
Detailed Answer: **391**

  ○ **A.** Increased thirst
  ○ **B.** Tachycardia
  ○ **C.** Polyuria
  ○ **D.** Hostility
  ○ **E.** Muscle weakness

14. A client with a fractured leg is exhibiting shortness of breath, pain upon deep breathing, and hemoptysis. What do these clinical manifestations indicate to the nurse?

Quick Answer: **388**
Detailed Answer: **391**

  ○ **A.** Congestive heart failure
  ○ **B.** Pulmonary embolus
  ○ **C.** Adult respiratory distress syndrome
  ○ **D.** Tension pneumothorax

15. A nurse is preparing to mix and administer chemotherapy. What equipment would be unnecessary to obtain?

Quick Answer: **388**
Detailed Answer: **391**

  ○ **A.** Surgical gloves
  ○ **B.** Luer lok fitting IV tubing
  ○ **C.** Surgical hat cover
  ○ **D.** Disposable long-sleeve gown

16. The charge nurse is assigning staff for the day. Staff consists of an RN, an LPN, and a certified nursing assistant. Which client assignment should be given to the nursing assistant?

Quick Answer: **388**
Detailed Answer: **391**

  ○ **A.** Exploratory laparotomy with a colon resection the previous shift
  ○ **B.** Client with a stroke who has been hospitalized for two days
  ○ **C.** A client with metastatic cancer on PCA morphine
  ○ **D.** A new admission with diverticulitis

17. The registered nurse is making shift assignments. Which client should be assigned to the licensed practical nurse (LPN)?

Quick Answer: **388**
Detailed Answer: **391**

- ○ **A.** A client who is a diabetic with a foot ulcer
- ○ **B.** A client with a deep vein thrombosis receiving intravenous heparin
- ○ **C.** A client being weaned from a tracheostomy
- ○ **D.** A post-operative cholecystectomy with a T-tube

18. A client with metastatic cancer of the lung has just been told the prognosis by the oncologist. The nurse hears the client state, "I don't believe the doctor; I think he has me confused with another patient." This is an example of which of Kubler-Ross' stages of dying?

Quick Answer: **388**
Detailed Answer: **391**

- ○ **A.** Denial
- ○ **B.** Anger
- ○ **C.** Depression
- ○ **D.** Bargaining

19. The surgical nurse is preparing a patient for surgery on the lower abdomen. In which position would the nurse most likely place the client for surgery on this area?

Quick Answer: **388**
Detailed Answer: **392**

- ○ **A.** Lithotomy
- ○ **B.** Sim's
- ○ **C.** Prone
- ○ **D.** Trendelenburg

20. The nurse is performing a history on a client admitted for surgery in the morning. Which long-term medication in the client's history would be most important to report to the physician?

Quick Answer: **388**
Detailed Answer: **392**

- ○ **A.** Prednisone
- ○ **B.** Lisinopril (Zestril)
- ○ **C.** Docusate (Colace)
- ○ **D.** Oscal D

21. A nurse is working in an endoscopy recovery area. Many of the clients are administered midazolam (Versed) to provide conscious sedation. Which medication is important to have available as an antidote for Versed?

Quick Answer: **388**
Detailed Answer: **392**

- ○ **A.** Diazepam (Valium)
- ○ **B.** Naloxone (Narcan)
- ○ **C.** Flumazenil (Romazicon)
- ○ **D.** Florinef (Fludrocortisone)

22. The nurse is caring for a client with a cerebrovascular accident (CVA) who is complaining of being nauseated and is requesting an emesis basin. Which action would the nurse take first?

    ○ **A.** Administer an ordered antiemetic.

    ○ **B.** Obtain an ice bag and apply to the client's throat.

    ○ **C.** Turn the client to one side.

    ○ **D.** Notify the physician.

Quick Answer: **388**
Detailed Answer: **392**

23. The nurse is assessing a client who had a colon resection two days ago. The client states, "I feel like my stitches have burst loose." Upon further assessment, dehiscence of the wound is noted. Which action should the nurse take?

    ○ **A.** Immediately place the client in the prone position.

    ○ **B.** Apply a sterile, saline-moistened dressing to the wound.

    ○ **C.** Administer atropine to decrease abdominal secretions.

    ○ **D.** Wrap the abdomen with an ACE bandage.

Quick Answer: **388**
Detailed Answer: **392**

24. A client with hepatitis C is scheduled for a liver biopsy. Which would the nurse include in the teaching plan for this client?

    ○ **A.** The client should lie on the left side after the procedure.

    ○ **B.** Cleansing enemas should be given the morning of the procedure.

    ○ **C.** Blood coagulation studies might be done before the biopsy.

    ○ **D.** The procedure is noninvasive and causes no pain.

Quick Answer: **388**
Detailed Answer: **392**

25. The nurse is caring for a client after a laryngectomy. The client is anxious, with a respiratory rate of 32 and an oxygen saturation of 88. What should be the initial nursing action?

    ○ **A.** Suction the client.

    ○ **B.** Increase the oxygen flow rate.

    ○ **C.** Notify the physician.

    ○ **D.** Recheck the O_2 saturation reading.

Quick Answer: **388**
Detailed Answer: **392**

26. The nurse is performing discharge teaching to a client who is on isoniazid (INH). Which diet selection by the client indicates to the nurse that further instruction is needed?

   ○ **A.** Tuna casserole

   ○ **B.** Ham salad sandwich

   ○ **C.** Baked potato

   ○ **D.** Broiled beef roast

Quick Answer: **388**
Detailed Answer: **392**

27. A client with a head injury has an intracranial pressure (ICP) monitor in place. Cerebral perfusion pressure calculations are ordered. If the client's ICP is 22 and the mean pressure reading is 70, what is the client's cerebral perfusion pressure?

   ○ **A.** 92

   ○ **B.** 72

   ○ **C.** 58

   ○ **D.** 48

Quick Answer: **388**
Detailed Answer: **392**

28. A student nurse is observing a neurological nurse perform an assessment. When the nurse asks the client to "stick out his tongue," the nurse is assessing the function of which cranial nerve?

   ○ **A.** II optic

   ○ **B.** I olfactory

   ○ **C.** X vagus

   ○ **D.** XII hypoglossal

Quick Answer: **388**
Detailed Answer: **392**

29. Which set of vital signs would best indicate to the nurse that a client has an increase in intracranial pressure?

   ○ **A.** BP 180/70, pulse 50, respirations 16, temperature 101°F

   ○ **B.** BP 100/70, pulse 64, respirations 20, temperature 98.6°F

   ○ **C.** BP 96/70, pulse 132, respirations 20, temperature 98.6°F

   ○ **D.** BP 130/80, pulse 50, respirations 18, temperature 99.6°F

Quick Answer: **388**
Detailed Answer: **393**

30. The nurse is assessing the laboratory results of a client scheduled to receive phenytoin sodium (Dilantin). The Dilantin level, drawn two hours ago, is 30mcg/mL. What is the appropriate nursing action?

Quick Answer: **388**
Detailed Answer: **393**

   ○ **A.** Administer the Dilantin as scheduled.

   ○ **B.** Hold the scheduled dose and notify the physician.

   ○ **C.** Decrease the dosage from 100mg to 50mg.

   ○ **D.** Increase the dosage to 200mg from 100mg.

31. A client with sickle cell disease is admitted in active labor. Which nursing intervention would be most helpful in preventing a sickling crisis?

Quick Answer: **388**
Detailed Answer: **393**

   ○ **A.** Obtaining blood pressures every two hours

   ○ **B.** Administering pain medication every three hours as ordered

   ○ **C.** Monitoring arterial blood gas results

   ○ **D.** Administering IV fluids at ordered rate of 200mL/hr

32. A client is admitted with a diagnosis of pernicious anemia. Which of the following signs or symptoms would indicate that the client has been noncompliant with ordered B12 injections?

Quick Answer: **388**
Detailed Answer: **393**

   ○ **A.** Hyperactivity in the evening hours

   ○ **B.** Weight gain

   ○ **C.** Paresthesia of hands and feet

   ○ **D.** Diarrhea stools

33. The nurse has performed nutritional teaching on a client with gout who is placed on a low-purine diet. Which selection by the client would indicate that teaching has been ineffective?

Quick Answer: **388**
Detailed Answer: **393**

   ○ **A.** Boiled cabbage

   ○ **B.** Apple

   ○ **C.** Peach cobbler

   ○ **D.** Spinach

34. The nurse is caring for a 70-year-old client with hypovolemia who is receiving a blood transfusion. Assessment findings reveal crackles on chest auscultation and distended neck veins. What is the nurse's initial action?

Quick Answer: **388**
Detailed Answer: **393**

   ○ **A.** Slow the transfusion.

   ○ **B.** Document the finding as the only action.

   ○ **C.** Stop the blood transfusion and turn on the normal saline.

   ○ **D.** Assess the client's pupils.

35. The orthopedic nurse should be particularly alert for a fat embolus in which of the following clients having the greatest risk for this complication after a fracture?

    ○ **A.** A 50-year-old with a fractured fibula

    ○ **B.** A 20-year-old female with a wrist fracture

    ○ **C.** A 21-year-old male with a fractured femur

    ○ **D.** An 8-year-old with a fractured arm

Quick Answer: **388**
Detailed Answer: **393**

36. The nurse has performed discharge teaching to a client in need of a high-iron diet. The nurse recognizes that teaching has been effective when the client selects which meal plan?

    ○ **A.** Hamburger, French fries, and orange juice

    ○ **B.** Sliced veal, spinach salad, and whole-wheat roll

    ○ **C.** Vegetable lasagna, Caesar salad, and toast

    ○ **D.** Bacon, lettuce, and tomato sandwich; potato chips; and tea

Quick Answer: **388**
Detailed Answer: **393**

37. An elderly female is admitted with a fractured right femoral neck. Which clinical manifestation would the nurse expect to find?

    ○ **A.** Free movement of the right leg

    ○ **B.** Abduction of the right leg

    ○ **C.** Internal rotation of the right hip

    ○ **D.** Shortening of the right leg

Quick Answer: **388**
Detailed Answer: **393**

38. The nurse is evaluating teaching effectiveness on a client with a gastrointestinal disorder prescribed a gluten-free diet. Which diet choice indicates that the client understands the instructions given?

    ○ **A.** Steamed broccoli

    ○ **B.** Wheat toast

    ○ **C.** Chocolate chip cookie

    ○ **D.** Bran cereal

Quick Answer: **388**
Detailed Answer: **393**

39. A client with asthma has an order to begin an aminophylline IV infusion. Which piece of equipment is essential for the nurse to safely administer the medication?

    ○ **A.** Large bore intravenous catheter

    ○ **B.** IV inline filter

    ○ **C.** IV infusion device

    ○ **D.** Cover to prevent exposure of solution to light

Quick Answer: **388**
Detailed Answer: **393**

40. The nurse caring for a client with anemia recognizes which clinical manifestation as the one that is specific for a hemolytic type of anemia?

Quick Answer: **388**
Detailed Answer: **394**

- ○ **A.** Jaundice
- ○ **B.** Anorexia
- ○ **C.** Tachycardia
- ○ **D.** Fatigue

41. A client with cancer who is receiving chemotherapeutic drugs has been given injections of pegfilgastrim (Neulasta). Which laboratory value reveals that the drug is producing the desired effect?

Quick Answer: **388**
Detailed Answer: **394**

- ○ **A.** Hemoglobin of 13.5g/dL
- ○ **B.** White blood cells count of 6,000/mm
- ○ **C.** Platelet count of 300,000/mm
- ○ **D.** Hematocrit of 39%

42. The nurse is performing discharge teaching on a client with polycythemia vera. Which would be included in the teaching plan?

Quick Answer: **388**
Detailed Answer: **394**

- ○ **A.** Avoid large crowds and exposure to people who are ill.
- ○ **B.** Keep the head of the bed elevated at night.
- ○ **C.** Wear socks and gloves when going outside.
- ○ **D.** Recognize clinical manifestations of thrombosis.

43. A client is being discharged after lithotripsy for removal of a kidney stone. Which statement by the client indicates understanding of the nurse's instructions?

Quick Answer: **388**
Detailed Answer: **394**

- ○ **A.** "I'll need to strain my urine starting in the morning."
- ○ **B.** "I will need to save all my urine."
- ○ **C.** "I will be careful to strain all the urine and save the stone."
- ○ **D.** "I won't need to strain my urine now that the procedure is complete."

44. The nurse is caring for a client with osteoporosis who is being discharged on alendronate (Fosamax). Which statement would indicate a need for further teaching?

- ○ **A.** "I should take the medication immediately before bedtime every night."
- ○ **B.** "I should remain in an upright position for 30 minutes after taking Fosamax."
- ○ **C.** "The medication should be taken by mouth with water."
- ○ **D.** "I should not have any food with this medication."

Quick Answer: **388**
Detailed Answer: **394**

45. A client is being evaluated for carpel tunnel syndrome. The nurse is observed tapping over the median nerve in the wrist and asking the client if there is pain or tingling. Which assessment is the nurse performing?

- ○ **A.** Phalen's maneuver
- ○ **B.** Tinel's sign
- ○ **C.** Kernig's sign
- ○ **D.** Brudzinski's sign

Quick Answer: **388**
Detailed Answer: **394**

46. The nurse is caring for a client who is recovering from a fractured femur. Which diet selection would be best for this client?

- ○ **A.** Loaded baked potato, fried chicken, and tea
- ○ **B.** Dressed cheeseburger, French fries, and a Diet Coke
- ○ **C.** Tuna fish salad on sourdough bread, potato chips, and skim milk
- ○ **D.** Mandarin orange salad, broiled chicken, and milk

Quick Answer: **388**
Detailed Answer: **394**

47. The nurse working in the emergency department realizes that it would be contraindicated to induce vomiting if someone had ingested which of the following?

- ○ **A.** Ibuprofen
- ○ **B.** Aspirin
- ○ **C.** Vitamins
- ○ **D.** Gasoline

Quick Answer: **388**
Detailed Answer: **394**

48. A client with AIDS has impaired nutrition due to diarrhea. The nurse teaches the client about the need to avoid certain foods. Which diet selection by the client would indicate a need for further teaching?

  ○ **A.** Tossed salad

  ○ **B.** Baked chicken

  ○ **C.** Broiled fish

  ○ **D.** Steamed rice

49. The nurse has just received a report from the previous shift. Which of the following clients should the nurse visit first?

  ○ **A.** A 50-year-old COPD client with a PCO_2 of 50

  ○ **B.** A 24-year-old admitted after an MVA complaining of shortness of breath

  ○ **C.** A client with cancer requesting pain medication

  ○ **D.** A one-day post-operative cholecystectomy with a temperature of 100°F

50. The nurse is performing a breast exam on a client when she discovers a mass. Which characteristic of the mass would best indicate a reason for concern?

  ○ **A.** Tender to the touch

  ○ **B.** Regular shape

  ○ **C.** Moves easily

  ○ **D.** Firm to the touch

51. The nurse is caring for a client after a motor vehicle accident. The client has a fractured tibia, and bone is noted protruding through the skin. Which action is of priority?

  ○ **A.** Provide manual traction above and below the leg.

  ○ **B.** Cover the bone area with a sterile dressing.

  ○ **C.** Apply an ACE bandage around the entire lower limb.

  ○ **D.** Place the client in the prone position.

52. The RN on the oncology unit is preparing to mix and administer amphoteracin B (Fungizone) to a client. Which action is contraindicated for administering this drug IV?

    ○ **A.** Mix the drug with normal saline solution.

    ○ **B.** Administer the drug over 4–6 hours.

    ○ **C.** Hydrate with IV fluids two hours before the infusion is scheduled to begin.

    ○ **D.** Premedicate the client with ordered acetaminophen (Tylenol) and diphenhydramine (Benadryl).

Quick Answer: **388**
Detailed Answer: **395**

53. A nurse is administering a blood transfusion to a client on the oncology unit. Which clinical manifestation indicates an acute hemolytic reaction to the blood?

    ○ **A.** Low back pain

    ○ **B.** Headache

    ○ **C.** Urticaria

    ○ **D.** Neck vein distention

Quick Answer: **388**
Detailed Answer: **395**

54. The nurse is caring for a client diagnosed with metastatic cancer of the bone. The client is exhibiting mental confusion and a BP of 150/100. Which laboratory value would correlate with the client's symptoms reflecting a common complication with this diagnosis?

    ○ **A.** Potassium 5.6 mEq/L

    ○ **B.** Calcium 13mg/dL

    ○ **C.** Inorganic phosphorus 1.7mEq/L

    ○ **D.** Sodium 138mEq/L

Quick Answer: **388**
Detailed Answer: **395**

55. A client with a stroke and malnutrition has been placed on Total Parenteral Nutrition (TPN). The nurse notes air entering the client via the central line. Which initial action is most appropriate?

    ○ **A.** Notify the physician.

    ○ **B.** Elevate the head of the bed.

    ○ **C.** Place the client in the left lateral decubitus position.

    ○ **D.** Stop the TPN and hang D5 1/2 NS.

Quick Answer: **388**
Detailed Answer: **395**

56. The nurse is preparing a client for cervical uterine radiation implant insertion. Which will be included in the teaching plan?

Quick Answer: **388**
Detailed Answer: **395**

   ○ **A.** TV or telephone use will not be allowed while the implant is in place.

   ○ **B.** A Foley catheter is usually inserted.

   ○ **C.** A high-fiber diet is recommended.

   ○ **D.** Excretions will be considered radioactive.

57. The nurse is caring for a client with a head injury who has an intracranial pressure monitor in place. Assessment reveals an ICP reading of 66. What is the nurse's best action?

Quick Answer: **388**
Detailed Answer: **395**

   ○ **A.** Notify the physician.

   ○ **B.** Record the reading as the only action.

   ○ **C.** Turn the client and recheck the reading.

   ○ **D.** Place the client supine.

58. The nurse is caring for a client with leukemia who is receiving the drug doxorubicin (Adriamycin). Which toxic effects of this drug would be reported to the physician immediately?

Quick Answer: **388**
Detailed Answer: **395**

   ○ **A.** Rales and distended neck veins

   ○ **B.** Red discoloration of the urine

   ○ **C.** Nausea and vomiting

   ○ **D.** Elevated BUN and dry, flaky skin

59. A client has developed diabetes insipidous after removal of a pituitary tumor. Which finding would the nurse expect?

Quick Answer: **388**
Detailed Answer: **395**

   ○ **A.** Polyuria

   ○ **B.** Hypertension

   ○ **C.** Polyphagia

   ○ **D.** Hyperkalemia

60. A client with cancer received platelet infusions 24 hours ago. Which of the following assessment findings would indicate the most therapeutic effect from the transfusions?

Quick Answer: **388**
Detailed Answer: **395**

   ○ **A.** Hemoglobin level increase from 8.9 to 10.6mg/dL

   ○ **B.** Temperature reading of 99.4°F

   ○ **C.** White blood cell count of 11,000/mm^3

   ○ **D.** Decrease in oozing of blood from IV site

61. A client is admitted with Parkinson's disease who has been taking Carbidopa/levodopa (Sinemet) for one year. Which clinical manifestation would be most important to report?

- ○ **A.** Dry mouth
- ○ **B.** Spasmodic eye winking
- ○ **C.** Dark urine color
- ○ **D.** Complaints of dizziness

Quick Answer: **388**
Detailed Answer: **396**

62. The nurse who is caring for a client with cancer notes a WBC of 500/mm^3 on the laboratory results. Which intervention would be most appropriate to include in the client's plan of care?

- ○ **A.** Assess temperature every four hours because of risk for hypothermia.
- ○ **B.** Instruct the client to avoid large crowds and people who are sick.
- ○ **C.** Instruct in the use of a soft toothbrush.
- ○ **D.** Assess for signs of bleeding.

Quick Answer: **388**
Detailed Answer: **396**

63. A client with Crohn's disease requires TPN to provide adequate nutrition. The nurse finds the TPN bag empty. What fluid would the nurse select to hang until another bag is prepared in the pharmacy?

- ○ **A.** Lactated Ringers
- ○ **B.** Normal saline
- ○ **C.** D10W solution
- ○ **D.** Normosol R

Quick Answer: **388**
Detailed Answer: **396**

64. The nurse is caring for a client with possible cervical cancer. What clinical data would the nurse most likely find in the client's history?

- ○ **A.** Post-coital vaginal bleeding
- ○ **B.** Nausea and vomiting
- ○ **C.** Foul-smelling vaginal discharge
- ○ **D.** Elevated temperature levels

Quick Answer: **388**
Detailed Answer: **396**

65. The nurse is preparing to receive a client from admitting with tumor lysis syndrome (TLS). Which of the following would the nurse expect to find on the laboratory and patient history sections of the chart?
Select all that apply.

- ○ **A.** Low blood pressure
- ○ **B.** Hyperactivity
- ○ **C.** Hyperkalemia
- ○ **D.** Hyperuricemia
- ○ **E.** Mental changes

66. A client is scheduled to undergo a bone marrow aspiration from the sternum. What position would the nurse assist the client into for this procedure?

- ○ **A.** Dorsal recumbent
- ○ **B.** Supine
- ○ **C.** High Fowler's
- ○ **D.** Lithotomy

67. The nurse is caring for a client with a head injury who has increased ICP. The physician plans to reduce the cerebral edema by constricting cerebral blood vessels. Which physician order would serve this purpose?

- ○ **A.** Hyperventilation per mechanical ventilation
- ○ **B.** Insertion of a ventricular shunt
- ○ **C.** Furosemide (Lasix)
- ○ **D.** Solu medrol

68. A client with a T6 injury six months ago develops facial flushing and a BP of 210/106. After elevating the head of the bed, which is the most appropriate nursing action?

- ○ **A.** Notify the physician.
- ○ **B.** Assess the client for a distended bladder.
- ○ **C.** Apply ordered oxygen via nasal cannula.
- ○ **D.** Increase the IV fluids.

69. The nurse is performing an admission history for a client recovering from a stroke. Medication history reveals the drug clopidogrel (Plavix). Which clinical manifestation alerts the nurse to an adverse effect of this drug?

Quick Answer: **388**
Detailed Answer: **396**

- ○ **A.** Epistaxis
- ○ **B.** Hypothermia
- ○ **C.** Nausea
- ○ **D.** Hyperactivity

70. The nurse caring for a client with a head injury would recognize which assessment finding as the most indicative of increased ICP?

Quick Answer: **388**
Detailed Answer: **396**

- ○ **A.** Vomiting
- ○ **B.** Headache
- ○ **C.** Dizziness
- ○ **D.** Papilledema

71. A client with angina is experiencing migraine headaches. The physician has prescribed Sumatriptan succinate (Imitrex). Which nursing action is most appropriate?

Quick Answer: **388**
Detailed Answer: **396**

- ○ **A.** Call the physician to question the prescription order.
- ○ **B.** Try to obtain samples for the client to take home.
- ○ **C.** Perform discharge teaching regarding this drug.
- ○ **D.** Consult social services for financial assistance with obtaining the drug.

72. A client with COPD is in respiratory failure. Which of the following results would be the most sensitive indicator that the client requires a mechanical ventilator?

Quick Answer: **388**
Detailed Answer: **396**

- ○ **A.** PCO_2 58
- ○ **B.** SaO_2 90
- ○ **C.** PH 7.23
- ○ **D.** HCO_3 30

73. The nurse in the emergency room is caring for a client with multiple rib fractures and a pulmonary contusion. Assessment reveals a respiratory rate of 38, a heart rate of 136, and restlessness. Which associated assessment finding would require immediate intervention?

  ○ **A.** Occasional small amounts of hemoptysis

  ○ **B.** Midline trachea with wheezing on auscultation

  ○ **C.** Subcutaneous air and absent breath sounds

  ○ **D.** Pain when breathing deeply, with rales in the upper lobes

74. The nurse is caring for a client with myasthenia gravis who is having trouble breathing. The nurse would encourage which of the following positions for maximal lung expansion?

  ○ **A.** Supine with no pillow, to maintain patent airway

  ○ **B.** Side-lying with back support

  ○ **C.** Prone with head turned to one side

  ○ **D.** Sitting or in high Fowler's

75. The nurse is caring for clients on a respiratory unit. Upon receiving the following client reports, which client should be seen first?

  ○ **A.** Client with emphysema expecting discharge

  ○ **B.** Bronchitis client receiving IV antibiotics

  ○ **C.** Bronchitis client with edema and neck vein distention

  ○ **D.** COPD client with abnormal PO_2

76. A client has sustained a severe head injury and damaged the preoccipital lobe. The nurse should remain particularly alert for which of the following problems?

  ○ **A.** Visual impairment

  ○ **B.** Swallowing difficulty

  ○ **C.** Impaired judgment

  ○ **D.** Hearing impairment

77. The nurse is caring for a client with epilepsy who is to receive phenytoin sodium (Dilantin) 100mg IV push. The client has an IV of D51/2NS infusing at 100mL/hr. When administering the Dilantin, which is the appropriate initial nursing action?

  ○ **A.** Obtain an ambu bag and put it at bedside.

  ○ **B.** Insert a 16g IV catheter.

  ○ **C.** Flush the IV line with normal saline.

  ○ **D.** Premedicate with promethiazine (phenergan) IV push.

78. A client with increased intracranial pressure is receiving Osmitrol (Mannitol) and Furosemide (Lasix). The nurse recognizes that these two drugs are given to reverse which effect?

- ○ **A.** Energy failure
- ○ **B.** Excessive intracellular calcium
- ○ **C.** Cellular edema
- ○ **D.** Excessive glutamate release

Quick Answer: **388**
Detailed Answer: **397**

79. The nurse is assessing a client upon arrival to the emergency department. Partial airway obstruction is suspected. Which clinical manifestation is a late sign of airway obstruction?

- ○ **A.** Rales in lungs
- ○ **B.** Restless behavior
- ○ **C.** Cyanotic ear lobes
- ○ **D.** Inspiratory stridor

Quick Answer: **388**
Detailed Answer: **397**

80. The nurse is working in the trauma unit of the emergency room when a 24-year-old female is admitted after an MVA. The client is bleeding profusely and a blood transfusion is ordered. Which would the nurse be prepared to administer without a type and crossmatch?

- ○ **A.** AB positive
- ○ **B.** AB negative
- ○ **C.** O positive
- ○ **D.** O negative

Quick Answer: **388**
Detailed Answer: **397**

81. When preparing a client for magnetic resonance imaging, the nurse should implement which of the following?

- ○ **A.** Obtain informed consent and administer atropine 0.4mg.
- ○ **B.** Scrub the injection site for 15 minutes.
- ○ **C.** Remove any jewelry and inquire about metal implants.
- ○ **D.** Administer Benadryl 50mg/mL IV.

Quick Answer: **388**
Detailed Answer: **397**

82. Upon admission to the hospital, a client reports having "the worst headache I've ever had." The nurse should give the highest priority to which action?

- ○ **A.** Administering pain medication
- ○ **B.** Starting oxygen
- ○ **C.** Performing neuro checks
- ○ **D.** Inserting a Foley catheter

Quick Answer: **388**
Detailed Answer: **397**

83. A client has an order to administer cisplatin (Platinol). Which drug would the nurse expect to be ordered to reduce renal toxicity from the cisplatin infusion?

Quick Answer: **388**
Detailed Answer: **397**

- ○ **A.** Amifostine (Ethyol)
- ○ **B.** Dexrazoxane (Zinecard)
- ○ **C.** Mesna (Mesenex)
- ○ **D.** Pamidronate (Aredia)

84. The client is admitted to the ER with multiple rib fractures on the right. The nurse's assessment reveals that an area over the right clavicle is puffy and that there is a "crackling" noise with palpation. The nurse should further assess the client for which of the following problems?

Quick Answer: **388**
Detailed Answer: **397**

- ○ **A.** Flail chest
- ○ **B.** Subcutaneous emphysema
- ○ **C.** Infiltrated subclavian IV
- ○ **D.** Pneumothorax

85. A client has an order for Demerol 75mg and atropine 0.4mg IM as a preoperative medication. The Demerol vial contains 50mg/mL, and atropine is available 0.4mg/mL. How much medication will the nurse administer in total?

Quick Answer: **388**
Detailed Answer: **398**

- ○ **A.** 1.0mL
- ○ **B.** 1.7mL
- ○ **C.** 2.5mL
- ○ **D.** 3.0 mL

86. Nimodipine (Nimotop) is ordered for the client with a ruptured cerebral aneurysm. What does the nurse recognize as a desired effect of this drug?

Quick Answer: **388**
Detailed Answer: **398**

- ○ **A.** Prevent the influx of calcium into cells.
- ○ **B.** Restore a normal blood pressure reading.
- ○ **C.** Prevent the inflammatory process.
- ○ **D.** Dissolve the clot that has formed.

87. A client is admitted to the hospital with seizures. The client has jerking of the right arm and twitching of the face, but is alert and aware of the seizure. This behavior is characteristic of which type of seizure?

Quick Answer: **388**
Detailed Answer: **398**

   ○ **A.** Absence

   ○ **B.** Complex partial

   ○ **C.** Simple partial

   ○ **D.** Tonic-clonic

88. The intensive care unit is full and the emergency room just called in a report on a ventilator-dependent client who is being admitted to the medical surgical unit. It would be essential that the nurse have which piece of equipment at the client's bedside?

Quick Answer: **388**
Detailed Answer: **398**

   ○ **A.** Cardiac monitor

   ○ **B.** Intravenous controller

   ○ **C.** Manual resuscitator

   ○ **D.** Oxygen by nasal cannula

89. The nurse is caring for a client on a ventilator that is set on intermittent mandatory ventilation (IMV). Assessment on the ventilator is IMV mode of eight breaths per minute. The nurse assesses the client's respiratory rate of 13 per minute. What do these findings indicate?

Quick Answer: **388**
Detailed Answer: **398**

   ○ **A.** The client is "fighting" the ventilator and needs medication.

   ○ **B.** Pressure support ventilation is being used.

   ○ **C.** Additional breaths are being delivered by the ventilator.

   ○ **D.** The client is breathing five additional breaths on his own.

90. The nurse has given instructions on pursed-lip breathing to a client with COPD. Which statement by the client would indicate effective teaching?

Quick Answer: **388**
Detailed Answer: **398**

   ○ **A.** "I should inhale through my mouth very deeply."

   ○ **B.** "I should tighten my abdominal muscles with inhalation."

   ○ **C.** "I should contract my abdominal muscles with exhalation."

   ○ **D.** "I should make inhalation twice as long as exhalation."

91. A client is receiving aminophylline IV. The nurse monitors the theophylline blood level and assesses that the level is within therapeutic range at which of the following levels?

- ○ **A.** 5ug/mL
- ○ **B.** 8ug/mL
- ○ **C.** 15ug/mL
- ○ **D.** 25ug/mL

Quick Answer: **388**
Detailed Answer: **398**

92. The nurse is assessing the arterial blood gases (ABG) of a chest trauma client with the results of pH 7.35, PO_2 85, PCO_2 55, and HCO_3 27. What do these values indicate?

- ○ **A.** Uncompensated respiratory acidosis
- ○ **B.** Uncompensated metabolic acidosis
- ○ **C.** Compensated respiratory acidosis
- ○ **D.** Compensated metabolic acidosis

Quick Answer: **388**
Detailed Answer: **398**

93. A pneumonectomy is performed on a client with lung cancer. Which of the following would probably be omitted from the client's plan of care?

- ○ **A.** Closed chest drainage
- ○ **B.** Pain-control measures
- ○ **C.** Supplemental oxygen administration
- ○ **D.** Coughing and deep-breathing exercises

Quick Answer: **388**
Detailed Answer: **398**

94. When planning the care for a client after a posterior fossa (infratentorial) craniotomy, which action is contraindicated?

- ○ **A.** Keeping the client flat on one side
- ○ **B.** Elevating the head of the bed 30°
- ○ **C.** Log-rolling or turning as a unit
- ○ **D.** Keeping the neck in a neutral position

Quick Answer: **388**
Detailed Answer: **398**

95. The nurse is performing discharge teaching on a client with ulcerative colitis who has been placed on a low-residue diet. Which food would need to be eliminated from this client's diet?

- ○ **A.** Roasted chicken
- ○ **B.** Noodles
- ○ **C.** Cooked broccoli
- ○ **D.** Roast beef

Quick Answer: **388**
Detailed Answer: **398**

96. The nurse is assisting a client with diverticulitis to select appropriate foods. Which food should be avoided?

Quick Answer: **388**
Detailed Answer: **398**

- ○ **A.** Bran
- ○ **B.** Fresh peach
- ○ **C.** Tomatoes
- ○ **D.** Dinner roll

97. A client is admitted with a possible bowel obstruction. Which question during the nursing history is least helpful in obtaining information regarding this diagnosis?

Quick Answer: **388**
Detailed Answer: **399**

- ○ **A.** "Tell me about your pain."
- ○ **B.** "What does your vomit look like?"
- ○ **C.** "Describe your usual diet."
- ○ **D.** "Have you noticed an increase in abdominal size?"

98. The nurse is caring for a client with epilepsy who is being treated with carbamazepine (Tegretol). Which laboratory value might indicate a serious side effect of this drug?

Quick Answer: **388**
Detailed Answer: **399**

- ○ **A.** BUN 10mg/dL
- ○ **B.** Hemoglobin 13.0gm/dL
- ○ **C.** WBC 4,000/mm^3
- ○ **D.** Platelets 200,000/mm^3

99. A client is admitted with a tumor in the parietal lobe. Which symptoms would be expected due to this tumor's location?

Quick Answer: **388**
Detailed Answer: **399**

- ○ **A.** Hemiplegia
- ○ **B.** Aphasia
- ○ **C.** Paresthesia
- ○ **D.** Nausea

100. A client weighing 150 pounds has received burns over 50% of his body at 1200 hours. Using the Parkland formula, calculate the expected amount of fluid that the client should receive by 2000 hours.

Quick Answer: **388**
Detailed Answer: **399**

- ○ **A.** 3,400
- ○ **B.** 6,800
- ○ **C.** 10,200
- ○ **D.** 13,600

101. The nurse is caring for a client post-op femoral popliteal bypass graft. Which post-operative assessment finding would require immediate physician notification?

   ○ **A.** Edema of the extremity and pain at the incision site

   ○ **B.** A temperature of 99.6°F and redness of the incision

   ○ **C.** Serous drainage noted at the surgical area

   ○ **D.** A loss of posterior tibial and dorsalis pedis pulses

Quick Answer: **388**
Detailed Answer: **399**

102. A client admitted with gastroenteritis and a potassium level of 2.9mEq/dL has been placed on telemetry. Which ECG finding would the nurse expect to find due to the client's potassium results?

   ○ **A.** A depressed ST segment

   ○ **B.** An elevated T wave

   ○ **C.** An absent P wave

   ○ **D.** A flattened QRS

Quick Answer: **388**
Detailed Answer: **399**

103. A client is experiencing acute abdominal pain. Which abdominal assessment sequence is appropriate for the nurse to use for examination of the abdomen?

   ○ **A.** Inspect, palpate, auscultate, percuss

   ○ **B.** Inspect, auscultate, percuss, palpate

   ○ **C.** Auscultate, inspect, palpate, percuss

   ○ **D.** Percuss, palpate, auscultate, inspect

Quick Answer: **388**
Detailed Answer: **399**

104. The nurse is to administer a cleansing enema to a client scheduled for colon surgery. Which client position would be appropriate?

   ○ **A.** Prone

   ○ **B.** Supine

   ○ **C.** Left Sim's

   ○ **D.** Dorsal recumbent

Quick Answer: **388**
Detailed Answer: **399**

105. The nurse is caring for a client following a crushing injury to the chest. Which finding would be most indicative of a tension pneumothorax?

   ○ **A.** Expectoration of moderate amounts of frothy hemoptysis

   ○ **B.** Trachea shift toward the unaffected side of the chest

   ○ **C.** Subcutaneous emphysema noted at the anterior chest

   ○ **D.** Opening chest wound with a whistle sound emitting from the area

Quick Answer: **388**
Detailed Answer: **399**

106. The nurse receives a report from the paramedic on four trauma victims. Which client would need to be treated first? A client with:

- ○ **A.** Lower rib fractures and a stable chest wall
- ○ **B.** Bruising on the anterior chest wall and a possible pulmonary contusion
- ○ **C.** Gun shot wound with open pneumothorax unstabilized
- ○ **D.** Dyspnea, stabilized with intubation and manual resuscitator

107. The nurse is discharging a client with asthma who has a prescription for zafirlukast (Accolate). Which comment by the client would indicate a need for further teaching?

- ○ **A.** "I should take this medication with meals."
- ○ **B.** "I need to report flu-like symptoms to my doctor."
- ○ **C.** "My doctor might order liver tests while I'm on this drug."
- ○ **D.** "If I'm already having an asthma attack, this drug will not stop it."

108. A client is four hours post-op left carotid endarterectomy. Which assessment finding would cause the nurse the most concern?

- ○ **A.** Temperature 99.4°F, heart rate 110, respiratory rate 24
- ○ **B.** Drowsiness, urinary output of 50mL in the past hour
- ○ **C.** BP 120/60, lethargic, right-sided weakness
- ○ **D.** Alert and oriented, BP 168/96, heart rate 70

109. The RN is making assignments on a 12-bed unit. Staff consists of one RN and two certified nursing assistants. Which client should be self-assigned?

- ○ **A.** A client receiving decadron for emphysema
- ○ **B.** A client with chest trauma and a new onset of hemoptysis
- ○ **C.** A client with rib fractures and an O_2 saturation of 93%
- ○ **D.** A client two days post-operative lung surgery with a pulse oximetry of 92%

110. The nurse is accessing a venous access port of a client about to receive chemotherapy.

Place the following steps in proper sequential order:

○ **A.** Apply clean gloves.

○ **B.** Clean the skin with antimicrobial and let air dry.

○ **C.** Insert needle into port at a 90° angle.

○ **D.** Connect 10mL NS into extension of huber needle and prime.

○ **E.** Instill heparin solution.

○ **F.** Stabilize the part by using middle and index fingers.

○ **G.** Wash hands and apply sterile gloves.

○ **H.** Inject saline and assess for infiltration.

○ **I.** Check placement of needle.

111. A client is being discharged on Coumadin after hospitalization for a deep vein thrombosis. The nurse recognizes that which food would be restricted while the client is on this medication?

○ **A.** Lettuce

○ **B.** Apples

○ **C.** Potatoes

○ **D.** Macaroni

112. Which assessment finding in a client with COPD indicates to the nurse that the respiratory problem is chronic?

○ **A.** Wheezing on exhalation

○ **B.** Productive cough

○ **C.** Clubbing of fingers

○ **D.** Generalized cyanosis

113. A client who has just undergone a laparoscopic cholecystectomy complains of "free air pain." What would be your best action?

○ **A.** Ambulate the client.

○ **B.** Instruct the client to breathe deeply and cough.

○ **C.** Maintain the client on bed rest with his legs elevated.

○ **D.** Insert an NG tube.

114. The RN is planning client assignments. Which is the least appropriate task for the nursing assistant?

Quick Answer: **388**
Detailed Answer: **400**

- ○ **A.** Assisting a COPD client admitted two days ago to get up in the chair.

- ○ **B.** Feeding a client with bronchitis who is paralyzed on the right side.

- ○ **C.** Accompanying a discharged emphysema client to the transportation area.

- ○ **D.** Assessing an emphysema client complaining of difficulty breathing.

115. When providing care for a client with pancreatitis, the nurse would anticipate which of the following orders?

Quick Answer: **388**
Detailed Answer: **401**

- ○ **A.** Force fluids to 3,000mL/24 hours.

- ○ **B.** Insert a nasogastric tube to low intermittent suction.

- ○ **C.** Place the client in reverse Trendelenburg position.

- ○ **D.** Place the client in enteric isolation.

116. The nurse is performing a neurological assessment on a client admitted with TIAs. Assessment findings reveal an absence of the gag reflex. The nurse suspects injury to which of the following cranial nerves?

Quick Answer: **388**
Detailed Answer: **401**

- ○ **A.** XII (hypoglossal)
- ○ **B.** X (vagus)
- ○ **C.** IX (glossopharyngeal)
- ○ **D.** VII (facial)

117. The nurse has been asked to present a lecture on the prevention of West Nile virus in the community setting. Which does the nurse include in the teaching plan?

Quick Answer: **388**
Detailed Answer: **401**

- ○ **A.** Wear protective clothing outside.
- ○ **B.** Avoid being outside in the middle of the day.
- ○ **C.** Avoid the use of insect repellant containing DEET.
- ○ **D.** The virus is more prevalent in people under 18 years old.

118. A client with gallstones and obstructive jaundice is experiencing severe itching. The physician has prescribed cholestyramine (Questran). The client asks, "How does this drug work?" What is the nurse's best response?

   ○ **A.** "It blocks histamine, reducing the allergic response."

   ○ **B.** "It inhibits the enzyme responsible for bile excretion."

   ○ **C.** "It decreases the amount of bile in the gallbladder."

   ○ **D.** "It binds with bile acids and is excreted in bowel movements with stool."

Quick Answer: **388**
Detailed Answer: **401**

119. A client with inflammatory bowel disease (IBD) requires an ileostomy. The nurse would instruct the client to do which of the following measures as an essential part of caring for the stoma?

   ○ **A.** Perform massage of the stoma three times a day.

   ○ **B.** Include high-fiber foods in the diet, especially nuts.

   ○ **C.** Limit fluid intake to prevent loose stools.

   ○ **D.** Cleanse the peristomal skin meticulously.

Quick Answer: **388**
Detailed Answer: **401**

120. Diphenoxylate hydrochloride and atropine sulfate (Lomotil) is prescribed for the client with ulcerative colitis. Which of the following nursing observations indicates that the drug is having a therapeutic effect?

   ○ **A.** There is an absence of peristalsis.

   ○ **B.** The number of diarrhea stools decreases.

   ○ **C.** Cramping in the abdomen has increased.

   ○ **D.** Abdominal girth size increases.

Quick Answer: **388**
Detailed Answer: **401**

121. A nurse is assisting the physician with chest tube removal. Which client instruction is appropriate during removal of the tube?

   ○ **A.** Take a deep breath or hum during removal.

   ○ **B.** Hold the breath for two minutes and exhale slowly.

   ○ **C.** Exhale upon actual removal of the tube.

   ○ **D.** Continually breathe deeply in and out during removal.

Quick Answer: **388**
Detailed Answer: **401**

122. A client with advanced Alzheimer's disease has been prescribed haloperidol (Haldol). What clinical manifestation suggests that the client is experiencing side effects from this medication?

   ○ **A.** Cough

   ○ **B.** Tremors

   ○ **C.** Diarrhea

   ○ **D.** Pitting edema

Quick Answer: **388**
Detailed Answer: **401**

123. A student in a cardiac unit is performing auscultation of a client's heart. Which stethoscope placement would indicate to the nurse that the student is performing pulmonic auscultation correctly?

- ○ **A.** Between the apex and the sternum
- ○ **B.** At the fifth intercostal space at the left midclavicular line
- ○ **C.** At the second intercostal space, left of the sternum
- ○ **D.** At the manubrium area of the chest

124. A client with Alzheimer's disease has been prescribed donepezil (Aricept). Which information should the nurse include in the teaching plan for a client on Aricept?

- ○ **A.** "Take the medication with meals."
- ○ **B.** "The medicine can cause dizziness, so rise slowly."
- ○ **C.** "If a dose is skipped, take two the next time."
- ○ **D.** "The pill can cause an increase in heart rate."

125. A client who had major abdominal surgery is having delayed healing of the wound. Which laboratory test result would most closely correlate with this problem?

- ○ **A.** Decreased albumin
- ○ **B.** Decreased creatinine
- ○ **C.** Increased calcium
- ○ **D.** Increased sodium

126. A client is admitted to the medical-surgical unit with a report of severe hematemesis. What is the priority nursing action?

- ○ **A.** Performing an assessment
- ○ **B.** Obtaining a blood permit
- ○ **C.** Initiating an IV
- ○ **D.** Inserting an NG tube

127. The nurse caring for a client with a suspected peptic ulcer recognizes which exam as the one most reliable in diagnosing the disease?

- ○ **A.** Upper-gastrointestinal x-ray
- ○ **B.** Gastric analysis
- ○ **C.** Endoscopy procedure
- ○ **D.** Barium studies x-ray

128. On the second post-operative day after a subtotal thyroidectomy, the client tells the nurse, "I feel numbness and my face is twitching." What is the nurse's best initial action?

Quick Answer: **389**
Detailed Answer: **402**

- ○ **A.** Offer mouth care.
- ○ **B.** Loosen the neck dressing.
- ○ **C.** Notify the physician.
- ○ **D.** Document the finding as the only action.

129. A client with adult respiratory distress syndrome has been placed on mechanical ventilation with PEEP. Which finding would indicate to the nurse that the client is experiencing the undesirable effect of an increase in airway and chest pressure?

Quick Answer: **389**
Detailed Answer: **402**

- ○ **A.** A PO_2 of 88
- ○ **B.** Rales on auscultation
- ○ **C.** Blood pressure decrease to 90/48 from 120/70
- ○ **D.** A decrease in spontaneous respirations

130. A nurse is teaching a group of teenagers the correct technique for applying a condom. Which point would the nurse include in the teaching plan?

Quick Answer: **389**
Detailed Answer: **402**

- ○ **A.** The condom can be reused one time.
- ○ **B.** Unroll the condom all the way over the erect penis.
- ○ **C.** Apply petroleum jelly to reduce irritation.
- ○ **D.** Place water in the tip of the condom before use.

131. A client with rheumatoid arthritis is being discharged with a prescription for etanercept (Enbrel). Which should the nurse teach the client to report immediately?

Quick Answer: **389**
Detailed Answer: **402**

- ○ **A.** Redness, itching, edema at injection site
- ○ **B.** Exposure to chickenpox or shingles
- ○ **C.** Headache
- ○ **D.** Vomiting

132. The nurse in the ER has received report of four clients en route to the emergency department. Which client should the nurse see first? A client with:

    ○ **A.** Third-degree burns to the face and neck area, with singed nasal hairs

    ○ **B.** Second-degree burns to each leg and thigh area, who is alert and oriented

    ○ **C.** A chemical burn that has been removed and liberally flushed before admission

    ○ **D.** An electrical burn entering and leaving on the same side of the body

Quick Answer: **389**
Detailed Answer: **402**

133. Which clinical manifestations would the nurse expect a client with a diagnosis of acute osteomyelitis to exhibit?
    Select all that apply.

    ○ **A.** Normal sedimentation rate

    ○ **B.** Pain and fever

    ○ **C.** Low blood count

    ○ **D.** Tenderness in affected area

    ○ **E.** Edema and pus from the wound

Quick Answer: **389**
Detailed Answer: **402**

134. The nurse recognizes which of the following clients as having the highest risk for pulmonary complications after surgery?

    ○ **A.** A 24-year-old with open reduction internal fixation of the ulnar

    ○ **B.** A 45-year-old with an open cholecystectomy

    ○ **C.** A 36-year-old after a hysterectomy

    ○ **D.** A 50-year-old after a lumbar laminectomy

Quick Answer: **389**
Detailed Answer: **402**

135. Which clinical manifestation is most indicative to the nurse that a possible carbon monoxide poisoning has occurred?

    ○ **A.** Pulse oximetry reading of 80%

    ○ **B.** Expiratory stridor and nasal flaring

    ○ **C.** Cherry red color to the mucous membranes

    ○ **D.** Presence of carbonaceous particles in the sputum

Quick Answer: **389**
Detailed Answer: **402**

136. A client is admitted with a ruptured spleen following a four-wheeler accident. In preparation for surgery, the nurse suspects that the client is in the compensatory stage of shock because of which clinical manifestation?

- ○ **A.** Blood pressure 120/70, confusion, heart rate 120
- ○ **B.** Crackles on chest auscultation, mottled skin, lethargy
- ○ **C.** Jaundice, urine output less than 30mL in the past hour, heart rate 170
- ○ **D.** Rapid shallow respirations, unconscious, petechiae anterior chest

137. A client reports to the nurse that he believes he has an ulcer and wants to be checked for *H. pylori*. Which of the following medications in the client's history could make the test invalid?

- ○ **A.** Omeprazole (Prilosec)
- ○ **B.** Furosemide (Lasix)
- ○ **C.** Propoxyphene napsylate (Darvocet)
- ○ **D.** Ibuprofen (Advil)

138. A client arrives in the emergency room with severe burns of the hands, right arm, face, and neck. The nurse needs to start an IV. Which site would be most suitable for this client?

- ○ **A.** Top of client's right hand
- ○ **B.** Left antecubital fossa
- ○ **C.** Top of either foot
- ○ **D.** Left forearm

139. Which client clinical manifestation during a bone marrow transplantation procedure alerts the nurse to the possibility of an adverse reaction?

- ○ **A.** Fever
- ○ **B.** Red colored urine
- ○ **C.** Hypertension
- ○ **D.** Shortness of breath

140. The nurse is assessing the integumentary system of a dark-skinned individual. Which area would be the most likely to show a skin cancer lesion?

- ○ **A.** Chest
- ○ **B.** Arms
- ○ **C.** Face
- ○ **D.** Palms

141. A client with a gastrointestinal bleed has an NG tube to low continuous wall suction. Which technique is the correct procedure for the nurse to utilize when assessing bowel sounds?

- ○ **A.** Obtain a sample of the NG drainage and test the pH.
- ○ **B.** Clamp the tube while listening to the abdomen with a stethoscope.
- ○ **C.** Irrigate the tube with 30mL of NS while auscultating the abdomen.
- ○ **D.** Turn the suction on high and auscultate over the naval area.

142. A burn client's care plan reveals an expected outcome of no localized or systemic infection. Which assessment by the nurse supports this outcome?

- ○ **A.** Wound culture results showing minimal bacteria
- ○ **B.** Cloudy, foul-smelling urine
- ○ **C.** White blood cell count of $14,000/mm^3$
- ○ **D.** Temperature elevation of 101°F

143. The nurse is discharging a client with a prescription of eyedrops. Which observation by the nurse would indicate a need for further client teaching?

- ○ **A.** Shaking of the suspension to mix the medication
- ○ **B.** Administering a second eyedrop medication immediately after the first one was instilled
- ○ **C.** Washing the hands before and after the administration of the drops
- ○ **D.** Holding the lower lid down without pressing the eyeball to instill the drops

144. The nurse is caring for a client with pneumonia who is allergic to penicillin. Which antibiotic is safest to administer to this client?

Quick Answer: **389**
Detailed Answer: **403**

- ○ **A.** Cefazolin (Ancef)
- ○ **B.** Amoxicillin
- ○ **C.** Erythrocin (Erythromycin)
- ○ **D.** Ceftriaxone (Rocephin)

145. The nurse notes the following laboratory test results on a 24-hour post-burn client. Which abnormality should be reported to the physician immediately?

Quick Answer: **389**
Detailed Answer: **403**

- ○ **A.** Potassium 7.5mEq/L
- ○ **B.** Sodium 131mEq/L
- ○ **C.** Arterial pH 7.34
- ○ **D.** Hematocrit 52%

146. The nurse is observing a student nurse administering ear drops to a two-year-old. Which observation by the nurse would indicate correct technique?

Quick Answer: **389**
Detailed Answer: **403**

- ○ **A.** Holds the child's head up and extended
- ○ **B.** Places the head in chin-tuck position
- ○ **C.** Pulls the pinna down and back
- ○ **D.** Irrigates the ear before administering medication

147. The nurse is caring for a client with scalding burns across the face, neck, upper half of the anterior chest, and entire right arm. Using the rule of nines, estimate the percentage of body burned.

Quick Answer: **389**
Detailed Answer: **403**

- ○ **A.** 18%
- ○ **B.** 23%
- ○ **C.** 32%
- ○ **D.** 36%

148. The nurse caring for a client in shock recognizes that the glomerular filtration rate of the kidneys will fail if the client's mean arterial pressure falls below which of the following levels?

Quick Answer: **389**
Detailed Answer: **404**

- ○ **A.** 140
- ○ **B.** 120
- ○ **C.** 100
- ○ **D.** 80

149. The nurse is caring for a child with a diagnosis of possible hydro-cephalus. Which assessment data on the admission history would be the most objective?

    ○ **A.** Anorexia

    ○ **B.** Vomiting

    ○ **C.** Head measurement

    ○ **D.** Temperature reading

Quick Answer: **389**
Detailed Answer: **404**

150. A client is admitted after a motor vehicle accident. Based on the following results, what physician's prescription will the nurse anticipate?

Quick Answer: **389**
Detailed Answer: **404**

CBC	Chemistry Profile	Arterial Blood Gases (ABGs)
Hgb 13.6g/dL	Potassium 3.9 mEq/L	pH 7.23
Hct 42%	Chloride 102 mEq/L	pCO_2 63
WBC 8000/mm^3	Glucose 100mg/dL	HCO_3 23mEq/L
Platelets 250,000		PO_2 50
		O_2 saturation 84

    ○ **A.** Blood transfusion

    ○ **B.** Potassium IVPB

    ○ **C.** Mechanical ventilator

    ○ **D.** Platelet transfusion

151. The nurse is caring for a client after a burn. Which assessment finding best indicates that the client's respiratory efforts are currently adequate?

    ○ **A.** The client is able to talk.

    ○ **B.** The client is alert and oriented.

    ○ **C.** The client's O_2 saturation is 97%.

    ○ **D.** The client's chest movements are uninhibited.

Quick Answer: **389**
Detailed Answer: **404**

152. The nurse is performing discharge teaching to the parents of a seven-year-old who has been diagnosed with asthma. Which sports activity would be most appropriate for this client?

    ○ **A.** Baseball

    ○ **B.** Swimming

    ○ **C.** Football

    ○ **D.** Track

Quick Answer: **389**
Detailed Answer: **404**

153. The leukemic client is prescribed a low-bacteria diet. Which does the nurse expect to be included in this diet?

   ○ **A.** Cooked spinach and sautéed celery

   ○ **B.** Lettuce and alfalfa sprouts

   ○ **C.** Fresh strawberries and whipped cream

   ○ **D.** Raw cauliflower or broccoli

Quick Answer: **389**
Detailed Answer: **404**

154. A child is to receive heparin sodium five units per kilogram of body weight by subcutaneous route every four hours. The child weighs 52.8 lb. How many units should the child receive in a 24-hour period?

   ○ **A.** 300

   ○ **B.** 480

   ○ **C.** 720

   ○ **D.** 960

Quick Answer: **389**
Detailed Answer: **405**

155. A client with cancer is experiencing a common side effect of chemotherapy administration. Which laboratory assessment finding would cause the most concern?

   ○ **A.** A sodium level of 50mg/dL

   ○ **B.** A blood glucose of 110mg/dL

   ○ **C.** A platelet count of $125,000/mm^3$

   ○ **D.** A white cell count of $5,000/mm^3$

Quick Answer: **389**
Detailed Answer: **405**

156. A client's admission history reveals complaints of fatigue, chronic sore throat, and enlarged lymph nodes in the axilla and neck. Which exam would assist the physician to make a tentative diagnosis of leukemia?

   ○ **A.** A complete blood count

   ○ **B.** An x-ray of the chest

   ○ **C.** A bone marrow aspiration

   ○ **D.** A CT scan of the abdomen

Quick Answer: **389**
Detailed Answer: **405**

157. A client is admitted with symptoms of vertigo and syncope. Diagnostic tests indicate left subclavian artery obstruction. What additional findings would the nurse expect?

   ○ **A.** Memory loss and disorientation

   ○ **B.** Numbness in the face, mouth, and tongue

   ○ **C.** Radial pulse differences over 10bpm

   ○ **D.** Frontal headache with associated nausea or emesis

Quick Answer: **389**
Detailed Answer: **405**

158. The nurse is performing discharge teaching on a client at high risk for the development of skin cancer. Which instruction should be included in the client teaching?

- ○ **A.** "You should see the doctor every six months."
- ○ **B.** "Sunbathing should be done between the hours of noon and 3 p.m."
- ○ **C.** "If you have a mole, it should be removed and biopsied."
- ○ **D.** "You should wear sunscreen when going outside."

Quick Answer: **389**
Detailed Answer: **405**

159. A client with pancreatitis has been transferred to the intensive care unit. The nurse assesses a pulmonary arterial wedge pressure (PAWP) of 14mmHg. Based on this finding, the nurse would want to further assess for what additional correlating wedge pressure data?

- ○ **A.** A drop in blood pressure
- ○ **B.** Rales on chest auscultation
- ○ **C.** A temperature elevation
- ○ **D.** Dry mucous membranes

Quick Answer: **389**
Detailed Answer: **405**

160. The nurse is caring for a client with a diagnosis of hepatitis who is experiencing pruritis. Which would be the most appropriate nursing intervention?

- ○ **A.** Suggest that the client take warm showers.
- ○ **B.** Add baby oil to the client's bath water.
- ○ **C.** Apply powder to the client's skin.
- ○ **D.** Suggest a hot-water rinse after bathing.

Quick Answer: **389**
Detailed Answer: **405**

161. A client is admitted to the emergency department with a loss of consciousness with unknown etiology. The nurse expects to perform which laboratory test to assist in determining etiology?

- ○ **A.** Total cholesterol
- ○ **B.** Alkaline phosphatese
- ○ **C.** Serum glucose
- ○ **D.** Urinalysis

Quick Answer: **389**
Detailed Answer: **405**

162. The physician has ordered a homocysteine blood level on a client. The nurse recognizes that the results will be increased in a client with a deficiency in which of the following:

   ○ **A.** Vitamin B12

   ○ **B.** Vitamin C

   ○ **C.** Vitamin A

   ○ **D.** Vitamin E

Quick Answer: **389**
Detailed Answer: **405**

163. The registered nurse is assigning staff for four clients on the 3–11 shift. Which client should be assigned to the LPN?

   ○ **A.** A client with a diagnosis of adult respiratory distress syndrome (ARDS) who was transferred from the critical care unit at 1400

   ○ **B.** A one-hour post-operative colon resection

   ○ **C.** A client with pneumonia expecting discharge in the morning

   ○ **D.** A client with cirrhosis of the liver experiencing bleeding from esophageal varices

Quick Answer: **389**
Detailed Answer: **405**

164. A client with multiple sclerosis has an order to receive Solu Medrol 200mg IV push. The available dose is Solu Medrol 250mg per mL. How much medication will the nurse administer?

   ○ **A.** 0.5 mL

   ○ **B.** 0.8 mL

   ○ **C.** 1.1 mL

   ○ **D.** 1.4 mL

Quick Answer: **389**
Detailed Answer: **405**

165. The nurse is obtaining a history on a 74-year-old client. Which statement made by the client would most alert the nurse to a possible fluid and electrolyte imbalance?

   ○ **A.** "My skin is always so dry."

   ○ **B.** "I often use a laxative for constipation."

   ○ **C.** "I have always liked to drink a lot of water."

   ○ **D.** "I sometimes have a problem with dribbling urine."

Quick Answer: **389**
Detailed Answer: **405**

166. The nurse is caring for a client in the acute care unit. Initial laboratory values reveal serum sodium of 156mEq/L. What behavior changes would the nurse expect the client to exhibit?

   ○ **A.** Hyporeflexia

   ○ **B.** Manic behavior

   ○ **C.** Depression

   ○ **D.** Muscle cramps

Quick Answer: **389**
Detailed Answer: **406**

167. The nurse is completing the preoperative checklist on a client scheduled for surgery and finds that the consent form has been signed, but the client is unclear about the surgery and possible complications. Which is the most appropriate action?

- ○ **A.** Call the surgeon and ask him to come see the client to clarify the information.
- ○ **B.** Explain the procedure and complications to the client.
- ○ **C.** Check in the physician's progress notes to see if understanding has been documented.
- ○ **D.** Check with the client's family to see if they understand the procedure fully.

168. When preparing a client for admission to the surgical suite, the nurse recognizes that which one of the following items is most important to remove before sending the client to surgery?

- ○ **A.** Hearing aid
- ○ **B.** Contact lenses
- ○ **C.** Wedding ring
- ○ **D.** Dentures

169. A client with cancer is to undergo a bone scan. The nurse should perform which of the following actions?

- ○ **A.** Force fluids 24 hours before the procedure is scheduled to begin.
- ○ **B.** Ask the client to void immediately before the study.
- ○ **C.** Hold medication that affects the central nervous system for 12 hours pre- and post-test.
- ○ **D.** Cover the client's reproductive organs with an x-ray shield during the procedure.

170. A client with suspected leukemia is to undergo a bone marrow aspiration. The nurse plans to include which statement in the teaching session?

- ○ **A.** "You will be lying on your abdomen for the examination procedure."
- ○ **B.** "Portions of the procedure will cause pain or discomfort."
- ○ **C.** "You will be given some medication to cause amnesia of the test."
- ○ **D.** "You will not be able to drink fluids for 24 hours before the study."

171. The nurse is caring for a client scheduled for a surgical repair of an abdominal aortic aneurysm. Which assessment is most crucial during the preoperative period?

   ○ **A.** Assessment of the client's level of anxiety

   ○ **B.** Evaluation of the client's exercise tolerance

   ○ **C.** Identification of peripheral pulses

   ○ **D.** Assessment of bowel sounds and activity

172. The nurse should carefully monitor the client for which common dysrhythmia that can occur during suctioning?

   ○ **A.** Bradycardia

   ○ **B.** Tachycardia

   ○ **C.** Ventricular ectopic beats

   ○ **D.** Sick sinus syndrome

173. The nurse is performing discharge instructions for a client with an implantable permanent pacemaker. What discharge instruction is an essential part of the plan?

   ○ **A.** "You cannot eat food prepared in a microwave."

   ○ **B.** "You should avoid moving the shoulder on the side of the pacemaker site for six weeks."

   ○ **C.** "You will have to learn to take your own pulse."

   ○ **D.** "You will not be able to fly on a commercial airliner with the pacemaker in place."

174. The nurse is completing admission on a client with possible esophageal cancer. Which finding would not be common for this diagnosis?

   ○ **A.** Foul breath

   ○ **B.** Dysphagia

   ○ **C.** Diarrhea

   ○ **D.** Chronic hiccups

175. A client arrives from surgery following an abdominal perineal resection with a permanent ileostomy. What should be the priority nursing care during the post-op period?

   ○ **A.** Teaching how to irrigate the ileostomy

   ○ **B.** Stopping electrolyte loss through the stoma

   ○ **C.** Encouraging a high-fiber diet

   ○ **D.** Facilitating perineal wound drainage

176. The nurse is making initial rounds on a client with a C5 fracture. The client is in a halo vest and is receiving O_2 at 40% via mask to a tracheostomy. Assessment reveals a respiratory rate of 40 and O_2 saturation of 88. The client is restless. Which initial nursing action is most indicated?

Quick Answer: **389**
Detailed Answer: **407**

- ○ **A.** Notifying the physician
- ○ **B.** Performing tracheal suctioning
- ○ **C.** Repositioning the client to the left side
- ○ **D.** Rechecking the client's O_2 saturation

177. A client has just finished her lunch, consisting of shrimp with rice, fruit salad, and a roll. The client calls for the nurse, stating, "My throat feels thick and I'm having trouble breathing." What action should the nurse implement first?

Quick Answer: **389**
Detailed Answer: **407**

- ○ **A.** Place the bed in Trendelenburg position and call the physician.
- ○ **B.** Take the client's vital signs and administer Benadryl 50mg PO.
- ○ **C.** Place the bed in high Fowler's position and call the physician.
- ○ **D.** Start an Aminophylline drip and call the physician.

178. The nurse is caring for a client with cirrhosis of the liver. Which is the best method to use for determining that the client has ascites?

Quick Answer: **389**
Detailed Answer: **407**

- ○ **A.** Inspection of the abdomen for enlargement
- ○ **B.** Bimanual palpation for hepatomegaly
- ○ **C.** Daily measurement of abdominal girth
- ○ **D.** Assessment for a fluid wave

179. A client arrives in the emergency room after a motor vehicle accident. Witnesses tell the nurse that they observed the client's head hit the side of the car door. Nursing assessment findings include BP 70/34, heart rate 130, and respirations 22. Based on the information provided, which is the priority nursing care focus?

Quick Answer: **389**
Detailed Answer: **407**

- ○ **A.** Brain tissue perfusion
- ○ **B.** Regaining fluid volume
- ○ **C.** Clearance of the client's airway
- ○ **D.** Measures to increase sensation

180. The home health nurse is visiting a 30-year-old with sickle cell disease. Assessment findings include spleenomegaly. What information obtained on the visit would cause the most concern? The client:

   ○   **A.** Eats fast food daily for lunch

   ○   **B.** Drinks a beer occasionally

   ○   **C.** Sometimes feels fatigued

   ○   **D.** Works as a furniture mover

181. The nurse on the oncology unit is caring for a client with a WBC of 1500/mm^3. During evening visitation, a visitor brings in a fruit basket. What action should the nurse take?

   ○   **A.** Encourage the client to eat small snacks of the fruit.

   ○   **B.** Remove fruits that are not high in vitamin C.

   ○   **C.** Instruct the client to avoid the high-fiber fruits.

   ○   **D.** Remove the fruits from the client's room.

182. The nurse is giving an end-of-shift report when a client with a chest tube is noted in the hallway with the tube disconnected. What is the most appropriate action?

   ○   **A.** Clamp the chest tube immediately.

   ○   **B.** Put the end of the chest tube into a cup of sterile normal saline.

   ○   **C.** Assist the client back to the room and place him on his left side.

   ○   **D.** Reconnect the chest tube to the chest tube system.

183. A client with deep vein thrombosis is receiving a continuous heparin infusion and Coumadin PO. INR lab test result is 8.0. Which intervention would be most important to include in the nursing care plan?

   ○   **A.** Assess for signs of abnormal bleeding.

   ○   **B.** Anticipate an increase in the heparin drip rate.

   ○   **C.** Instruct the client regarding the drug therapy.

   ○   **D.** Increase the frequency of vascular assessments.

184. Which breakfast selection by a client with osteoporosis indicates that the client understands the dietary management of the disease?

- ○ **A.** Scrambled eggs, toast, and coffee
- ○ **B.** Bran muffin with margarine
- ○ **C.** Granola bar and half of a grapefruit
- ○ **D.** Bagel with jam and skim milk

Quick Answer: **389**
Detailed Answer: **407**

185. A client with hepatitis C who has cirrhosis changes has just returned from a liver biopsy. The nurse will place the client in which position?

- ○ **A.** Trendelenburg
- ○ **B.** Supine
- ○ **C.** Right side-lying
- ○ **D.** Left Sim's

Quick Answer: **389**
Detailed Answer: **407**

186. The nurse is caring for a client who was admitted to the burn unit four hours after the injury with second-degree burns to the trunk and head. Which finding would the nurse least expect to find during this time period?

- ○ **A.** Hypovolemia
- ○ **B.** Laryngeal edema
- ○ **C.** Hypernatremia
- ○ **D.** Hyperkalemia

Quick Answer: **389**
Detailed Answer: **407**

187. The nurse is evaluating nutritional outcomes for a client with anorexia nervosa. Which one of the following is the most objective favorable outcome for the client?

- ○ **A.** The client eats all the food on her tray.
- ○ **B.** The client requests that family bring special foods.
- ○ **C.** The client's weight has increased.
- ○ **D.** The client weighs herself each morning.

Quick Answer: **389**
Detailed Answer: **407**

188. The client who is two weeks post-burn with a 40% deep partial-thickness injury still has open wounds. The nurse's assessment reveals the following findings: temperature 96.5°F, BP 87/40, and severe diarrhea stools. What problem does the nurse most likely suspect?

- ○ **A.** Findings are normal, not suspicious of a problem
- ○ **B.** Systemic gram—positive infection
- ○ **C.** Systemic gram—negative infection
- ○ **D.** Systemic fungal infection

Quick Answer: **389**
Detailed Answer: **408**

189. The nurse assesses a new order for a blood transfusion. The order is to transfuse one unit of packed red blood cells (contains 250mL) in a two-hour period. What will be the hourly rate of infusion?

Quick Answer: **389**
Detailed Answer: **408**

   ○ **A.** 50mL/hr

   ○ **B.** 62mL/hr

   ○ **C.** 125mL/hr

   ○ **D.** 137mL/hr

190. A client has signs of increased intracranial pressure. Which one of the following is an early indicator of deterioration in the client's condition?

Quick Answer: **389**
Detailed Answer: **408**

   ○ **A.** Widening pulse pressure

   ○ **B.** Decrease in the pulse rate

   ○ **C.** Dilated, fixed pupils

   ○ **D.** Decrease in level of consciousness

191. Which of the following statements by a client with a seizure disorder who is taking topiramate (Topamax) indicates that the client has understood the nurse's instruction?

Quick Answer: **389**
Detailed Answer: **408**

   ○ **A.** "I will take the medicine before going to bed."

   ○ **B.** "I will drink 8 to 10 ten-ounce glasses of water a day."

   ○ **C.** "I will eat plenty of fresh fruits."

   ○ **D.** "I must take the medicine with a meal or snack."

192. A client with terminal lung cancer is admitted to the unit. A family member asks the nurse, "How much longer will it be?" Which response by the nurse is most appropriate?

Quick Answer: **389**
Detailed Answer: **408**

   ○ **A.** "This must be a terrible situation for you."

   ○ **B.** "I don't know. I'll call the doctor."

   ○ **C.** "I cannot say exactly. What are your concerns at this time?"

   ○ **D.** "Don't worry, from the way things look, it will be very soon."

193. A client with a history of colon cancer is admitted to the oncology unit. Laboratory results reveal a WBC of 1600/mm^3. What plans will the nurse add to the care plan because of the WBC reading? Select all that apply.

   ○ **A.** No sick visitors

   ○ **B.** Private room necessary

   ○ **C.** No aspirin products

   ○ **D.** Low bacteria diet

   ○ **E.** Electric razors only

Quick Answer: **389**
Detailed Answer: **408**

194. The nurse is caring for a client with a closed head injury. Fluid is assessed leaking from the ear. What is the nurse's first action?

   ○ **A.** Irrigate the ear canal gently.

   ○ **B.** Notify the physician.

   ○ **C.** Test the drainage for glucose.

   ○ **D.** Apply an occlusive dressing.

Quick Answer: **389**
Detailed Answer: **408**

195. The nurse has inserted an NG tube for enteral feedings. Which assessment result is the best indicator of the tube's stomach placement?

   ○ **A.** Aspiration of tan-colored mucus

   ○ **B.** Green aspirate with a pH of 3

   ○ **C.** A swish auscultated with the injection of air

   ○ **D.** Bubbling noted when the end of the tube is placed in liquid

Quick Answer: **389**
Detailed Answer: **408**

196. The nurse would identify which one of the following assessment findings as a normal response in a craniotomy client post-operatively?

   ○ **A.** A decrease in responsiveness the third post-op day

   ○ **B.** Sluggish pupil reaction the first 24–48 hours

   ○ **C.** Dressing changes three to four times a day for the first three days

   ○ **D.** Temperature range of 98.8°F to 99.6°F the first 2–3 days

Quick Answer: **389**
Detailed Answer: **408**

197. A client with alcoholism has been instructed to increase his intake of thiamine. The nurse knows the client understands the instructions when he selects which food?

   ○ **A.** Roast beef

   ○ **B.** Broiled fish

   ○ **C.** Baked chicken

   ○ **D.** Sliced pork

Quick Answer: **389**
Detailed Answer: **408**

198. The nurse would expect to find which drug prescribed for a patient diagnosed with ALS?

Quick Answer: **389**
Detailed Answer: **408**

- ○ **A.** Amantadine hydrochloride (Symmetrel)
- ○ **B.** Riluzole (Rilutek)
- ○ **C.** Lisinopril (Zestril)
- ○ **D.** Estrodial (Estrogel)

199. A client has a CVP monitor in place via a central line. Which would be included in the nursing care plan for this client?

Quick Answer: **389**
Detailed Answer: **408**

- ○ **A.** Notify the physician of readings less than 3cm or more than 8cm of water.
- ○ **B.** Use the clean technique to change the dressing at the insertion site.
- ○ **C.** Elevate the head of the bed to 90° to obtain CVP readings.
- ○ **D.** The 0 mark on the manometer should align with the client's right clavicle for the readings.

200. A client is admitted to the chemical dependency unit for poly-drug abuse. The client states, "I don't know why you are all so worried; I am in control. I don't have a problem." Which defense mechanism is being utilized?

Quick Answer: **389**
Detailed Answer: **409**

- ○ **A.** Rationalization
- ○ **B.** Projection
- ○ **C.** Dissociation
- ○ **D.** Denial

201. A client scheduled for a carotid endarterectomy requires insertion of an intra-arterial blood pressure-monitoring device. The nurse plans to perform the Allen test. Which observation indicates patency of the ulnar artery?

Quick Answer: **389**
Detailed Answer: **409**

- ○ **A.** Blanching of the hand on compression and release of the ulnar artery
- ○ **B.** Muscular twitching of the bicep muscle with use of a tourniquet at the wrist
- ○ **C.** Hand turning pink after the nurse releases the pressure on the ulnar artery
- ○ **D.** Flexion of the wrist when tapping the ulnar artery with a reflex hammer

202. A client's chest tube drainage device has continuous bubbling in the water seal chamber. What is the nurse checking for when she clamps different areas of the tube to find out where the bubbling stops?

○ **A.** An air leak in the system

○ **B.** The suction being too high

○ **C.** The suction being too low

○ **D.** A tension pneumothorax

203. The nurse should be particularly alert for which one of the following problems in a client with barbiturate overdose?

○ **A.** Oliguria

○ **B.** Cardiac tamponade

○ **C.** Apnea

○ **D.** Hemorrhage

204. A client taking the drug disulfiram (Antabuse) is admitted to the ER. Which clinical manifestations are most indicative of recent alcohol ingestion?

○ **A.** Vomiting, heart rate 120, chest pain

○ **B.** Nausea, mild headache, bradycardia

○ **C.** Respirations 16, heart rate 62, diarrhea

○ **D.** Temp 101°F, tachycardia, respirations 20

205. A client with cancer and metastasis to the bone is admitted to the hospital. Which symptom of hypercalcemia causes the nurse the most concern?

○ **A.** Weakness

○ **B.** Anorexia

○ **C.** Flaccid muscles

○ **D.** Cardiac changes

206. The nurse expects that a client with cocaine addiction would most likely be placed on which medication?

○ **A.** Bromocriptine (Parlodel)

○ **B.** Methadone

○ **C.** THC

○ **D.** Disulfiram (Antabuse)

207. The nurse is reviewing the laboratory values of a client with a myocardial infarction. Which laboratory test is used to identify injury to the myocardium and can remain elevated for up to three weeks?

Quick Answer: **389**
Detailed Answer: **409**

- ○ **A.** Total CK
- ○ **B.** CK-MB
- ○ **C.** Myoglobulin
- ○ **D.** Troponin T or I

208. A client with newly diagnosed epilepsy tells the nurse, "If I keep having seizures, I'm scared my husband will feel differently toward me." Which response by the nurse would be most appropriate?

Quick Answer: **389**
Detailed Answer: **409**

- ○ **A.** "You don't know if you'll ever have another seizure. Why don't you wait and see what happens?"
- ○ **B.** "You seem to be concerned that there could be a change in the relationship with your husband."
- ○ **C.** "You should focus on your children. They need you."
- ○ **D.** "Let's see how your husband reacts before getting upset."

209. While interviewing a client who abuses alcohol, the nurse learns that the client has experienced "blackouts." The wife asks what this means. What is the nurse's best response at this time?

Quick Answer: **389**
Detailed Answer: **409**

- ○ **A.** "Your husband has experienced short-term memory amnesia."
- ○ **B.** "Your husband has experienced loss of remote memory."
- ○ **C.** "Your husband has experienced a loss of consciousness."
- ○ **D.** "Your husband has experienced a fainting spell."

210. Which would the nurse include in the nursing care plan of a client experiencing severe delirium tremens?

Quick Answer: **389**
Detailed Answer: **409**

- ○ **A.** Placing the client in a darkened room
- ○ **B.** Keeping the closet and bathroom doors closed
- ○ **C.** Administering a diuretic to decrease fluid excess
- ○ **D.** Checking vital signs every eight hours

211. The nurse is caring for a client admitted with a diagnosis of epilepsy. The client begins to have a seizure. Which action by the nurse is contraindicated?

   ○ **A.** Turning the client to the side-lying position

   ○ **B.** Inserting a padded tongue blade and oral airway

   ○ **C.** Loosening restrictive clothing

   ○ **D.** Removing the pillow and raising padded side rails

Quick Answer: **389**
Detailed Answer: **410**

212. A client has been placed on the drug valproic acid (Depakene). Which would indicate to the nurse that the client is experiencing an adverse reaction to this medication?

   ○ **A.** Photophobia

   ○ **B.** Poor skin turgor

   ○ **C.** Lethargy

   ○ **D.** Reported visual disturbances

Quick Answer: **389**
Detailed Answer: **410**

213. A client has an order for vancomycin (Vancocin) 1 gram IVPB in 250 mL normal saline to infuse over 60 minutes. The nurse would set the IV drop rate to deliver how many drops per minute if the IV set delivers 15gtts/mL? Fill in the blank.

   _____Gtts/minute

Quick Answer: **389**
Detailed Answer: **410**

214. The nurse is performing fluid resuscitation on a burn client. Which piece of assessment data is the best indicator that it is effective?

   ○ **A.** Respirations 24, unlabored

   ○ **B.** Urine output of 30ml/hr

   ○ **C.** Capillary refill < 4 seconds

   ○ **D.** Apical pulse of 110/min

Quick Answer: **389**
Detailed Answer: **410**

215. A client diagnosed with COPD is receiving theophylline (Theodur). Morning laboratory values reveal a theophylline level of 38mcg/mL. Which is the most appropriate nursing action?

   ○ **A.** Take no action; this is within normal range.

   ○ **B.** Notify the physician of the level results.

   ○ **C.** Administer Narcan 2mg IV push stat.

   ○ **D.** Give the client an extra dose of the medication.

Quick Answer: **389**
Detailed Answer: **410**

216. A client has suffered a severe electrical burn. Which medication would the nurse expect to have ordered for application to the burned area?

- ○ **A.** Mafenide acetate (Sulfamylon)
- ○ **B.** Silver nitrate
- ○ **C.** Providone-iodine ointment
- ○ **D.** Silver sulfadiazine (Silvadene)

Quick Answer: **389**
Detailed Answer: **410**

217. A client with a head injury develops syndrome of inappropriate antidiuretic hormone (SIADH). Which physician prescription would the nurse question?

- ○ **A.** D5W at 200mL/hr
- ○ **B.** Demeclocycline (Declomycin) 150mg Q6h
- ○ **C.** Daily weights
- ○ **D.** Monitor intake and output

Quick Answer: **389**
Detailed Answer: **410**

218. A client with essential tremors has been prescribed the drug primidone (Mysoline). Which of the following will the nurse teach the patient about the drug?

- ○ **A.** Avoid alcohol while taking the drug.
- ○ **B.** The drug causes hyperactivity.
- ○ **C.** The drug can be stopped abruptly without effects.
- ○ **D.** Euphoria is a side effect of taking the drug.

Quick Answer: **389**
Detailed Answer: **410**

219. The nurse is caring for a postpartum client two hours post-delivery who is unable to void. Which of the following nursing interventions should be considered first?

- ○ **A.** Insert a straight catheter for residual.
- ○ **B.** Encourage oral intake of fluids.
- ○ **C.** Check perineum for swelling or hematoma.
- ○ **D.** Palpate bladder for distention and position.

Quick Answer: **389**
Detailed Answer: **410**

220. A client is admitted to the intensive care unit after falling on an icy sidewalk and striking the right side of the head. An MRI revealed a right-sided epidural hematoma. Which physical force explains the location of the client's injury?

- ○ **A.** Coup
- ○ **B.** Contrecoup
- ○ **C.** Deceleration
- ○ **D.** Acceleration

Quick Answer: **389**
Detailed Answer: **410**

221. The nurse is preparing to teach a client about phenytoin sodium (Dilantin). Which fact would be most important to teach the client regarding why the drug should not be stopped suddenly?

- ○ **A.** Physical dependence can develop over time.
- ○ **B.** Status epilepticus can develop.
- ○ **C.** A hypoglycemic reaction can develop.
- ○ **D.** Heart block can develop.

Quick Answer: **389**
Detailed Answer: **410**

222. The nurse on the neurological unit admits a patient with a newly diagnosed amyotrophic lateral sclerosis (ALS) disorder. Which does the nurse expect to assess in this patient? Select all that apply.

- ○ **A.** Drooling
- ○ **B.** Weakness
- ○ **C.** Spasticity
- ○ **D.** Diarrhea
- ○ **E.** Depression
- ○ **F.** Pain

Quick Answer: **389**
Detailed Answer: **410**

223. A client is admitted with suspected Guillain-Barre syndrome. The nurse would expect the cerebrospinal fluid (CSF) analysis to reveal which of the following to confirm the diagnosis?

- ○ **A.** CSF protein of 10mg/dL and WBC 2 cells/mm^3
- ○ **B.** CSF protein of 60mg/dL and WBC 0 cells/mm^3
- ○ **C.** CSF protein of 50mg/dL and WBC 20 cells/mm^3
- ○ **D.** CSF protein of 5mg/dL and WBC 20 cells/mm^3

Quick Answer: **389**
Detailed Answer: **411**

224. A client with burns is admitted and fluid resuscitation has begun. The client's CVP reading is 14cm/H_2O. Which evaluation by the nurse would be most accurate?

- ○ **A.** The client has received enough fluid.
- ○ **B.** The client's fluid status is unaltered.
- ○ **C.** The client has inadequate fluids.
- ○ **D.** The client has a volume excess.

Quick Answer: **389**
Detailed Answer: **411**

225. The nurse is working on a neurological unit. If the following events occur simultaneously, which would receive RN priority?

Quick Answer: **389**
Detailed Answer: **411**

- ○ **A.** A client with a cerebral aneurysm complains of sudden weakness on the right side.
- ○ **B.** A client with a suspected brain tumor complains of a frontal type headache.
- ○ **C.** A client post-op lumbar laminectomy vomits.
- ○ **D.** A client with Guillain-Barré syndrome has a temperature elevation.

226. The nurse assesses a client's fundal height every 15 minutes during the first hour postpartum. What should the height of the fundus be during this hour ?

Quick Answer: **389**
Detailed Answer: **411**

- ○ **A.** 1–2 fingerbreadths under the umbilicus
- ○ **B.** Four fingerbreadths under the umbilicus
- ○ **C.** One fingerbreadth above the umbilicus
- ○ **D.** Four fingerbreadths above the umbilicus

227. A patient arrives in the ER with a possible Zika virus diagnosis. Which clinical manifestation(s) would the nurse expect the patient to exhibit? Select all that apply.

Quick Answer: **389**
Detailed Answer: **411**

- ○ **A.** Hypothermia
- ○ **B.** Abdominal pain
- ○ **C.** Headache
- ○ **D.** Conjunctivitis
- ○ **E.** Diplopia

228. A client with chronic obstructive pulmonary disease (COPD) is admitted to the respiratory unit. Which physician prescription should the nurse question?

Quick Answer: **389**
Detailed Answer: **411**

- ○ **A.** O_2 at 5L/min by nasal cannula
- ○ **B.** Solu Medrol 125mg IV push every six hours
- ○ **C.** Ceftriaxone (Rocephin) 1gram IVPB daily
- ○ **D.** Darvocet N 100 po prn pain

229. A burn client begins treatments with silver sulfadiazine (Silvadene) applied to the wounds. The nurse should carefully monitor for which adverse affect associated with this drug?

- ○ **A.** Hypokalemia
- ○ **B.** Leukopenia
- ○ **C.** Hyponatremia
- ○ **D.** Thrombocytopenia

Quick Answer: **389**
Detailed Answer: **411**

230. The nurse is presenting a workshop on the Zika virus infection. Which is included in the teaching plan? Select all that apply.

- ○ **A.** The virus is spread primarily by rodent contact.
- ○ **B.** Sexual transmission can spread the virus.
- ○ **C.** The virus can cause brain defects to the fetus of pregnant women.
- ○ **D.** There is no specific treatment for Zika.
- ○ **E.** Zika virus should be nationally reported.

Quick Answer: **389**
Detailed Answer: **411**

231. The nurse is assessing a client for tactile fremitus. Which of the following diagnoses would most likely reveal a decrease in tactile fremitus?

- ○ **A.** Emphysema
- ○ **B.** Bronchial pneumonia
- ○ **C.** Tuberculosis
- ○ **D.** Lung tumor

Quick Answer: **389**
Detailed Answer: **411**

232. A client who has been diagnosed with lung cancer is starting a smoking-cessation program. Which of the following drugs would the nurse expect to be included in the program's plan?

- ○ **A.** Bupropion SR (Zyban)
- ○ **B.** Metaproterenol (Alupent)
- ○ **C.** Oxitropuim (Oxivent)
- ○ **D.** Alprazolam (Xanax)

Quick Answer: **389**
Detailed Answer: **411**

233. A client delivered a nine-pound infant two hours ago. The client has an IV of D5W with oxytocin. The nurse determines that the medication is achieving the desired effect when which of the following is assessed?

- ○ **A.** A rise in blood pressure
- ○ **B.** A decrease in pain
- ○ **C.** An increase in lochia rubra
- ○ **D.** A firm uterine fundus

Quick Answer: **389**
Detailed Answer: **411**

234. The nurse is evaluating cerebral perfusion outcomes for a client with a subdural hematoma. The nurse evaluates which of the following as a favorable outcome for this client?

    ○   **A.** Arterial blood gas PO_2 of 98

    ○   **B.** Increase in lethargy

    ○   **C.** Pupils slow to react to light

    ○   **D.** Temperature of 101°F

Quick Answer: **389**
Detailed Answer: **412**

235. The nurse is caring for a client with a chronic airway disease. Which of the associated disorders has changes that are reversible?

    ○   **A.** Bronchiectasis

    ○   **B.** Emphysema

    ○   **C.** Asthma

    ○   **D.** Chronic bronchitis

Quick Answer: **389**
Detailed Answer: **412**

236. A client experienced a major burn over 55% of his body 36 hours ago. The client is restless and anxious, and states, "I am in pain." There is a physician prescription for intravenous morphine. What should the nurse do first?

    ○   **A.** Administer the morphine.

    ○   **B.** Assess respirations.

    ○   **C.** Assess urine output.

    ○   **D.** Check serum potassium levels.

Quick Answer: **389**
Detailed Answer: **412**

237. The nurse is caring for a client seven days post-burn injury with 60% body surface area involved. What should be the primary focus of nursing care during this time period?

    ○   **A.** Meticulous infection-control measures

    ○   **B.** Fluid-replacement evaluation

    ○   **C.** Psychological adjustment to the wound

    ○   **D.** Measurement and application of a pressure garment

Quick Answer: **389**
Detailed Answer: **412**

238. The nurse is preparing a teaching plan for a client beginning external radiation treatments. Which of the following will be included in the teaching plan?
Select all that apply.

    ○   **A.** Space activities with rest periods.

    ○   **B.** Avoid spicy and hot foods.

    ○   **C.** Expose radiated areas to sunlight daily.

    ○   **D.** Wash the skin with plain water.

    ○   **E.** Expect to have difficulty swallowing.

Quick Answer: **389**
Detailed Answer: **412**

239. The nurse is performing discharge teaching for a client after a cardiac catheterization. Which statement by the client indicates a need for further teaching?

Quick Answer: 389
Detailed Answer: 412

    ○ **A.** "I should not bend, strain, or lift heavy objects for one day."

    ○ **B.** "If bleeding occurs, I should place an ice bag on the site for 10 minutes."

    ○ **C.** "I need to call the doctor if my temperature goes above 101°F."

    ○ **D.** "I should talk to the doctor to find out when I can go back to work."

240. A burn client is in the acute phase of burn care. The nurse assesses jugular vein distention, edema, urine output of 20 mL in two hours, and crackles on auscultation. Which order would the nurse anticipate from the physician?

Quick Answer: 389
Detailed Answer: 412

    ○ **A.** Furosemide (Lasix) 40 mg IV push

    ○ **B.** Irrigate the Foley catheter

    ○ **C.** Increase the IV fluids to 200mL/hr

    ○ **D.** Place the client in Trendelenburg position

241. The nurse is suctioning a tracheostomy, what is the maximum suction pressure the nurse should use?

Quick Answer: 389
Detailed Answer: 412

    ○ **A.** 120mmHg

    ○ **B.** 145mmHg

    ○ **C.** 160mmHg

    ○ **D.** 185mmHg

242. A client admitted with transient ischemia attacks has returned from a cerebral arteriogram. The nurse performs an assessment and finds a newly formed hematoma in the right groin area. What is the nurse's initial action?

Quick Answer: 389
Detailed Answer: 412

    ○ **A.** Apply direct pressure to the site.

    ○ **B.** Check the pedal pulses on the right leg.

    ○ **C.** Notify the physician.

    ○ **D.** Turn the client to the prone position.

243. The nurse is assessing an ECG strip of a 42-year-old client and finds a regular rate greater than 100, a normal QRS complex, a normal P wave in front of each QRS, a PR interval between 0.12 and 0.20 seconds, and a P: QRS ratio of 1:1. What is the nurse's interpretation of this rhythm?

Quick Answer: **389**
Detailed Answer: **412**

- ○ **A.** Premature atrial complex
- ○ **B.** Sinus tachycardia
- ○ **C.** Atrial flutter
- ○ **D.** Supraventricular tachycardia

244. A nurse is caring for a client in the critical care unit who is complaining of chest pain. Nursing assessment reveals a BP of 78/40, shortness of breath, and third-degree AV block on the heart monitor. What is the most appropriate initial action?

Quick Answer: **389**
Detailed Answer: **413**

- ○ **A.** Provide trancutaneous pacing.
- ○ **B.** Turn the client on his side.
- ○ **C.** Reassess the blood pressure.
- ○ **D.** Consult with cardiology.

245. The nurse is discussing cigarette smoking with an emphysema client. The client states, "I don't know why I should worry about smoking." The nurse's response is based on the fact that smoking has which of the following negative effects to the emphysematous lung?

Quick Answer: **389**
Detailed Answer: **413**

- ○ **A.** Affects peripheral blood vessels
- ○ **B.** Causes vasoconstriction to occur
- ○ **C.** Destroys the lung parenchyma
- ○ **D.** Paralyzes ciliary activity

246. The nurse is caring for a client admitted with congestive heart failure. Which finding would the nurse expect if the failure was on the right side of the heart?

Quick Answer: **389**
Detailed Answer: **413**

- ○ **A.** Jugular vein distention
- ○ **B.** Dry, nonproductive cough
- ○ **C.** Dyspneic when supine
- ○ **D.** Crackles on chest auscultation

247. A client with chest pain is scheduled for a heart catheterization. Which of the following would the nurse include in the client's care plan?

- ○ **A.** Keep the client NPO for 12 hours afterward.
- ○ **B.** Inform the client that general anesthesia will be administered throughout the procedure.
- ○ **C.** Assess the site for bleeding or hematoma once per shift.
- ○ **D.** Instruct the client that he might be asked to cough and breathe deeply during the procedure.

Quick Answer: **389**
Detailed Answer: **413**

248. The nurse is caring for a COPD client who is discharged on p.o. Theophylline. Which of the following statements by the client would indicate a correct understanding of discharge instructions?

- ○ **A.** "A slow, regular pulse could be a side effect."
- ○ **B.** "Take the pill with antacid or milk and crackers."
- ○ **C.** "The doctor might order it intravenously if symptoms worsen."
- ○ **D.** "Hold the drug if symptoms decrease."

Quick Answer: **389**
Detailed Answer: **413**

249. The nurse has just admitted a client with emphysema. Arterial blood gas results indicate hypoxia. Which physician prescription would the nurse implement for the best improvement in the client's hypoxia?

- ○ **A.** Elevate the head of the bed 45°.
- ○ **B.** Encourage diaphragmatic breathing.
- ○ **C.** Initiate an Alupent nebulizer treatment.
- ○ **D.** Start O_2 at 2L/min.

Quick Answer: **389**
Detailed Answer: **413**

250. The nurse is assessing the chart of a client with a stroke. MRI results reveal a hemorrhagic stroke to the brain. Which physician prescription would the nurse question?

- ○ **A.** Normal saline IV at 50mL/hr
- ○ **B.** O_2 at 3L/min by nasal cannula
- ○ **C.** Heparin infusion per pharmacist protocol
- ○ **D.** Insert a Foley catheter to bedside drainage

Quick Answer: **389**
Detailed Answer: **413**

Quick Answers

1. B	32. C	63. C	94. B
2. D	33. D	64. A	95. C
3. C	34. A	65. C, D, and E	96. C
4. D	35. C	66. C	97. C
5. B	36. B	67. A	98. C
6. A	37. D	68. B	99. C
7. B	38. A	69. A	100. B
8. A	39. C	70. D	101. D
9. B	40. A	71. A	102. A
10. D	41. B	72. C	103. B
11. C	42. D	73. C	104. C
12. A	43. C	74. D	105. B
13. B, D, E	44. A	75. C	106. C
14. B	45. B	76. A	107. A
15. C	46. D	77. C	108. C
16. B	47. D	78. C	109. B
17. A	48. A	79. C	110. A, B, D, G, F, C, I, H, E
18. A	49. B	80. D	111. A
19. D	50. D	81. C	112. C
20. A	51. B	82. C	113. A
21. C	52. A	83. A	114. D
22. C	53. A	84. D	115. B
23. B	54. B	85. C	116. B
24. C	55. C	86. A	117. A
25. A	56. B	87. C	118. D
26. A	57. A	88. C	119. D
27. D	58. A	89. D	120. B
28. D	59. A	90. C	121. A
29. A	60. D	91. C	122. B
30. B	61. B	92. C	123. C
31. D	62. B	93. A	

124. B	**156.** A	**188.** C	**220.** A
125. A	**157.** C	**189.** C	**221.** B
126. A	**158.** D	**190.** D	**222.** A, B, C, E, and F
127. C	**159.** B	**191.** B	**223.** B
128. C	**160.** B	**192.** C	**224.** D
129. C	**161.** C	**193.** A, B, and D	**225.** A
130. B	**162.** A	**194.** C	**226.** C
131. B	**163.** C	**195.** B	**227.** C
132. A	**164.** B	**196.** D	**228.** A
133. B, D, and E	**165.** B	**197.** D	**229.** B
134. B	**166.** B	**198.** B	**230.** B, C, D, and E
135. C	**167.** A	**199.** A	**231.** A
136. A	**168.** D	**200.** D	**232.** A
137. A	**169.** B	**201.** C	**233.** D
138. B	**170.** B	**202.** A	**234.** A
139. D	**171.** C	**203.** C	**235.** C
140. D	**172.** A	**204.** A	**236.** B
141. B	**173.** C	**205.** D	**237.** A
142. A	**174.** C	**206.** A	**238.** A, B, and D
143. B	**175.** D	**207.** D	**239.** B
144. C	**176.** B	**208.** B	**240.** A
145. A	**177.** C	**209.** A	**241.** A
146. C	**178.** C	**210.** B	**242.** A
147. B	**179.** B	**211.** B	**243.** B
148. D	**180.** D	**212.** C	**244.** A
149. C	**181.** D	**213.** 63 gtts/minute	**245.** D
150. C	**182.** B	**214.** B	**246.** A
151. C	**183.** A	**215.** B	**247.** D
152. B	**184.** D	**216.** A	**248.** B
153. A	**185.** C	**217.** A	**249.** D
154. C	**186.** C	**218.** A	**250.** C
155. A	**187.** C	**219.** D	

Answers and Rationales

1. **Answer B is correct**. The nurse would be prepared to administer Cipro in combination with rifampin (Rifadin) for all others exposed or in contact with a patient who had meningococcal meningitis. Answers A, C, and D medications are given to the patient with Meningococcal meningitis.

2. **Answer D is correct**. Activity, exercise, and repositioning the client will increase circulation and improve tissue perfusion. Answer A will help to identify problem areas but will not improve the perfusion of the tissue. Answer B should be avoided because it could increase the damage if trauma was present. Answer C should be done to prevent irritation of the skin, but this action does not improve perfusion.

3. **Answer C is correct**. This client needs a balanced nutritional diet with protein and vitamin C. Answers A and B both lack protein, which is very important in maintaining a positive nitrogen balance. Answer D has protein but is lacking in vitamin C.

4. **Answer D is correct**. Rales would indicate lung congestion and the need for follow-up. Answers A, B, and C are all normal health-related changes associated with aging.

5. **Answer B is correct**. Respiratory depression can occur from the administration of opioids. Naloxone should be available as an antagonist for these drugs. Answers A, C, and D might also be needed, but the most important problem that could occur would be the respiratory depression. These clients might also develop itching and nausea, and would likely use Benadryl and Phenergan, respectively, for treatment. Toradol is classified as an NSAID and is useful for its anti-inflammatory properties.

6. **Answer A is correct**. Hematocrit levels are elevated with hypovolemia. Answers B, C, and D are all normal levels. Potassium (normal 3.5–5.3mEq/L) levels can be either increased or decreased with hypovolemia; BUN (normal 5–25mg/dL) and specific gravity (1.005–1.030) levels would be elevated with hypovolemia.

7. **Answer B is correct**. Athletes can sometimes consume large amounts of water when competing. This can lead to decreased sodium levels. Symptoms of hyponatremia include an altered mental status, anorexia, muscle cramps, and exhaustion. Answers A, C, and D do not correlate with the history or the symptoms given.

8. **Answer A is correct**. If the nurse suspects a leaking or a ruptured abdominal aortic aneurysm, the first action is to improve blood flow to the brain and elevate the blood pressure. This can be accomplished quickly with the change in position. Answers B and C would be appropriate, but not before answer A. Answer D would not be required at this time.

9. **Answer B is correct**. Clients with cardiogenic shock often have chest pain. This symptom is not related to anaphylactic shock. Answers A and C can occur with both types of shock, but are not specific to the cardiogenic type. Answer D is a normal temperature reading.

10. **Answer D is correct.** This is the correct classification for the primary tumor of T1, N1, and M0. The letter T denotes the extent of the primary tumor, N indicates the absence or presence and extent of regional lymph nodes, and M denotes the absence or presence of distant metastasis. Answer A is correct for T1, N0, and M0. Answer B is correct for the classification of TX, NX, MX. Answer C is the correct classification for T1, N1, and M1.

11. **Answer C is correct.** Daunorubicin can damage the heart muscle and is the most serious of the ones listed. It can also cause bone marrow suppression. Answers A, B, and D are all common, but not as life-threatening as answer C.

12. **Answer A is correct.** The organ donor must have a BP of 90 or greater to ensure tissue perfusion. Answers B, C, and D are not related to adequate tissue maintenance for an organ donation.

13. **Answers B, D, and E are correct.** These clients will have loss of thirst and decreased urinary output making choices A and C incorrect. The client may also exhibit irritability in addition to the answers given.

14. **Answer B is correct.** Hemoptysis is a hallmark symptom of a pulmonary embolus, and this client's fracture history and other clinical manifestations lead to this conclusion. The clinical manifestations do not correlate with the diagnoses in answers A, C, and D.

15. **Answer C is correct.** A surgical hat cover is not necessary to mix or administer chemotherapy. OSHA (Occupational Safety and Health Administration) and ONS (Oncology Nurse Society) recommend answers A, B, and D when mixing or administering chemotherapy. The nurse should dispose of all equipment used in chemotherapy preparation and administration as hazardous waste in leak-proof, puncture-proof containers.

16. **Answer B is correct.** The client who had a stroke is the most stable client of the ones listed. The client in answer A needs extensive assessment. The client in answer C has a patient-controlled analgesic (PCA) pump and requires an RN because of the intravenous infusion. The client in answer D is a new admission with an infected diverticulum and would be less stable with more unknowns.

17. **Answer A is correct.** The diabetic with the foot ulcer is the most stable client and should be assigned to the LPN. Answer B requires assessments for clotting and bleeding complications, as well as monitoring of the IV heparin. Weaning from a tracheostomy could constitute an airway problem, making answer C incorrect. A postoperative client would be less stable and require more extensive care, so answer D is incorrect.

18. **Answer A is correct.** Kubler-Ross identified five stages of dying as ways that people cope with death. The stage of denial can be used as a buffer and a way to adapt. When dealing with these clients, the nurse would need to use open-ended statements, such as, "Tell me more." Other examples of statements made by the client in this stage are "This can't be true" and "I want another opinion." Answers B, C, and D are a few of the other stages of dying. In order, the stages are denial, anger, bargaining, depression, and acceptance.

19. **Answer D is correct.** The Trendelenburg position is used for surgeries on the lower abdomen and pelvis. This position helps to displace intestines into the upper abdomen and out of the surgical area. Answer A is reserved for vaginal, perineal, and some rectal surgeries. Answer B is used for renal surgery, and answer C is used for back surgery and some rectal surgeries.

20. **Answer A is correct.** Abrupt withdrawal of steroids can lead to collapse of the cardiovascular system; therefore, the physician should be notified for drug coverage. The medications in answers B, C, and D would not be as important as the maintenance of the steroids. Answer B is an ace inhibitor used as an antihypertensive. Answer C is a stool softener, and answer D is a calcium and vitamin agent.

21. **Answer C is correct.** Versed is used for conscious sedation and is an antianxiety agent. The antidote for this drug is Romazicon, a benzodiazepine. Answers A, B, and D are not utilized as antagonists for Versed; however, answer B is the antagonist for narcotics.

22. **Answer C is correct.** Turning the client to the side will allow any vomit to drain from the mouth and decrease the risk for aspiration. Answers A, B, and D are all appropriate nursing interventions, but a patent airway and prevention of aspiration are priorities.

23. **Answer B is correct.** When dehiscence and/or evisceration of a wound occurs, the nurse should apply a sterile saline dressing before notifying the physician. Answer A is not the appropriate position; the client should be placed in low Fowler's position. Answers C and D will not help in this situation.

24. **Answer C is correct.** There is a risk of bleeding with a liver biopsy; therefore, laboratory tests are done to determine any problems with coagulation before the biopsy. Answers A, B, and D are incorrect statements. The client lies on the right side, not the left; no enemas are given; and the test is invasive and can cause some pain.

25. **Answer A is correct.** Obstruction of the tracheostomy can cause anxiety, increased respiratory rate, and an O_2 saturation decrease. The nurse should first suction the client. If this doesn't work, she should notify the physician, as in answer C. Answer B would not help if the tube was obstructed. Answer D would be done to assess for improvement after the suctioning was performed.

26. **Answer A is correct.** Clients who are taking INH should avoid tuna, red wine, soy sauce, and yeast extracts because of the side effects that can occur, such as headaches and hypotension. Answers B, C, and D are all allowed with this drug.

27. **Answer D is correct.** The cerebral perfusion pressure is obtained by subtracting the ICP from the mean arterial pressure (MAP). A client must have a CPP of 70–100 to have a normal reading and adequate cerebral perfusion. Answers A, B, and C are all incorrect calculations.

28. **Answer D is correct.** The XII hypoglossal cranial nerve deals with the function of the tongue and its movement. Clients can exhibit weakness and deviation with impairment of this cranial nerve. Answers A, B, and C are not tested by this procedure. Cranial nerve I is involved with smelling, cranial nerve II is involved with visual function, and cranial nerve X deals with the gag reflex.

29. **Answer A is correct.** Increased intracranial pressure vital sign changes include an elevated BP with a widening pulse pressure, decreased heart rate, and temperature elevation. Answer C could occur with shock or hypovolemia. Answer B does not correlate with increased ICP. Answer D is not as evident of increased intracranial pressure as answer A.

30. **Answer B is correct.** The normal Dilantin level is 10–20mcg/mL; a level of 30 exceeds the normal. The appropriate action is to notify the physician for orders. Answer A would be inappropriate with a high level, and answers C and D would require changing the physician's prescription.

31. **Answer D is correct.** Hydration is needed to prevent slowing of blood flow and occlusion. It is important to perform assessments in answers A, B, and C, but answer D is the best intervention for preventing the crisis.

32. **Answer C is correct.** B12 is an essential component for proper functioning of the peripheral nervous system. Clients who have a B12 deficit will have symptoms such as paresthesia. Answers A and D do not occur with pernicious anemia; the client in answer B would have weight loss rather than weight gain.

33. **Answer D is correct.** Spinach should be avoided on a low-purine diet; other foods to avoid include poultry, liver, lobster, oysters, peas, fish, and oatmeal. Answers A, B, and C are all foods included on a low-purine diet.

34. **Answer A is correct.** The client is exhibiting symptoms of fluid volume excess; slowing the rate is the proper action. The nurse would not stop the infusion of blood, as in answer C, and answers B and D would not help.

35. **Answer C is correct.** Fat emboli occur more frequently with long bone or pelvic fractures and usually in young adults ages 20–30. Answers A, B, and D are not high-risk groups for this complication.

36. **Answer B is correct.** Sliced veal, a spinach salad, and a whole-wheat roll is the selection with the highest iron content. Other foods high in iron include cream of wheat, oatmeal, liver, collard greens, mustard greens, clams, chili with beans, brown rice, and dried apricots. Answers A, C, and D are not high in iron.

37. **Answer D is correct.** Symptoms of a fractured femoral neck include shortening, adduction, and external rotation of the affected limb. Answer A is incorrect because the patient usually is unable to move the leg because of pain. Answers B and C are incorrect because the leg would be adducted and externally rotated if a fracture was present.

38. **Answer A is correct.** Fresh vegetables and fruits are allowed on a gluten-free diet. The answers in options B, C, and D contain gluten so they are incorrect.

39. **Answer C is correct.** Aminophylline must be regulated by an infusion device to prevent improper infusion rates. Answers A, B, and D are not necessary for administration of this drug, so they are incorrect.

40. **Answer A is correct.** Hemolytic anemia involves the destruction of red blood cells that prompt the release of bilirubin, leading to a yellow hue of the skin. Answers C and D occur with several types of anemia but are not specific to hemolytic anemia. Answer B is not related to anemia.

41. **Answer B is correct.** Neulasta is given to increase the white blood cell count in patients with leucopenia. This white blood cell count is within the normal range for showing an improvement. Answers A, C, and D are not specific to the drug's desired effect.

42. **Answer D is correct.** Clients with a diagnosis of polycythemia have an increased risk for thrombosis and must be aware of the symptoms. Answers A, B, and C are not related to this disorder.

43. **Answer C is correct.** The client should strain all urine after the procedure and save any stones for examination. The statements in answers A, B, and D indicate a misunderstanding of how to provide proper self-care after the lithotripsy procedure.

44. **Answer A is correct.** The medication should be taken in the morning before food or other medications are ingested, with water as the only liquid. Answers B, C, and D are correct administrations. Answer B is an important choice for preventing esophageal problems with Fosamax administration.

45. **Answer B is correct.** Assessing for Tinel's sign is done to check for paresthesia in the median nerve. An abnormal result would be pain or tingling as this procedure is done. This test can also be performed by inflating a blood pressure cuff to the client's systolic pressure, resulting in pain and tingling. Answer A is another test in which the nurse asks the client to place the backs of the hands together and flex them at the same time. If the client experiences paresthesia within 60 seconds of performing the test, it is a positive result indicating carpel tunnel syndrome. Answers C and D are both assessment procedures for meningeal irritation.

46. **Answer D is correct.** A diet of mandarin orange salad, broiled chicken, and milk is the most balanced and best selection for promoting healing. Answers A, B, and C are not as inclusive of the food groups that promote healing.

47. **Answer D is correct.** Vomiting would be contraindicated with an acid, alkaline, or petroleum product. Answers A, B, and C do not contain any of these solutions, so vomiting would be a possible treatment.

48. **Answer A is correct.** Clients with AIDS who are experiencing diarrhea should avoid bowel irritants such as raw vegetables, nuts, and fatty and fried foods. Answers B, C, and D would not serve as irritants to the bowels.

49. **Answer B is correct.** The nurse should prioritize these clients and decide to see the client with the shortness of breath because this could be a possible alteration in breathing. The client in answer A has an abnormal PCO_2 (normal 35–45), but this would be expected in a client with COPD. The client's condition in answer C can be corrected by pain medication that someone else could administer. Answer D is incorrect because a temperature elevation of this level would not be a reason for great concern in a client after gallbladder surgery.

50. **Answer D is correct.** A malignant mass is usually firm and hard, typically is located in one breast, is not movable, and has an irregular shape. Answers A, B, and C are not characteristics of a malignancy.

51. **Answer B is correct.** The client has an open fracture, so the priority would be to cover the wound and prevent further contamination. Swelling usually occurs with a fracture, making answer C incorrect. Manual traction should not be attempted, as in answer A. Placing the client in the prone position, as in answer D, provides excessive movement and is an inappropriate action.

52. **Answer A is correct.** The drug can be mixed with D5W only. Mixing with normal saline can cause precipitates to form. The answers in B, C, and D are appropriate implementations for administering amphoteracin B, so they are incorrect.

53. **Answer A is correct.** This clinical manifestation is due to the hemolysis of the red blood cells in the kidney. Answer B doesn't occur in a hemolytic reaction. A rash or urticaria occurs with an allergic reaction, making answer C incorrect. Answer D is incorrect because this clinical manifestation usually occurs with circulatory overload.

54. **Answer B is correct.** Hypercalcemia is a common occurrence with cancer of the bone. Clinical manifestations of hypercalcemia include mental confusion and an elevated blood pressure. The potassium level in answer A is elevated, but this is not related to the diagnosis. Answers C and D are both normal levels.

55. **Answer C is correct.** The client is at risk for an air embolus. Placing the client in a left lateral decubitus position will displace air from the right ventricle. Answers B and D would not help, and answer A would not be done first.

56. **Answer B is correct.** A catheter will allow urine elimination without disrupting the implant. There is usually no restriction on TV or phone use, as in answer A. The client is placed on a low-residue diet, not a high-fiber diet, as stated in answer C. Even though the implant is internally placed, neither the patient nor her secretions are radioactive, but the applicator is. Because secretions are not radioactive, answer D is incorrect.

57. **Answer A is correct.** Normal ICP is 10–20. A reading of 66 is high, and the physician should be notified. Answers C and D would not be appropriate actions. Answer B would be the action if the reading was normal.

58. **Answer A is correct.** Doxorubicin (Adriamycin) can cause cardiotoxicity exhibited by changes in the ECG and congestive heart failure. Rales and distended neck veins are clinical manifestations of congestive heart failure. Answer B is incorrect because the reddish discoloration of the urine is a harmless side effect of doxorubicin. Answer D is not specific to this drug, and answer C is common and not a reason to immediately notify the physician.

59. **Answer A is correct.** Clients with diabetes insipidous have excessive urinary output because of the lack of antidiuretic hormone. Answers B, C, and D are not exhibited with diabetes insipidous so they are incorrect.

60. **Answer D is correct.** Platelets deal with the clotting of blood, and a lack of platelets can cause bleeding. Answers A, B, and C do not directly relate to platelets.

61. **Answer B is correct.** Spasmodic eye winking could indicate a toxicity or overdose of the drug Carbidopa/levodopa (Sinemet) and should be reported to the physician. Other signs of toxicity include involuntary twitching of muscles, facial grimaces, and severe tongue protrusion. Answers A, C, and D are side effects but do not indicate toxicity of the drug.

62. **Answer B is correct.** With neutropenia, the client is at risk for infection; therefore, this client would need to avoid crowds and people who are ill. Answer A would not be appropriate, and answers C and D correlates with a risk for bleeding.

63. **Answer C is correct.** D10W is the preferred solution to prevent complications from a sudden lack of glucose. Answers A, B, and D do not have glucose.

64. **Answer A is correct.** Vaginal bleeding or spotting is a common symptom of cervical cancer. Nausea, vomiting, and foul-smelling discharge, in answers B and C, are not specific or common to cervical cancer. Hyperthermia, in answer D, is not related to the diagnosis.

65. **Answers C, D, and E are correct.** TLS is a complication of chemotherapy that causes cells (especially potassium and purines) to be overabundant. Answers C, D, and E are all associated with TLS. Other symptoms associated with TLS include hypertension and fatigue; therefore, answers A and B would not be selected.

66. **Answer C is correct.** A bone marrow aspiration is usually done by the physician with specimens obtained from the sternum or the iliac crest. The high Fowler's position is the best position in which to obtain a specimen from the client's sternum. Answers A, B, and D are inappropriate positions for getting a bone marrow biopsy.

67. **Answer A is correct.** Hyperventilation is utilized to decrease the PCO_2, producing cerebral blood vessel constriction. Answers B, C, and D can decrease cerebral edema, but not by constriction of cerebral blood vessels.

68. **Answer B is correct.** The client is experiencing autonomic hyperreflexia, which can be caused by a full bowel or bladder or a wrinkled sheet. Answer A is not the appropriate action before performing the assessment of the bladder; answers C and D are not appropriate actions in this situation.

69. **Answer A is correct.** Plavix is an antiplatelet. Bleeding from the nose (epistaxis) could indicate a severe effect. Answers B, C, and D are not associated with the undesired effects of Plavix.

70. **Answer D is correct.** Papilledema is a hallmark symptom of increased intracranial pressure. Answers A, B, and C are not as conclusive.

71. **Answer A is correct.** Imitrex results in cranial vasoconstriction to reduce pain, but it can also cause vasoconstrictive effects systemically. Therefore, it is contraindicated in clients with angina, and the physician should be notified. Answers B and D are inappropriate actions from the information given. Answer C is appropriate, but answer A is the most appropriate.

72. **Answer C is correct.** The pH is an accurate indicator of acute ventilatory failure and a need for mechanical ventilation. An elevated PCO_2, as in answer A, is not an adequate criterion for instituting ventilator support. Answer B, oxygen saturation of 90, would not be very abnormal for a COPD client. Answer D is normal.

73. **Answer C is correct.** The absence of breath sounds and subcutaneous air, increased heart rate, dyspnea, and restlessness indicate a pneumothorax, which would require immediate intervention. Answer A could occur with the pulmonary contusion and would be expected. Answer D would be expected with fractured ribs. Answer B is not a cause for great concern because the midline trachea is a normal finding.

74. **Answer D is correct.** A position of sitting or high Fowler's is the best choice for assisting the client to use respiratory muscles to breathe and lift the diaphragm from the abdominal area. Answer A is contraindicated, and answers B and C would not help as much as answer D for breathing.

75. **Answer C is correct.** This client is exhibiting symptoms of heart failure that happen commonly in clients with a COPD disorder. The client in answer A is being discharged, and the client in answer D with an abnormal PO_2 would not be cause for alarm in a COPD client. The client in answer B would not require immediate attention.

76. **Answer A is correct.** The occipital lobe is the visual lobe. If the client were having problems with the occipital lobe, it would mean that the edema and bleeding were increasing in that area. Answers B, C, and D are not related to the occipital lobe.

77. **Answer C is correct.** Flushing of the line is required when giving Dilantin IV push because Dilantin crystallizes in the tubing if D5W is present. Answers A, B, and D would not be appropriate or necessary for this procedure.

78. **Answer C is correct.** Lasix and Mannitol are given for their diuretic effects in decreasing cerebral edema. Answers A, B, and D are not the effects of the drugs in this situation.

79. **Answer C is correct.** Cyanosis and loss of consciousness will occur later as the obstruction worsens. Answers B and D are both earlier symptoms of obstruction, and answer A is not a definite clinical manifestation of obstruction.

80. **Answer D is correct.** O negative blood type is universal blood type for females of childbearing age. Answers A, B, and C are not to be given to females of childbearing age if this is not their blood type. A blood type of O positive is given to males and postmenopausal women in emergencies.

81. **Answer C is correct.** An MRI uses a powerful magnetic force; therefore, any metal or jewelry should be removed before this test. Answers A, B, and D are not appropriate for this test.

82. **Answer C is correct.** The nurse should pay particular attention to any complaints of a headache when it is described in this way. The client could have a cerebral aneurysm. Pain medications are contraindicated in undiagnosed neurological clients, so answer A is not appropriate. No criterion in the stem makes answers B or D appropriate.

83. **Answer A is correct.** Ethyol is used to reduce renal toxicity with cisplatin administration. The drugs in answers B, C, and D are cytoprotectants not used for cisplatin administration, so they are incorrect.

84. **Answer D is correct.** The nurse should further assess the client for the cause of the symptoms, usually a pneumothorax. Answer A is another type of chest trauma not associated with the symptoms. Answer B is simply a term used to describe the symptoms, and answer C is not an appropriate assessment for these symptoms.

85. **Answer C is correct.** The calculated dosage of Atropine is 1.0mL, and the calculated dosage of Demerol is 1.5mL, making a total of 2.5mL the correct answer. Answers A, B, and D are incorrect calculations.

86. **Answer A is correct.** Nimotop is a calcium channel blocker and is used to prevent calcium influx. The etiology of vasospasm of the blood vessel has been thought to relate to this calcium influx; therefore, the drug is given to prevent this. Answers B, C, and D do not describe the action of this drug.

87. **Answer C is correct.** A simple partial seizure is characterized by jerking of extremities, twitching of the face, and mental alertness. Answers A, B, and D are not characterized with these clinical manifestations. Answer B is differentiated by the client's awareness of the seizure.

88. **Answer C is correct.** The essential piece of equipment is the ambu bag (manual resuscitator). Ventilator clients must always have another means of ventilation in case of a problem, such as a power failure. Answers A and B may be needed, but not as much as answer C. Answer D is inappropriate for a client on the ventilator.

89. **Answer D is correct.** If the ventilator is set for eight breaths per minute and the client's rate is 13 per minute, subtract 8 from 13 to find that the client is actually breathing five breaths on his own. Answers A, B, and C are incorrect information for the description provided in the stem, so they are wrong.

90. **Answer C is correct.** Contracting the abdominal muscles with exhalation is the proper technique for pursed-lip breathing. Answers A, B, and D are all incorrect techniques. The goal is to increase the exhalation phase.

91. **Answer C is correct.** A level of 15ug/mL is within the normal therapeutic theophylline level of 10–20ug/mL. Answers A, B, and D are not within the therapeutic range.

92. **Answer C is correct.** Readings of pH 7.35, PO_2 85, PCO_2 55, and HCO_3 27 represent compensated respiratory acidosis with increased PCO_2 (normal 35–45), low pH of less than 7.4 (normal 7.35–7.45), and high HCO_3 with compensation (normal 22–26). Answers A, B, and D are not reflected in the blood gas results listed in the stem.

93. **Answer A is correct.** Closed chest drainage is not usually used because it is helpful for serous fluid to accumulate in the space to prevent mediastinal shift. Answers B, C, and D are all involved in care of a client with lung surgery.

94. **Answer B is correct.** Any posterior craniotomy requires the client to lie flat and on one side as in answer A, rather than with the head of the bed elevated, as stated in answer B. A posterior fossa procedure would be at the lower back of the head. Answer C would not be contraindicated, and answer D would help to decrease intracranial pressure.

95. **Answer C is correct.** Raw or cooked vegetables are not allowed on a low-residue diet. Answers A, B, and D are all allowed foods.

96. **Answer C is correct.** A client with diverticulitis should avoid high-fiber foods containing seeds or nuts. Other foods to avoid include corn, popcorn, celery, figs, and strawberries. Answers A, B, and D are foods that do not contain nuts or seeds and would not need to be avoided.

97. **Answer C is correct.** Asking the client about his usual diet is the least helpful information in identifying the problem. Answer A is important because the pain sometimes decreases as obstruction worsens. The distention in answer D indicates obstruction, and answer B is useful because a description of the vomit can help differentiate the type of obstruction.

98. **Answer C is correct.** Tegretol can cause bone marrow depression, which is evident by the low WBC of 4,000 (normal 5,000–10,000). It can also cause problems with the liver that would raise the BUN (normal 5–25mg/dL). Answers A, B, and D are not related to the adverse effects of this drug.

99. **Answer C is correct.** The parietal lobe deals with sensation; therefore, anyone with a problem in this area of the brain can have problems with sensation. Answers A, B, and D are not directly associated with this part of the brain.

100. **Answer B is correct.** Every nurse must know military times, Parkland formula, and how to calculate the amount of fluid needed for replacement therapy. The Parkland formula is 4mL × Weight in kilograms × Percentage of body surface area burned = Amount of fluid to be given in 24 hours. The nurse is to give half this amount in the first eight hours.

    4mL × 68kg × 50% BSA = 13,600ml (amount to be given in 24 hours)

    Give half this amount in the first eight hours.

    13,600 ÷ 2 = 6,800

    Answers A, C, and D are incorrect calculations.

101. **Answer D is correct.** A loss of pulse could indicate an occlusion in the graft that requires surgical intervention. Answers A and C are expected post-operative occurrences with this surgical procedure, which makes them incorrect. Answer B is not an immediate concern, so it is incorrect.

102. **Answer A is correct.** ECG changes associated with hypokalemia are peaked P waves, flat T waves, depressed ST segments, and prominent U waves. Answers B, C, and D are not associated with low potassium levels, so they are incorrect.

103. **Answer B is correct.** Inspect, auscultate, percuss, and palpate is the correct sequence of assessing the abdomen. The initial step is to inspect the abdomen. Auscultation must be accomplished before touching because movement could make auscultation inaccurate. Answers A, C, and D are incorrect assessment sequences.

104. **Answer C is correct.** Left Sim's position is the best position because it follows the natural direction of the colon. In answer A, the client would be placed on the abdomen. In answers B and D, the client would be placed on the back, so these answers are incorrect.

105. **Answer B is correct.** Trachea shift differentiates this clinical manifestation as a tension pneumothorax. When a person has a tension pneumothorax, air enters but cannot escape, causing a pressure buildup and shifting of the great vessels, the heart, and the trachea to the unaffected side. Answer A correlates with a pulmonary contusion, so it is incorrect. Answers C and D are associated with a pneumothorax; this makes them nonspecific for a tension pneumothorax and, thus, incorrect.

106. **Answer C is correct.** A client with an open pneumothorax is in distress and should be seen by the nurse first. The key word in this correct response is *unstable*. The clients in answers A, B, and D are more stable clients or those that are not as severely ill as the client in C, so they are incorrect.

107. **Answer A is correct.** Accolate should be taken one hour before or two hours after eating, to prevent slow absorption of the drug when taken with meals; therefore, this statement is incorrect and requires further teaching by the nurse. Answers B, C, and D are all true statements regarding this drug and are correct statements made by the client.

108. **Answer C is correct.** The assessment finding that causes the most concern is the one indicating a possible stroke. Right-sided weakness would mean that there is a loss of muscular functioning on the side opposite the surgical procedure. Answers A, B, and D might indicate a need for reassessments but are not a cause for immediate concern or intervention, so they are incorrect.

109. **Answer B is correct.** This client is the least stable of the ones listed. The key term in this answer is the word *new*. Bleeding would also give this client a priority status because of the possible deficit in maintaining circulation. The clients in answers A, C, and D are more stable, so they can be assigned to other personnel.

110. The correct answer sequence is as follows:

    A. Apply clean gloves.

    B. Clean the skin with antimicrobial and let air dry.

    D. Connect 10mL NS into extension of huber needle and prime.

    G. Wash hands and apply sterile gloves.

    F. Stabilize the part by using middle and index fingers.

    C. Insert needle into port at a 90° angle.

    I. Check placement of needle.

    H. Inject saline and assess for infiltration.

    E. Instill heparin solution.

111. **Answer A is correct.** Vitamin K decreases the effects of Coumadin. The client should be taught to avoid green, leafy vegetables, such as broccoli, cabbage, turnip greens, and lettuce. Answers B, C, and D are food choices that are low in vitamin K, so they are incorrect.

112. **Answer C is correct.** The clinical manifestation of clubbing of the fingers takes time, indicating that the condition is chronic and not acute. Answers A, B, and D are all non-specific for chronicity, so they are incorrect.

113. **Answer A is correct.** Ambulating the client should help to pass the air. The air is used during the surgical procedure to assist in performance of the surgery. Answers B and C would not help, and answer D is not necessary or appropriate at this time.

114. **Answer D is correct.** Assessment is not within the role of a nurse's assistant, which makes this the least appropriate of the tasks listed. Answers A, B, and C are all appropriate tasks for an assistant, so they are incorrect.

115. **Answer B is correct.** An NG is inserted to decrease the secretion of pancreatic juices and assist in pain relief. Answer A is incorrect because these clients are held NPO. Clients are placed in semi-Fowler's position, which makes answer C incorrect. Answer D is not appropriate because the wastes are not contaminated.

116. **Answer B is correct.** To test for vagus nerve problems, the nurse uses a tongue blade and depresses the back of the throat to elicit a gag reflex. Another way to test for damage to the vagus nerve is to have the client say "Ah" while observing for uniform rising of the uvula and the soft palate. The absence of this reflex could indicate damage to the X cranial nerve. Answers A, C, and D are not tested in this manner, so they are incorrect.

117. **Answer A is correct.** People should wear protective clothing outside, such as long sleeves and pants, to prevent mosquito bites. People should limit being outside during dawn and dusk and use insect repellants that contain DEET, making B and C incorrect options. The virus is more prevalent in the senior population group, so option D is incorrect.

118. **Answer D is correct.** Questran works by binding the bile acid in the GI tract and eliminating it, decreasing the itching associated with jaundice. Answers A, B, and C are not how Questran works to decrease itching.

119. **Answer D is correct.** Careful cleansing is necessary to prevent skin breakdown and skin irritation. Answer A is not an intervention used for ileostomies. Clients should avoid the high-fiber and gas-producing foods in answer B. Answer C is incorrect because these clients are not on fluid restriction.

120. **Answer B is correct.** Lomotil's desired effect is to decrease GI motility and the number of diarrhea stools. Answers A and D do not occur with the use of Lomotil. The drug should decrease cramping instead of increasing it, as in answer C.

121. **Answer A is correct.** During chest tube removal this procedure prevents air entrance into the chest cavity. Answers B and C are inappropriate actions for chest tube removal. Answer D could allow the air to enter the thoracic cavity, so it is incorrect.

122. **Answer B is correct.** Tremors are an extrapyramidal side effect that can occur when taking Haldol. Answers A, C, and D are not side or adverse effects of Haldol so are incorrect.

123. **Answer C is correct.** The pulmonic area is found in the second intercostal space, left of the sternum. Answer B is the correct location of the tricuspid area. Answers A and D are not assessment locations for heart auscultation.

124. **Answer B is correct.** A side effect of Aricept is dizziness; therefore, the client should be reminded to move slowly when rising from a lying or sitting position. Answer A is incorrect because it should be taken at bedtime, with no regard to food. Increasing the number of pills can increase the side effects, so answer C is incorrect. Another effect of the drug is bradycardia, making answer D incorrect.

125. **Answer A is correct.** Protein is a necessary component of wound healing. An inadequate amount of protein would correlate with the client's wound not healing properly. Answers B, C, and D do not directly relate to wound healing, so they are incorrect.

126. **Answer A is correct.** The first step is to assess the client, noting any signs or symptoms of a fluid volume deficit. Answers B, C, and D might all be required interventions at some point, but assessment is needed before any other actions, so they are incorrect.

127. **Answer C is correct.** All of the tests listed can be used to diagnose an ulcer, but an endoscopic exam is the only way to obtain accurate visual evidence. Answers A, B, and D are not as accurate or reliable, which makes them incorrect.

128. **Answer C is correct.** The parathyroid gland can be inadvertently removed or injured with thyroid removal. This can cause hypocalcemia and symptoms of tetany, which requires notifying the physician. Answers A and B are ineffective for treating or obtaining treatment for hypocalcemia, and answer D would allow the condition to progress; thus, these are incorrect.

129. **Answer C is correct.** PEEP can compress thoracic blood vessels, resulting in a decreased cardiac output and low BP. Answers A, B, and D don't relate to PEEP and are not the result of increased thoracic pressure.

130. **Answer B is correct.** This is the accurate instruction for application of the condom. The condom can be used once, so answer A is incorrect. K-Y jelly and glycerin are the only solutions that can be safely used with condoms, making answer C incorrect. Answer D is incorrect because the air should be squeezed out and nothing should be in the tip of the condom before application.

131. **Answer B is correct**. This information is important to report to the doctor when taking this drug. The answers in A, C, and D are side effects, but do not warrant immediate doctor notification, so they are incorrect.

132. **Answer A is correct.** Clients with face and neck burns and singed nasal hairs are more serious because of the likely respiratory and airway involvement. The clients in answers B and C are more stable. The danger of heart damage from an electrical burn occurs more often when the current enters and leaves on opposite sides of the body, which makes answer D incorrect.

133. **Answers B, D, and E are correct**. These answers are all symptoms of osteomyelitis. The answers in A and C are not associated with osteomyelitis, so they are incorrect.

134. **Answer B is correct.** The client with the most risk factors for pulmonary complications is the 45-year-old with an open cholecystectomy. These include abdominal surgery and prolonged bed rest. The clients in answers A, C, and D do not have as high of a risk factor, so these are incorrect.

135. **Answer C is correct.** The hallmark symptom of carbon monoxide poisoning is the cherry red color. The answers in A, B, and D are not specific to carbon monoxide poisoning.

136. **Answer A is correct.** When a person is in the compensatory stage of shock, the BP remains within normal limits. Increased heart rate occurs, allowing cardiac output to be maintained. The client also exhibits confusion and cold, clammy skin. Answer B correlates with the progressive stage of shock, so it is incorrect. Answers C and D both indicate that the client is past compensation, so they are incorrect.

137. **Answer A is correct**. This drug could make the test read false negative. The drugs in B, C, and D do not affect *H. pylori* testing, so they are incorrect.

138. **Answer B is correct.** Burn clients need large veins to administer the volume of fluid necessary for fluid-replacement therapy. Answer A is contraindicated because of the area burned. Answer C is an area that is not recommended because of the possibility of deep vein thrombosis. The vein in the forearm is smaller than the antecubital; therefore, answer D is incorrect.

139. **Answer D is correct.** Shortness of breath signifies an adverse reaction to the transplant procedure. Answers A and C can occur with the transplant process but do not signify an adverse reaction. Answer B is a normal finding with the bone marrow transplant.

140. **Answer D is correct.** Palms of the hands and soles of the feet are areas in dark-skinned clients where skin cancer is more likely to develop because of the decreased pigmentation found in these areas. Answers A, B, and C are not areas where low pigmentation occurs, so they are incorrect.

141. **Answer B is correct.** It is important to clamp the tube while auscultating because the sound from the suction interferes with the auscultation process. Answer A is one measure used to determine whether the NG is in the stomach. Answers C and D are not the correct procedure for assessing bowel sounds, so they are incorrect.

142. **Answer A is correct.** A culture result that shows minimal bacteria is a favorable outcome. The answers in B, C, and D are abnormal and negative outcomes, so they are incorrect.

143. **Answer B is correct.** The client should wait at least five minutes before instilling a second eye medication. Answers A, C, and D are correct procedures for eyedrop administration, so there is no need for further instruction with these observations.

144. **Answer C is correct.** Erythromycin is the only drug listed that is not penicillin based. Answers A, B, and D are in the same family as penicillin, so they are not as safe to administer; this makes them incorrect.

145. **Answer A is correct.** A normal potassium level is 3.5–5.5. Severe life-threatening complications can occur with hyperkalemia, requiring physician notification of any abnormality. Answers B, C, and D are normal results, making them incorrect.

146. **Answer C is correct.** Pulling the pinna down and back is correct for administering ear drops to a child because a child's ear canal is short and straight. The pinna is pulled up and back for adults. Answers A and B are improper techniques that would make it harder for the drops to be administered. Answer D would be incorrect because this is not a necessary part of the administration of ear drops, even though irrigation might be done to cleanse the ear before assessment.

147. **Answer B is correct.** The picture that follows depicts the percentages for each body part according to the Rule of Nines.

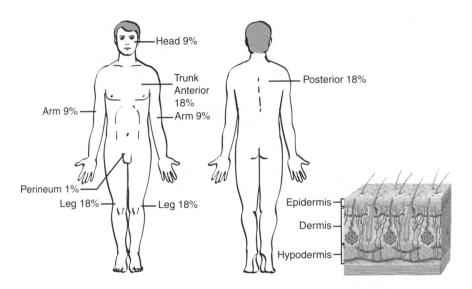

FIGURE 5.1   Rule of Nines

The percentages in Figure 5.1 total 100% of the body surface area.

The burned areas in the question are 4.5%, 9%, and 9% equal to 22.5%, with the closest estimate at 23%. The answers in A, C, and D are not correctly calculated sums of the burned areas.

148. **Answer D is correct.** Acute renal failure can occur with a lack of functioning in filtration when the MAP drops below 80. The mean arterial pressures in answers A, B, and C allow for proper functioning of the kidneys, which makes them incorrect.

149. **Answer C is correct.** An increase in head growth is used as a diagnostic gauge for hydrocephalus. Answers A and B can also occur with hydrocephalus, but they are not as specific or diagnostic as head circumference. Answer D is not related to hydrocephalus, so it is incorrect.

150. **Answer C is correct.** The arterial blood gases are abnormal indicating respiratory collapse with acidosis, making mechanical ventilation necessary. The Hgb, Hct, potassium, and platelets are all normal, making A, B, and D incorrect options.

151. **Answer C is correct.** Oxygen saturation is the best indicator of respiratory status because it is more objective. Answers A, B, and D are subjective and nonspecific, so they are incorrect.

152. **Answer B is correct.** Because of the moisturized air inhaled with swimming, it is an ideal sport for children with respiratory conditions. Answers A, C, and D can trigger an attack with asthma and would not be recommended.

153. **Answer A is correct.** Clients requiring low-bacteria foods cannot have raw fruits and vegetables. These types of foods must be cooked. Answers B, C, and D are raw fruits and vegetables, so they are incorrect.

154. **Answer C is correct.** The child weighs 24kg and should receive 5 units/kg, or 120 units every four hours. This would be 720 units in 24 hours. The answers in A, B, and D are incorrect dosages.

155. **Answer A is correct.** Hyponatremia can result from anorexia and nausea and vomiting caused by chemotherapy drugs. Normal sodium is 135–145mEq/L, so 50mg/dL is a low blood level that should be reported. Answers B, C, and D are normal or near-normal readings, so they are incorrect.

156. **Answer A is correct.** CBC results would indicate an elevated WBC count with leukemia. Answers B and D would not assist with the diagnosis, and answer C would be utilized to confirm leukemia; thus, they are incorrect.

157. **Answer C is correct.** Radial pulse differences over 10bpm are findings that relate to the location of the subclavian artery. Obstruction of the artery would also show a decrease in radial heart rate on the side of the obstruction. Answers A, B, and D are related to neurological problems as deficits, which makes them incorrect.

158. **Answer D is correct.** Everyone should wear sunscreen when going outside, to protect them from ultraviolet exposure. Answer A is not necessary. Answer B is the period of day when the sun's rays are most detrimental to the skin. Answer C is incorrect because only moles that are suspicious require removal and biopsy.

159. **Answer B is correct.** Normal pulmonary arterial wedge pressure is 4–12. This reading is elevated, indicating hypervolemia. The nurse should further assess for other indications of volume excess. Answers A and D correlate with hypovolemia. Answer C does not relate to the wedge pressure result.

160. **Answer B is correct.** Applying baby oil could help soothe the itchy skin. Answers A, C, and D would increase dryness and worsen the itching.

161. **Answer C is correct.** A glucose level would assist in determining the cause of the loss of consciousness. The tests in options A, B, and D would not assist in determination of the patient's loss of consciousness, so they are incorrect.

162. **Answer A is correct.** Homocysteine levels are increased when a client has B12 deficiency. The answers in B, C, and D are incorrect because homocysteine levels are not increased by these disorders.

163. **Answer C is correct.** The pneumonia client is the most stable of the four. The clients in answers A and B are recent arrivals to the unit, indicating extensive assessments. The client in answer D is in danger of fluid volume deficit, requiring RN interventions.

164. **Answer B is correct.** The calculated dosage is 0.8mL. Answers A, C, and D are inaccurate dosages for the amount of medication ordered, making them incorrect.

$$\frac{200}{250} \times mL = 0.8\ mL$$

165. **Answer B is correct.** The misuse and overuse of laxatives can cause serious fluid and electrolyte imbalances in the elderly. Answers A and D can be normal occurrences associated with the physiological changes of aging. Answer C is an incorrect response because the client states that increased fluid intake is not a new occurrence.

166. **Answer B is correct.** The normal sodium level is 135–145mEq/L. When hypernatremia occurs, the client can exhibit manic and hyperactivity behaviors. Other symptoms of increased sodium include restlessness, twitching, seizures, and hyperreflexia. Answers A, C, and D are not symptoms of high sodium levels. Answer D is associated with low sodium levels.

167. **Answer A is correct.** It is not a nursing responsibility to give detailed information about surgical procedures. The nurse can reinforce, but if the nurse feels that the client is not adequately informed, she can serve as an advocate and request that the surgeon visit the client to explain the procedure. Answer B is not the role of the nurse, so this is incorrect. Answers C and D are not appropriate and will not help in increasing or verifying patient understanding.

168. **Answer D is correct.** Safety and prevention of aspiration is the first priority. Answers A, B, and C would not be priority removals, so they are incorrect.

169. **Answer B is correct.** The client is asked to void before the procedure to prevent blurring of the pelvic bones. Answer A is incorrect because, although the client does need fluids to distribute and eliminate the isotope, this is not necessary 24 hours before the procedure. Answers C and D are not appropriate actions for the bone scan exam.

170. **Answer B is correct.** There will be a sensation of pulling during the aspiration. This feeling is painful. Answer A is incorrect because the position is inappropriate for bone marrow aspiration. Answer D is not a required preprocedure diet change. Although the client might receive a local anesthetic and/or pain medication, amnesic medications such as Versed are not usually administered, so answer C is incorrect.

171. **Answer C is correct.** It is most important to identify the pulses pre-operatively to have a baseline for post-operative evaluation. The answers in A, B, and D are not priorities for the client pre-operatively.

172. **Answer A is correct.** Excessive vagal stimulation causes bradycardia because of parasympathetic stimulation. Answers B, C, and D are not common arrhythmias associated with suctioning, so they are incorrect.

173. **Answer C is correct.** The client must be able to check the heart rate and report any rate that differs from the preset rate. Answers A and D are not required or have no effect on the pacemaker. Answer B would be contraindicated because the lack of movement could cause an inability to move the shoulder.

174. **Answer C is correct.** Diarrhea is not associated with esophageal cancer. Answers A, B, and D are clinical manifestations of esophageal cancer, so they are incorrect. The nurse would also assess for weight loss, regurgitation, and vomiting associated with esophageal cancer.

175. **Answer D is correct.** Perineal wound drainage is important to prevent abscess formation and infection. Answer A is incorrect because ileostomies produce liquid stools and do not require irrigation. Answer B cannot be done, and answer C would be inappropriate.

176. **Answer B is correct.** The client could have a mucus plug, so tracheal suctioning is the initial action most indicated. If suctioning doesn't work, notifying the doctor, as in answer A, is the next appropriate action. Answer C would not help, and answer D would be appropriate after the suctioning is done, to see if there has been any improvement.

177. **Answer C is correct.** High Fowler's is the best position for facilitating breathing. The nurse would suspect an allergic reaction to the shrimp. Answers B and D would both require an order from the physician. Answer A would worsen the client's respiratory efforts, so it is incorrect.

178. **Answer C is correct.** A measurement that reveals a numerical value would be the most accurate to detect changes in the size of the abdomen. Answers A, B, and D are less objective, so they are incorrect.

179. **Answer B is correct.** The stem gives objective assessment data that indicates a fluid volume deficit, a low BP with an elevated heart rate. Answer A is incorrect because of the lack of objective information that supports this as a problem. Answers C and D have no supportive data, so they are incorrect.

180. **Answer D is correct.** A client with an enlarged spleen has an increased risk for rupture; therefore, heavy lifting is contraindicated. Answers A, B, and C are not a cause for concern with an enlarged spleen.

181. **Answer D is correct.** A client who is immuno-suppressed is not allowed fresh fruit. Answers A, B, and C would still allow the client to eat raw fruit, which makes them incorrect.

182. **Answer B is correct.** The nurse must provide a water seal. Answer A could cause a tension pneumothorax if the client had no escape for the air. Answer C serves no purpose, and answer D would not allow maintenance of a sterile system.

183. **Answer A is correct.** An INR greater than 6.0 could result in spontaneous bleeding, so this would be a priority. Answers B, C, and D are not associated with the high INR result, so they are incorrect.

184. **Answer D is correct.** The highest calcium level is in the bagel with jam and skim milk. The client also needs to know that calcium in combination with high fiber and caffeine decreases the absorption; therefore, answers A, B, and C are incorrect.

185. **Answer C is correct.** Hemorrhage can occur with liver biopsies. The client is positioned on the right side to keep pressure on the area and prevent bleeding. Answers A, B, and D are not correct positions because of the location of the liver.

186. **Answer C is correct.** Hypernatremia is not an expected finding because hyponatremia is the likely occurrence when sodium moves out of the cell during the "fluid shift" phase of burn injury. The answers in A, B, and D are more of a priority for this client, which makes them incorrect.

187. **Answer C is correct.** Increased weight is the most objective answer. Answers A, B, and D also show favorable outcomes of anorexia nervosa but are not as objective, making them incorrect.

188. **Answer C is correct.** Gram negative infection invasion reveals clinical manifestations of severe diarrhea, hypothermia, and hypotension. Answer A is incorrect because the symptoms are abnormal. The infections identified in answers B and D are not consistent with the clinical manifestations identified in the question, so they are incorrect.

189. **Answer C is correct.** A 250mL infusion of packed cells to infuse over two hours is calculated by 250 divided by 2 = 125mL/hr. The answers in A, B, and D are incorrect calculations for infusion of the blood in two hours.

190. **Answer D is correct.** The nurse observes for sluggishness or lethargy, for early indications of increased ICP. A change in vital signs and papillary changes, as in answers A, B, and C, are late signs of increased ICP.

191. **Answer B is correct.** There is an increased risk for kidney stones with the use of topiramate (Topamax), so fluids are an important part of problem prevention. The drug is administered without regard to food and is not an hour-of-sleep medication, making answers A and D incorrect. Answer C is not required with the use of this medication.

192. **Answer C is correct.** The nurse responds appropriately by answering the question honestly and attempting to assess for more information, allowing the person to ventilate feelings. Answer A is an appropriate response but not as appropriate as answer C. Answers B and D are nontherapeutic communication techniques.

193. **Answers A, B, and D are correct.** The WBC count is below normal making the client at risk for infection. The correct answers decrease a clients' risk of infection. Answers C and E are related to platelet counts and a risk for bleeding, so they are incorrect.

194. **Answer C is correct.** The initial action is to test the drainage for glucose because this could indicate the presence of cerebrospinal fluid. The next action is to notify the physician, as stated in answer B. Answers A and D are contraindicated, so they are incorrect.

195. **Answer B is correct.** The aspirate of gastric content should be green, brown, clear, or colorless, with a gastric pH of between 1 and 5. Answer A would likely be from the lungs, so it is incorrect. Answers C and D are not as accurate as color and pH for confirming gastric location, so they are incorrect.

196. **Answer D is correct.** A slight elevation in temperature would be expected from surgical intervention and would not be a cause for concern. Answers A, B, and C could indicate a progressing complication, so they are incorrect.

197. **Answer D is correct.** Pork has more thiamine than beef, fish, or chicken, which makes answers A, B, and C incorrect.

198. **Answer B is correct.** Rilutek is used as a treatment for ALS. Symmetrel is a drug used for Parkinson's disease, Lisinopril is an antihypertensive, and estrogel is a hormone, so Answers A, C, and D are incorrect options.

199. **Answer A is correct.** The normal reading for central venous pressure is 3–8cm of H_2O. The doctor should be notified of any abnormal readings. Answer B is incorrect because a sterile technique should be utilized. Answer C is incorrect because of the 90° angle; the angle should be supine up to 45°. The zero should align at the phlebostatic axis, fourth intercostals space midaxillary, instead of the right clavicle, so answer D is incorrect.

200. **Answer D is correct.** The statement in answer D reflects the use of denial as a means of coping with the illness. Answers A, B, and C are defense mechanisms not reflected by the statement, so they are incorrect.

201. **Answer C is correct.** The Allen test is performed by having the client make a fist while the radial and ulnar arteries are compressed. When the hand blanches, the client is asked to release the fist while the nurse maintains pressure on the radial artery. Patency is indicated by the hand turning pink. Answers A, B, and D are incorrect for the Allen test procedure.

202. **Answer A is correct.** Clamping various areas of the tube allows the nurse to assess for a leak in the tubing. When the bubbling stops, the leak has been located. Answers B and C are assessed by reading the suction gauge and observing the bubbling in the suction-control chamber. Answer D is a diagnosis confirmed by client symptoms and x-ray not related to the chest tube system.

203. **Answer C is correct.** Respiratory depression is a sign of overdose. Other symptoms of overdose include seizures, shock, coma, and cardiovascular collapse. Answers A, B, and D lack any symptoms of overdose, so they are incorrect.

204. **Answer A is correct.** Vomiting, a heart rate of 120, and chest pain are symptoms of drinking alcohol while taking Antabuse. Additional symptoms include severe headache, nausea, cardiac collapse, respiratory collapse, convulsions, and death. Answers B, C, and D contain incomplete or inaccurate clinical signs of the combination of alcohol and Antabuse.

205. **Answer D is correct.** Clients with hypercalcemia can have dysrhythmias (heart block). This is the priority of the symptoms listed in A, B, and C, so they are incorrect. Remember prioritization—airway, breathing, and circulation.

206. **Answer A is correct.** Bromocriptine (Parlodel) is the drug used for addiction to cocaine. It is classified as an anti-Parkinsonism drug and gives clients with this addiction a substitute for the neurotransmitter dopamine. Answer B is used for opioid addiction. Answer C is marijuana and is not used for replacement therapy. Answer D is used for alcohol abuse.

207. **Answer D is correct.** Troponin, T or I, is a protein found in the myocardium. Testing for protein is frequently used to identify an acute myocardial infarction. Answers A, B, and C return to normal in less than four days, which makes them incorrect.

208. **Answer B is correct.** The correct response uses the therapeutic technique of identifying the client's feelings. Answers A, C, and D are nontherapeutic, closed statements that reflect judgment and opinions by the nurse, so they are incorrect.

209. **Answer A is correct.** The most appropriate response is to answer the request of the client's spouse and define blackouts. Answers B, C, and D are not accurate definitions of blackouts, so they are incorrect.

210. **Answer B is correct.** Closing the doors can prevent shadows and help with the client's paranoia and hallucinations. A darkened room, as in answer A, would increase the client's anxiety. Answer C is an inappropriate intervention that does not usually occur with DTs, and vital signs would be assessed more frequently than in answer D.

211. **Answer B is correct.** Nothing should be put in the mouth of a client during a seizure. Answers A, C, and D are important nursing interventions to maintain a patent airway and prevent injury during a seizure, so they are incorrect.

212. **Answer C is correct.** Lethargy could indicate hepatatoxicity. The nurse should also observe for jaundice, nausea and vomiting, anorexia, facial edema, and unusual bleeding or bruising. Answers A, B, and D are not clinical manifestations of adverse effects of the drug Depakene.

213. 63 gtts/minute is correct:

$$\frac{250mL \times 15gtts/mL}{60 \ min} = \frac{3750}{60} = 62.5 \ or \ 63 \ gtts/min$$

214. **Answer B is correct.** Adequate output would be an accurate assessment of fluid volume. If the client was hypovolemic, the body would compensate by retaining fluids and decreasing the urinary output. Answers A, C, and D do not relate to the fluid volume, and heart rate increase occurs with fluid volume deficit, so they are incorrect.

215. **Answer B is correct.** The therapeutic theophylline level is 10–20mcq/mL; therefore, notifying the physician is most appropriate. Answers A and D are not appropriate actions at this time, and answer C is a narcotic antagonist that is not used to reverse the effects of theophylline.

216. **Answer A is correct.** Sulfamylon is the topical agent of choice for electrical burns because of its ability to penetrate thick eschar. Answers B, C, and D have little or no penetration through eschar tissue, making them incorrect.

217. **Answer A is correct.** Fluid restriction is part of the treatment plan for clients with SIADH. This prescription gives the client too much fluid volume; therefore, the nurse should question this order. Answer B is a common medication for these clients. The weight and I and O are closely monitored, making answers C and D incorrect.

218. **Answer A is correct.** Patients taking Primidone should avoid alcohol. The drug causes drowsiness, so B and D are incorrect options. Serious effects can occur when the drug is stopped abruptly, so C is incorrect.

219. **Answer D is correct.** Before taking any action, an assessment is necessary to further investigate the situation. Answers A and B are appropriate actions, but not initially. Assessing the perineum, as in answer C, will not help the client to void or help assess for bladder distention, so it is incorrect.

220. **Answer A is correct.** A coup type of injury occurs when the brain damage is directly under the site of impact. When the injury is opposite the side of impact, it is identified as contrecoup, as in answer B. Answers C and D relate to the movement of brain tissue inside the head.

221. **Answer B is correct.** Abruptly discontinuing seizure medications can cause status epilepticus to occur. This disorder is life threatening, so this would be most important to tell the client. Answers A, C, and D are not correct statements about Dilantin, so they are incorrect.

222. **Answer: A, B, C, E, F.** Answers A, B, C, E, and F are correct symptoms associated with ALS. The patient could have constipation, so Answer D would not be selected.

223. **Answer B is correct.** CSF evaluations are used to diagnose Guillain-Barré (GB) syndrome. An elevated protein without an increase in other cells is indicative of GB, which makes answers A, C, and D incorrect.

224. **Answer D is correct.** The normal CVP is 3–8cm of water. An elevation in CVP indicates a fluid volume excess. Answers A, B, and C indicate that the reading is normal or low, so they are incorrect.

225. **Answer A is correct.** A change in a client's neurological status requires further immediate intervention to prevent rapid deterioration. Answers B, C, and D would not be a cause for immediate concern.

226. **Answer C is correct.** The correct location of the fundus for this time period is one fingerbreadth above the umbilicus. Answer B occurs on the fourth day post-delivery, and answer A is the location for 12 hours after delivery. Answer D could indicate a distended bladder; therefore, answers A, B, and D are incorrect.

227. **Answers C and D are correct.** Answers C and D should be selected. Other clinical manifestations include arthralgia, maculopapular rash, and myalgia. The patient also might have an acute onset of fever, so A would not be a correct selection. Options B and E are not symptoms of Zika Virus, so they should not be selected.

228. **Answer A is correct.** The client with COPD uses hypoxemia as a stimulus to breathe. Raising the client's O_2 blood level can suppress the respiratory drive; therefore, this is the prescription the nurse should question. Answers B, C, and D are correct physician prescriptions for COPD clients and would not need to be questioned.

229. **Answer B is correct.** A decreased WBC count can occur with the application of Silvadene. The nurse would need to assess the laboratory test results for this adverse effect. Decreased potassium, sodium, and platelets are not associated with Silvadene administration, which makes answers A, C, and D incorrect.

230. **Answers: B, C, D, E.** Answers B, C, D, and E are choices that should be selected. These choices are true about the Zika Virus and should be included in the teaching plan. The virus is spread primarily by mosquito bites, so A should not be selected.

231. **Answer A is correct.** Tactile fremitus is checked by asking the client to repeat terms such as *one*, *two*, *three* as the nurse's hands move down the thorax. Air does not conduct sound as well as a solid substance, so fremitus is increased with a solid substance and decreased when air is present, as with emphysema. Answers B and D are solid-tissue illnesses that would result in increased, not decreased, tactile fremitus. Answer C is incorrect because bronchopneumonia usually develops with tuberculosis, causing increased fremitus.

232. **Answer A is correct.** Zyban and Wellbutrin are classified as antidepressants and have been proven to increase long-term smoking abstinence. Answers B and C are bronchodilator drugs and are not used for smoking cessation. Answer D is a short-acting benzodiazepine and is not used for smoking-cessation therapy.

233. **Answer D is correct.** Pitocin is administered post-delivery to contract the uterus, resulting in a firm uterus and less chance of hemorrhage. Answers A and C are not desired effects of this drug. The contraction of the uterus is painful, which makes answer B incorrect.

234. **Answer A is correct.** Arterial blood gas PO_2 of 98 indicates adequate oxygenation and a favorable outcome. Answers B, C, and D are undesirable negative assessment findings, which makes them incorrect.

235. **Answer C is correct.** Asthma is the only disorder that is reversible with treatment or spontaneously after the attack. Answers A, B, and D can produce permanent damage to parts of the respiratory system, so they are incorrect.

236. **Answer B is correct.** The client's respirations would be assessed before administering morphine because morphine can cause respiratory depression. Answers C and D have no correlation with morphine administration, so they are incorrect. Answer A would be the next action after the assessment of a normal respiratory rate, but it would not be the first action.

237. **Answer A is correct.** The main cause of death after the immediate post-burn time frame is sepsis; therefore, preventing infection is a priority for this time period. Answer B would be emphasized earlier, and answer D requires a healed wound before it can be implemented. Answer C would be a necessary intervention during care, but it is not the primary focus.

238. **Answers A, B, and D are correct.** These answers are all teaching points for clients using external radiation therapy. Clients should avoid exposure of the area to sunlight during treatment and up to 12 months after the treatments; therefore, answer C is incorrect. Answer E could indicate damage to the esophagus from the therapy and the physician should be notified.

239. **Answer B is correct.** If there is any bleeding, new bruising, or pain at the puncture site, the physician should be notified. The information in answers A, C, and D are correct discharge teaching statements, so these answers are incorrect.

240. **Answer A is correct.** The nurse suspects congestive heart failure and anticipates an order for a diuretic to remove excess fluid. Answer B has insufficient data to support the need. Answer C would increase the client's fluid volume. Lowering the head, in answer D, would be an expectation for a client with a fluid volume deficit.

241. **Answer A is correct.** The suction source should not exceed 120mmHg when performing trachial suctioning. Answers B, C, and D exceed this amount and could cause damage to the trachea, so they are incorrect.

242. **Answer A is correct.** Bleeding at the site requires pressure to stop it. Answers B and C would be correct actions to take, but eliminating the bleeding process would take priority. Answer D is an inappropriate action, and the movement could increase the bleeding, so it is incorrect.

243. **Answer B is correct.** The systemic analysis of the electrocardiogram shows the information in the question as criteria for sinus tachycardia. Answer A would reveal an irregular rhythm and an early or different P wave. Answer C is incorrect because the P waves would be saw-toothed and the P: QRS ratio would be 2:1, 3:1, or 4:1. Answer D requires an unidentifiable P wave and a PR interval of less than 0.12 seconds, so it is incorrect.

244. **Answer A is correct.** This is the most appropriate initial action for heart block. Turning the patient on the side (answer B) is an inappropriate action. Answers C and D are appropriate, but should not be the initial action.

245. **Answer D is correct.** Cigarette smoking directly affects the sweeping action of the cilia, which interferes with the ability to remove mucus and clear the airway. Answers A and B are accurate statements but do not relate to emphysema. Answer C is not a direct effect of smoking.

246. **Answer A is correct.** The increase in venous pressure causes the jugular veins to distend. Other symptoms of right-sided heart failure include ascites, weakness, anorexia, dependent edema, and weight gain. Answers B, C, and D result from the left ventricle's inability to pump blood out of the ventricle to the body and are specific for left-sided, not right-sided, heart failure.

247. **Answer D is correct.** The client might be asked to cough and breathe deeply at certain times during the procedure. Answer A is incorrect because fluids are encouraged, to increase urine output and flush out the dye. The client will receive mild to moderate sedation, which makes answer B incorrect. Assessment of the site and pedal pulses are performed every 15 minutes for the first hour and then every 1–2 hours until pulses are stable, which makes answer C incorrect.

248. **Answer B is correct.** Theophylline should be taken with food to prevent GI irritation. Because this drug can cause tachycardia, answer A is incorrect. The IV drug is aminophylline and may not be ordered with worsening symptoms, so answer C is incorrect. Answer D is incorrect because the client should continue to take the drug when symptoms get better.

249. **Answer D is correct.** The delivery of oxygen is the best measure to correct hypoxia. Answers A, B, and C should also improve the client's hypoxia, but oxygen is the prescription that would deliver immediate relief.

250. **Answer C is correct.** Delivering an anticoagulant to a client with a hemorrhagic stroke is contraindicated because of the likelihood of increasing the bleed and worsening the client's condition. Answers A, B, and D are necessary positive treatments for clients with strokes, so they would not be questioned.

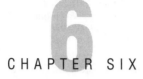

CHAPTER SIX

Alternative Items: Questions and Rationales

1. Which actions should be utilized prior to performing a tub bath on the 80 year-old client?
   Select all that apply.

   ○ **A.** Fill the tub one-half full of water at should be 46°C.

   ○ **B.** Put a rubber mat on the bottom of the tub.

   ○ **C.** Maintain water flow pressure during the bath.

   ○ **D.** Check water temperature using a bath thermometer.

   ○ **E.** Wash and dry the client's back moving from shoulders to buttocks.

   ○ **F.** Perform back massage upon completion of the bath.

2. Which tasks should not be delegated to the unlicensed assistive personnel?
   Select all that apply.

   ○ **A.** Bathing a client with a closed head injury

   ○ **B.** Performing a tube feeding on a client with an established line

   ○ **C.** Administering parenteral medications

   ○ **D.** Performing basic life support

   ○ **E.** Providing perineal care to a client with an indwelling urinary catheter

Quick Check

3. The nurse is teaching a group of staff members regarding the need for changes in the IV site care procedure. Which guidelines would hamper staff learning and compliance?
Select all that apply.

Quick Answer: **446**
Detailed Answer: **447**

   ○ **A.** Provide scientific information regarding nosocomial infections.

   ○ **B.** Clarify information with staff during each session.

   ○ **C.** Acknowledge resistance of staff to changes in policies.

   ○ **D.** Utilize diagrams to provide information.

   ○ **E.** Provide all information needed to the staff on the first session.

   ○ **F.** Tell the staff that changes were mandated by hospital policy.

   ○ **G.** Send a memo regarding errors in IV site care procedure.

4. The nurse is assessing the client with metabolic alkalosis. Which findings would likely be observed in this client?
Select all that apply.

Quick Answer: **446**
Detailed Answer: **447**

   ○ **A.** Kussmaul's respirations

   ○ **B.** Numbness of the extremities

   ○ **C.** Vomiting and nausea

   ○ **D.** Warm flushed skin

   ○ **E.** Circumoral paresthesia

   ○ **F.** Hypertonic muscle contractions

Quick Answer: **446**
Detailed Answer: **447**

5. The nurse is observing the sign in the following diagram.

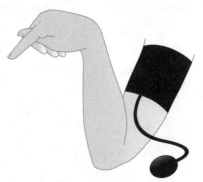

The nurse is assessing the client for which of the following conditions?

○ **A.** Hypomagnesemia

○ **B.** Hypocalcemia

○ **C.** Hypokalemia

○ **D.** Hyponatremia

Quick Answer: **446**
Detailed Answer: **447**

6. A pulse oximeter is ordered for a neonate. To obtain a reliable reading, the nurse should apply the sensor to which of the following?
Select all that apply.

○ **A.** Finger

○ **B.** Toe

○ **C.** Hand

○ **D.** Forehead

○ **E.** Earlobe

○ **F.** Foot

7. The client with right-sided congestive heart failure is admitted to the medical unit. Utilizing the following chart, the nurse would document which of the following?

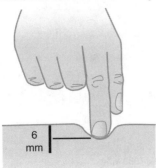

- ○ **A.** 1+ edema
- ○ **B.** 2+ edema
- ○ **C.** 3+ edema
- ○ **D.** 4+ edema

Quick Answer: **446**
Detailed Answer: **447**

8. The nurse is teaching the client with hepatitis B regarding transmission. The nurse should instruct the client to do which of the following?
Select all that apply.

- ○ **A.** Refrain from eating fresh fruits and vegetables.
- ○ **B.** Avoid using another family member's toothbrush.
- ○ **C.** Clean the commode after each bowel movement.
- ○ **D.** Boil water prior to drinking and place open containers in the refrigerator.
- ○ **E.** Inform the dentist of his diagnosis.

Quick Answer: **446**
Detailed Answer: **448**

9. Which of the following diagnoses require droplet precautions?
Select all that apply.

- ○ **A.** Varicella
- ○ **B.** Rubella
- ○ **C.** Streptococcal pharyngitis
- ○ **D.** Scarlet fever
- ○ **E.** Shigella
- ○ **F.** Hepatitis A

Quick Answer: **446**
Detailed Answer: **448**

10. Place in sequence the correct method of removal of contaminated personal protective equipment.

    ○ **A.** Mask

    ○ **B.** Gloves

    ○ **C.** Gown

    ○ **D.** Eyewear

Quick Answer: **446**
Detailed Answer: **448**

11. Which laboratory values should be reported to the physician?
Select all that apply.

    ○ **A.** Magnesium of 2.6mEq/L

    ○ **B.** Potassium 4.6mEq/L

    ○ **C.** Sodium 90mEq/L

    ○ **D.** Calcium 12.0mg/dL

    ○ **E.** Chloride 95mEq/L

Quick Answer: **450**
Detailed Answer: **448**

12. The client is admitted with a possible myocardial infarction. The nurse would anticipate an order from the physician for which laboratory test?
Select all that apply.

    ○ **A.** Creatine kinase

    ○ **B.** Ammonia

    ○ **C.** Myoglobin

    ○ **D.** Troponin T

    ○ **E.** Gamma-glutamyl transferase

    ○ **F.** Bilirubin

Quick Answer: **446**
Detailed Answer: **448**

13. The client is scheduled for a cardiac CTA. Prior to the cardiac CTA, the nurse should do which of the following?
Select all that apply.

    ○ **A.** Check the client's creatinine.

    ○ **B.** Question the client regarding allergies to shellfish.

    ○ **C.** Obtain a consent from the client or responsible person.

    ○ **D.** Question the client regarding difficulty hearing.

    ○ **E.** Instruct the client to drink 8 glasses of water the day prior to the exam.

Quick Answer: **446**
Detailed Answer: **448**

Quick Check

14. The nurse is preparing to collect a sputum specimen from the client suspected of having tuberculosis. What is the correct method for obtaining a sputum specimen?
Select all that apply.

○ **A.** Collect the specimen in the morning prior to breakfast.

○ **B.** Collect the specimen on three consecutive days.

○ **C.** Transport the collected specimen to the laboratory immediately.

○ **D.** Offer mouth care after collecting the sputum specimen.

○ **E.** Allow the client to rinse his mouth with an antiseptic solution prior to the sputum collection.

Quick Answer: **446**
Detailed Answer: **448**

15. Which method of transmission would most likely result in contamination with botulism?
Select all that apply.

○ **A.** Close contact with a family member with botulism

○ **B.** Eating foods from a perforated can

○ **C.** Being bitten by a mosquito

○ **D.** Wound contamination with C- botulism

○ **E.** Contact with goat saliva

○ **F.** Breathing dust from contaminated cat litter

Quick Answer: **446**
Detailed Answer: **448**

16. The elderly client is being discharged following a total knee replacement. To facilitate independence, the nurse should instruct the client/family to do which of the following?
Select all that apply.

○ **A.** Use an elevated commode seat.

○ **B.** Remove throw rugs from the floor.

○ **C.** Install grab bars in the bathroom.

○ **D.** Wear a medic alert monitor.

○ **E.** Leave the nightlight on during resting hours.

○ **F.** Apply foot protectors to the heels.

○ **G.** Place the walker at the bedside.

○ **H.** Elevate the side rails and instruct the client to ask for help.

Quick Answer: **446**
Detailed Answer: **448**

17. The nurse is bathing the elderly client. If the nurse observes the following diagram, he would chart the finding as a stage _____ decubitus ulcer.

Quick Answer: **446**
Detailed Answer: **449**

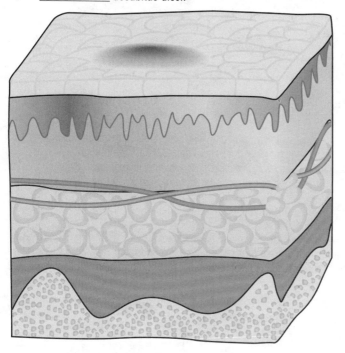

18. Which action can be delegated to the licensed practical nurse? Select all that apply.

Quick Answer: **446**
Detailed Answer: **449**

○ **A.** Inserting an indwelling urinary catheter

○ **B.** Performing tracheostomy care

○ **C.** Initiating a blood transfusion

○ **D.** Irrigating a peripherally inserted central catheter

○ **E.** Performing a sterile dressing change

Quick Check

Quick Answer: **446**
Detailed Answer: **449**

19. The obstetric client is admitted with a prolapsed umbilical cord. Identify from the diagrams the correct position for the client to assume at this time.

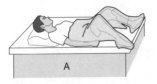

A

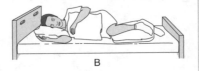

B

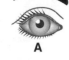

C

D

Quick Answer: **446**
Detailed Answer: **449**

20. The nurse is examining the eyes of the client with anisocoria. Which illustration demonstrates anisorcoria?

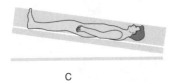

A

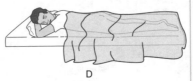

B

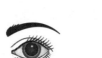

C

D

Quick Answer: **446**
Detailed Answer: **449**

21. The clinic nurse is teaching a co-worker regarding medication administration. The nurse is aware that which of the following medications are category X medications and should not be taken by the client during pregnancy?

○ **A.** Menocycline

○ **B.** Tazorac

○ **C.** Devonex

○ **D.** Levothyroxine

○ **E.** Cefozolin

22. The nurse is preparing to administer both regular and NPH insulin to a client with diabetes. Place in sequence the correct method for completing this task.

    ___Withdraw the NPH insulin.

    ___Withdraw the regular insulin.

    ___Inject air into the vial of regular insulin.

    ___Inject air into the vial of NPH insulin.

Quick Answer: **446**
Detailed Answer: **449**

23. The client has an order to resume a full liquid diet. Calculate the intake in milliliters. Round to whole numbers.

    750ml IV D5W

    _____

    60ml pudding

    _____

    1 scrambled egg

    _____

    8 ounces of orange juice

    _____

    4 ounces of pudding

    _____

Quick Answer: **446**
Detailed Answer: **449**

24. A Rapid Plasma Reagin (RPR) is performed for the client seen in the family planning clinic. The nurse is aware that the client may have a false positive if the client has which of the following? Select all that apply.

    ○ **A.** Tuberculosis

    ○ **B.** Systemic Lupus Erythematosis

    ○ **C.** Viral Hepatitis

    ○ **D.** Guillain–Barré

    ○ **E.** Osteoarthritis

    ○ **F.** Mononucleosis

Quick Answer: **446**
Detailed Answer: **449**

25. The nurse has an order to begin one unit of Packed Red Blood Cells at 1600 hours. If she starts the infusion at 2ml per minute, what time will the infusion be completely infused? One unit equals 250ml.

    _____

Quick Answer: **446**
Detailed Answer: **449**

26. Which task should be delegated to the licensed practical nurse? Select all that apply.

Quick Answer: **446**
Detailed Answer: **449**

- ○ **A.** Administering heparin subcutaneously
- ○ **B.** Feeding the client with a percutaneous endoscopy gastrostomy tube
- ○ **C.** Removing a peripherally inserted central line
- ○ **D.** Monitoring chest tube drainage
- ○ **E.** Performing tracheostomy care

27. The nurse notes the following ECG monitor strip.

Quick Answer: **446**
Detailed Answer: **449**

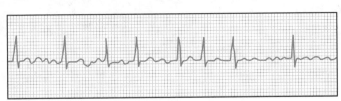

The nurse would anticipate an order for which medication?

- ○ **A.** Aspirin (ASA)
- ○ **B.** Acetaminophen (Tylenol)
- ○ **C.** Ibuprofen (Motrin)
- ○ **D.** Indomethacin (Indocin)

28. The client is admitted to the intensive care unit following a coronary artery bypass graft. The nurse checks the vital signs and notes a heart rate of 120 beats per minute, blood pressure of 70/40, and respiration of 32 breaths per minute. The nurse suspects hypovolemic shock. Which assessment tools would contribute to a diagnosis of hypovolemic shock? Select all that apply.

Quick Answer: **446**
Detailed Answer: **449**

- ○ **A.** Hemoglobin of 5g
- ○ **B.** Central venous pressure of 2mm of mercury
- ○ **C.** Pulmonary artery wedge pressure of 16mm of mercury
- ○ **D.** Hematocrit of 22%
- ○ **E.** Troponin (T 1) level of 4mcg/L

Quick Check

29. The client is admitted to the family-planning clinic with a desire to use a diaphragm as her method of contraception. Which instructions should be included in the teaching plan?
Select all that apply.

Quick Answer: **446**
Detailed Answer: **450**

- ○ **A.** Wash the diaphragm with hot water after use.
- ○ **B.** Insert contraceptive gel into the diaphragm prior to intercourse.
- ○ **C.** Douche following intercourse.
- ○ **D.** The diaphragm should be resized and replaced every six months.
- ○ **E.** Leave the diaphragm in place for six hours after intercourse.

30. A client is admitted with a blood glucose level of 740mg/dl. Which actions should the nurse take at this time?
Select all that apply.

Quick Answer: **446**
Detailed Answer: **450**

- ○ **A.** Assess the client for peripheral neuropathy.
- ○ **B.** Prepare to administer an IV of dextrose.
- ○ **C.** Call the physician.
- ○ **D.** Prepare to administer IV NPH insulin.
- ○ **E.** Prepare to administer sliding scale regular insulin.
- ○ **F.** Assess the client's level of consciousness.

31. Which of the following statements applies to the care of the client hospitalized with influenza?
Select all that apply.

Quick Answer: **446**
Detailed Answer: **450**

- ○ **A.** The nurse should wear an N-95 mask when caring for the client.
- ○ **B.** The client may cohort with another client hospitalized with the same diagnosis.
- ○ **C.** Equipment used in the client's care should remain in the room until the client is discharged.
- ○ **D.** The door to the client's room may remain open to the hallway.
- ○ **E.** The nurse should wear a mask when direct care of the client is required.

Quick Check

Quick Answer: **446**
Detailed Answer: **450**

32. Which of the following factors affects the accuracy of pulse oximetry readings?
Select all that apply.

○ **A.** Diminished peripheral circulation

○ **B.** Placement of the oximetry probe

○ **C.** Environmental lighting

○ **D.** Dark skin color

Quick Answer: **446**
Detailed Answer: **450**

33. Place in correct sequence the steps from 1–7 used when performing tracheostomy suctioning.

_____ **A.** Suction the oral cavity.

_____ **B.** Auscultate breath sounds for effectiveness.

_____ **C.** Set suction control at 80–120 mm Hg.

_____ **D.** Ambu or oxygenate at 100% O_2.

_____ **E.** Apply suction while withdrawing the suction catheter.

_____ **F.** Turn the head toward the side to be suctioned.

_____ **G.** Auscultate breath sounds prior to suctioning.

Quick Answer: **446**
Detailed Answer: **450**

34. Identify the following patient conditions as emergent (E), urgent (U), or non-urgent (NU).

_____ **A.** 2-month-old with a temperature of 102°F

_____ **B.** 23-year-old with blunt trauma to the right upper quadrant of the abdomen

_____ **C.** 30-year-old with full thickness burns to the anterior chest and neck

_____ **D.** 68-year-old with abrasions of the left forearm

_____ **E.** 16-year-old with closed fracture of the right tibia

_____ **F.** 52-year-old with chest pain

Quick Check

35. Which statements apply to the care of the client receiving hemodialysis?
Select all that apply.

Quick Answer: **446**
Detailed Answer: **450**

- ○ **A.** The client's blood pressure should be checked in the standing and lying position.

- ○ **B.** A signed permit is required before each hemodialysis procedure.

- ○ **C.** The nurse should wear personal protective garb during the procedure.

- ○ **D.** The blood should be placed in a warmer before placing in the dialyzer.

- ○ **E.** The nurse should monitor the client's partial thomboplastin time or other standard lab studies.

- ○ **F.** The nurse should pre-medicate the client with acetaminophen and diphenhydramine.

36. The nurse is caring for a client with mitral valve stenosis related to a history of rheumatic fever. Place an X in the following diagram to show the location of the mitral valve.

Quick Answer: **446**
Detailed Answer: **451**

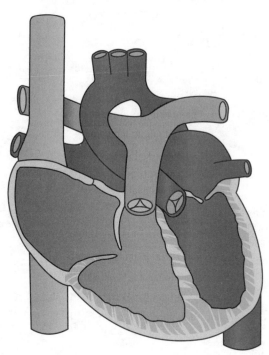

37. Joint Commission has established protocols for preventing surgical errors. Which steps are parts of that protocol? Select all that apply.

Quick Answer: **446**
Detailed Answer: **451**

   ○ **A.** Circle the surgical site with a marker.
   ○ **B.** Verify patient information with a designated patient representative.
   ○ **C.** Designate operative site with a facility designated mark.
   ○ **D.** Include a copy of the Advanced Directives on the chart before surgery.
   ○ **E.** Verify patient information three times.
   ○ **F.** Observe pre-op time out before proceeding with surgery.

38. The nurse is providing dietary teaching to a client with recurrent urinary calculi. To prevent the recurrence of oxylate stones, the client should be told to limit the intake of which foods? Select all that apply.

Quick Answer: **446**
Detailed Answer: **451**

   ○ **A.** Almonds
   ○ **B.** Chocolate
   ○ **C.** Beets
   ○ **D.** Cheese
   ○ **E.** Whole grains
   ○ **F.** Cranberries
   ○ **G.** Rhubarb
   ○ **H.** Eggs
   ○ **I.** Cabbage
   ○ **J.** Nuts

39. A client's arterial blood gas reveals the following results: pH 7.2 PCO2 50mm Hg HCO3 28mEq/L. From these results, the nurse determines that the client is in _____. (Fill in the blank.)

Quick Answer: **446**
Detailed Answer: **452**

40. The nurse is caring for a toddler with Tetralogy of Fallot. Place an X to identify each of the four defects associated with the disorder.

Quick Answer: **446**
Detailed Answer: **452**

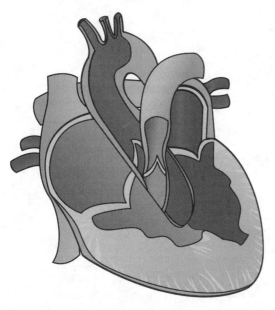

41. The nurse is caring for a client with a closed chest drainage system. Place an X on the suction control chamber.

Quick Answer: **446**
Detailed Answer: **453**

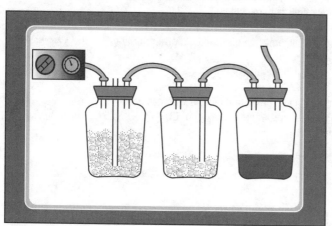

42. Which of the following activities have been associated with an increase in lead exposure?
Select all that apply.

    ○ **A.** Working with stained glass

    ○ **B.** Drinking from disposable water bottles

    ○ **C.** Restoring collectible toys

    ○ **D.** Drinking coffee and tea from decorative ceramic mugs

    ○ **E.** Using non-stick cookware

    ○ **F.** Residing in a home constructed before 1950

Quick Answer: **446**
Detailed Answer: **453**

43. Which of the following age-related changes affect the vision of the elderly client?
Select all that apply.

    ○ **A.** Increased ability of the pupil to dilate

    ○ **B.** Decreased elasticity of the lens

    ○ **C.** Discoloration of the lens

    ○ **D.** Increased eye mobility

    ○ **E.** Development of enophthalmos

Quick Answer: **446**
Detailed Answer: **453**

44. The nurse is caring for a client with full thickness burns of both legs. The client's admission weight was 182 pounds. Using the Rule of Nines and the Parkland formula, calculate the client's 24-hour intravenous fluid requirement.

Quick Answer: **446**
Detailed Answer: **453**

45. Following a parathyroidectomy, the nurse should give priority to assessing the patient for _____ and _____. (Fill in the blanks.)

Quick Answer: **446**
Detailed Answer: **454**

46. Which instruction should be given to the client who has been prescribed a dry powder inhaler for treatment of COPD?
Select all that apply.

    ○ **A.** Remove the mouthpiece cap and shake before using.

    ○ **B.** Rinse the inhaler mouthpiece and spacer after each use.

    ○ **C.** Use a spacer or hold the canister two fingerbreadths away from the mouth.

    ○ **D.** Place the mouthpiece directly in the mouth.

    ○ **E.** Clean the mouthpiece weekly using a dry cloth.

Quick Answer: **446**
Detailed Answer: **454**

Quick Check

Quick Answer: **446**
Detailed Answer: **454**

47. Place an X on the diagram that depicts an accurately administered tuberculin skin test.

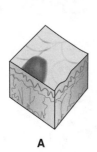

A

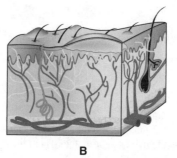

B

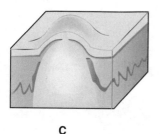

C

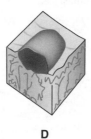

D

48. A sweat test has been ordered for an infant suspected of having cystic fibrosis. A diagnosis of cystic fibrosis is confirmed if the sweat chloride level is greater than _____. (Fill in the blank.)

Quick Answer: **446**
Detailed Answer: **454**

49. Which of the following statements applies to the nurse's collection of forensic evidence in the emergency room? Select all that apply.

Quick Answer: **446**
Detailed Answer: **454**

   ○ **A.** Items of clothing should be collected and placed in a plastic bag.

   ○ **B.** Valuables should be collected and placed in the hospital safe or given to family with appropriate documentation.

   ○ **C.** Clothing may be cut without regard for blood stains, tears, or dirt.

   ○ **D.** In case of homicide, paper bags should be used to cover the hands.

   ○ **E.** Wounds and clothing should be photographed.

50. A client taking Cymbalta (duloxetine) tells the nurse that he has also been taking St. John's wort. Use of these substances together should be discouraged since _____ _____ can occur. (Fill in the blank.)

Quick Answer: **446**
Detailed Answer: **454**

51. Place in sequence from 1–5 the proper order for introducing items to the infant's diet.

    _____ **A.** Strained meats

    _____ **B.** Whole milk

    _____ **C.** Rice cereal

    _____ **D.** Fruits

    _____ **E.** Vegetables

52. A newborn weighing 7 pounds at birth should be expected to weigh _____ pounds by one year of age. (Fill in the blank.)

53. Place an X on the diagram depicting the sign commonly observed in the patient with Duchenne muscular dystrophy.

A   **B**

C   **D**

54. The nurse monitors a client with SIADH for weight loss. A loss of 6 pounds since admission indicates a loss of _____ liters of fluid. (Fill in the blank.)

55. Which of the following are sources of dietary iron? Select all that apply.

    ○ **A.** Cheese

    ○ **B.** Molasses

    ○ **C.** Carrots

    ○ **D.** Raisins

    ○ **E.** Peanut butter

    ○ **F.** Collards

56. Which nursing interventions are included in the post-operative care of the client following the repair of a retinal detachment with instillation of silicone oil?
Select all that apply.

- ○ **A.** Placing the client in a prone position
- ○ **B.** Maintaining strict bed rest for 24 hours
- ○ **C.** Offering a clear liquid diet
- ○ **D.** Instructing the client to keep his head bowed when sitting upright
- ○ **E.** Applying an eye patch to protect the affected eye from light

Quick Answer: **446**
Detailed Answer: **456**

57. Which emergency interventions should be carried out for the patient with a venomous snake bite of the right hand?
Select all that apply.

- ○ **A.** Have the patient lie down.
- ○ **B.** Administer an oral antihistamine.
- ○ **C.** Obtain a complete history to include previous history of snake bite.
- ○ **D.** Perform a skin or eye test dose of anti-venin.
- ○ **E.** Immobilize affected area below level of the heart.

Quick Answer: **446**
Detailed Answer: **456**

58. A client with BPH has undergone a TURP. Which nursing interventions are parts of the client's post-operative care?
Select all that apply.

- ○ **A.** Monitoring the client's vital signs
- ○ **B.** Maintaining constant bladder irrigation
- ○ **C.** Limiting fluid intake to 1000mL per day
- ○ **D.** Checking for post-operative bleeding
- ○ **E.** Maintaining bed rest for 48 hours

Quick Answer: **446**
Detailed Answer: **456**

59. Which toys are suited to the developmental skills of the 2–3 year old?
Select all that apply.

- ○ **A.** Soap bubbles
- ○ **B.** Skates
- ○ **C.** Riding toys
- ○ **D.** Bicycle
- ○ **E.** Talking toys

Quick Answer: **446**
Detailed Answer: **456**

60. Which behaviors are expected to be observed in the 18-month old?
Select all that apply.

Quick Answer: 446
Detailed Answer: 456

- ○ **A.** Has a vocabulary of 900 words
- ○ **B.** Removes clothes
- ○ **C.** Points to at least one named body part
- ○ **D.** Asks many questions
- ○ **E.** Can kick a ball forward

61. The nurse working in a clinic is reviewing the chart of a client with a probable anemia. Which would most likely indicate a deficiency in Vitamin B12?
Select all that apply.

Quick Answer: 446
Detailed Answer: 456

- ○ **A.** Night cramps
- ○ **B.** Splenomegaly
- ○ **C.** Nausea
- ○ **D.** Cheilosis
- ○ **E.** Petechiae
- ○ **F.** Anorexia

62. The home care nurse is preparing a teaching plan for a client with deficiencies in folic acid. Which foods will increase the clients' folic acid level?
Select all that apply.

Quick Answer: 446
Detailed Answer: 456

- ○ **A.** Broccoli
- ○ **B.** Cabbage
- ○ **C.** Chicken
- ○ **D.** Dried fruit
- ○ **E.** White bread
- ○ **F.** Milk

63. The nurse is preparing to visit a newly admitted client with a diagnosis of polycythemia vera. Which nursing action is most appropriate?

   Assess the information included in the following exhibit to assist in answering the question.

Quick Answer: **446**
Detailed Answer: **456**

Chart Information

Vital Signs	Notes	Medication	Laboratory Values
BP 140/80, pulse 80, respirations 20, temperature 99°F	Complained of a headache on admission	Aspirin 325mg daily

Diphenhydramine (Benadryl) 50mg as needed for itching | White blood cells (WBCs) 7500uL

Hematocrit (Hct) 60% |

   ○ **A.** Notify the healthcare provider of the vital signs.

   ○ **B.** Gather equipment for therapeutic phlebotomy.

   ○ **C.** Collect and dispense pamphlets on smoking cessation.

   ○ **D.** Administer aspirin as prescribed for headache.

64. An adult client is admitted to the orthopedic unit with a history of thalassemia. What clinical manifestations does the nurse expect the client to exhibit?
   Select all that apply.

Quick Answer: **446**
Detailed Answer: **456**

   ○ **A.** Splenomegaly

   ○ **B.** Mild anemia

   ○ **C.** Jaundice

   ○ **D.** Headache complaints

   ○ **E.** Epistaxis

65. A caregiver providing care to a client receiving chemotherapy for breast cancer asks the nurse, "What can I do to prevent or relieve nausea and vomiting for her?" The nurse would include which measures in the response?
Select all that apply.

- ○ **A.** "Make sure she eats, but not immediately before her chemotherapy treatment."
- ○ **B.** "Let her suck on hard candy or soda crackers."
- ○ **C.** "Try to control environmental strong, smelly foods."
- ○ **D.** "Serve hot and spicy foods to prevent or decrease the amount of nausea."
- ○ **E.** "Assist her to lie down after each meal."

66. The nurse is evaluating the evidence-based practice used for the units' client care standards. Which of the following provides the most support for evidence-based practice?
Select all that apply.

- ○ **A.** Client preference
- ○ **B.** Practice guidelines
- ○ **C.** Care plans
- ○ **D.** Research journal articles
- ○ **E.** Systematic literature reviews

67. A new nurse is observing an advanced practice nurse assess a client with possible carpel tunnel syndrome. Which assessment technique does the nurse expect to see performed?
Please select from the following images.

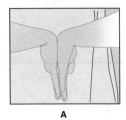

A

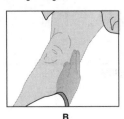

B

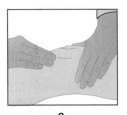

C

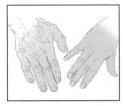

D

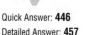

Quick Answer: **446**
Detailed Answer: **457**

68. The nurse is caring for a client with the device depicted in the following image. Which nursing intervention(s) are appropriate for clients using this device?
Select all that apply.

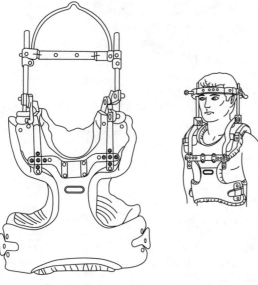

- ○ **A.** Ensure weights hang freely when client is in bed.
- ○ **B.** Perform frequent neurovascular assessments.
- ○ **C.** Assess pin sites and provide pin site care per policy.
- ○ **D.** Report any signs of infection at sites to the physician.
- ○ **E.** Keep wire cutters at bedside for emergency use.

69. The nurse receives report on the group of clients listed here. Place the client list in sequential priority order for the nurse to assess. (Most important for the nurse to assess first, second, third, and fourth.)

Quick Answer: **446**
Detailed Answer: **457**

- _____ **A.** Client admitted from the emergency room previous shift with unrelieved migraine headache.

- _____ **B.** Client transferred from surgical intensive care after traumatic brain injury. Pulse oximetry reading 94%.

- _____ **C.** Client with a Glasgow coma scale (GCS) of 5 with evidence of cerebral aneurysm rupture on CT scan.

- _____ **D.** Client admitted from the emergency room after a motor vehicle accident and GCS of 13.

Quick Check

70. After reviewing the chart of a client with a fractured femur, the nurse places highest priority on performing which assessment?

Quick Answer: **446**
Detailed Answer: **457**

See the following information to assist in answering the question.

Laboratory Values	Nurse's Notes	Patient History
Hemoglobin (hgb) 7.0g/dL	20-year-old male admitted from the emergency room after a motor vehicle accident	History of sickle cell trait diagnosed at age of 6
Hematocrit (HCT) 28%		
White blood cells (WBC) 10,000		

- ○ **A.** Vital signs
- ○ **B.** Lung sounds
- ○ **C.** Neurovascular checks
- ○ **D.** Pupil equality

71. The nurse is determining the intravenous (IV) intake of fluids for a client with congestive heart failure during an 8-hour period from 0700 until 1500. The following data is recorded:

Quick Answer: **446**
Detailed Answer: **457**

IV Record

D5 1/2 NS @ 75mL per hour

Vancocin (Vancomycin) in 250mL at 09:00

Pantoprazole (Protonix) in 50mL every 6 hours at 0800 and 1400

How many mL should the nurse document? (Record an answer that is a whole number.)

Answer _____ mL

72. The charge nurse of a medical surgical unit is assigning tasks for the day. Which client care assignments are most appropriate for the unlicensed assistive personnel?
Select all that apply.

Quick Answer: **446**
Detailed Answer: **457**

- ○ **A.** Feeding a client with a hand in a cast
- ○ **B.** Performing vital signs on an unstable client
- ○ **C.** Ambulating a client to the bathroom
- ○ **D.** Checking stools for blood
- ○ **E.** Bathing a client with arthritis

Quick Check

73. The nurse is evaluating the laboratory value results of a client after a craniotomy for a pituitary tumor. Which values cause the nurse to suspect a diabetes insipidus complication?
Select all that apply.

Quick Answer: **446**
Detailed Answer: **457**

- ○ **A.** Low urine specific gravity
- ○ **B.** Serum sodium of 158mEq/L
- ○ **C.** Serum potassium of 4.0mEq/L
- ○ **D.** Hemoglobin of 13.6g/dL
- ○ **E.** Normal serum chloride level

74. The nurse is caring for a client with an ischemic stroke and is assessing the chart for information on admission. What data is most important for the nurse to report to the healthcare provider?

Quick Answer: **446**
Detailed Answer: **457**

See the following table to assist in answering the question.

Physician's Orders	Medication History	Laboratory Values	Health History
Begin TPA infusion	Lisinopril (Zestril) 10mg daily	Hgb 14g/dL WBC 6,000	Active gastric ulcer disease with GI bleeding
Neurological checks every 15 minutes	Fish oil 2 capsules daily		
Monitor BP every 30 minutes			

- ○ **A.** Health history
- ○ **B.** Lisinopril (Zestril) dosage
- ○ **C.** Laboratory values
- ○ **D.** Medication history

75. A client is admitted to the emergency room with a head injury resulting from a fall. After reviewing the client's record, the nurse anticipates which medication to be prescribed by the emergency room physician?

See the following exhibit to assist in answering the question.

Nursing Documentation	Medication History	Vital Signs
Client admitted to the ER trauma room by stretcher. Unable to respond to verbal or tactile stimuli. Paramedics reported seizure activity en route to the facility.	Birth control pills.	BP 140/72, pulse 60, temperature 101.4, respirations 20.

○ **A.** Demerol 100mg IM now and Q4H prn pain

○ **B.** Aspirin X gr temperature above 100°F

○ **C.** Furosemide (Lasix) 80mg PO

○ **D.** Phenytoin sodium (Dilantin) 100mg IV push

76. The nurse is explaining to an adult client with an ulcer diagnosis about the drug esomeprazole (Nexium). Which side effect(s) will the nurse want to include in the discussion?
Select all that apply.

○ **A.** Headache

○ **B.** Diarrhea

○ **C.** Flushing

○ **D.** Dizziness

○ **E.** Nausea

77. The nurse is educating the caregiver of a client with dysphagia, due to a stroke, in ways to ensure safety and avoid aspiration during meals. Which information should be included?
Select all that apply.

○ **A.** Position sitting upright for meals.

○ **B.** Place the food on unaffected side.

○ **C.** Give solid foods.

○ **D.** Swallowing should be one bite at a time.

○ **E.** Liquids should be thin.

78. A client has viral encephalitis and has been prescribed IV acyclovir (Zovirax). What nursing interventions should be used when administering the drug?
    Select all that apply.

    Quick Answer: **446**
    Detailed Answer: **458**

    - ○ **A.** Administer at a slow rate.
    - ○ **B.** Assure the client is well hydrated before giving the drug.
    - ○ **C.** Observe for neurotoxicity.
    - ○ **D.** Check the apical heart rate prior to administration.
    - ○ **E.** Infuse cautiously in clients with renal insufficiency.

79. The nurse is teaching a client with ulcerative colitis who has been prescribed sulfasalazine (Azulfidine). What clinical manifestations will the nurse tell the client to be particularly alert for when taking this drug?
    Select all that apply.

    Quick Answer: **446**
    Detailed Answer: **458**

    - ○ **A.** Flu-like symptoms
    - ○ **B.** Purplish rash
    - ○ **C.** Skin blisters
    - ○ **D.** Anorexia
    - ○ **E.** Nausea

80. The nurse is caring for a client with a brain tumor who has been prescribed levofloxacin (Levaquin) for a sinus infection. What specific instructions should be included when educating the client regarding taking this drug?
    Select all that apply.

    Quick Answer: **446**
    Detailed Answer: **458**

    - ○ **A.** Avoid direct sunlight.
    - ○ **B.** Report unexplained joint pain.
    - ○ **C.** No antacids should be taken within 2 hours of taking the drug.
    - ○ **D.** Take the medication on an empty stomach.
    - ○ **E.** Keep the head of the bed elevated for 30 minutes after taking.

81. The nurse is preparing a teaching session for a client with hepatitis B who has been prescribed lamivudine (Epivir). Which does the nurse include as adverse effects of the drug?

Quick Answer: **446**
Detailed Answer: **458**

- ○ **A.** Nausea
- ○ **B.** Vomiting
- ○ **C.** Steatorrhea
- ○ **D.** Neutropenia
- ○ **E.** Amnesia

82. The nurse is educating a group of caregivers about the West Nile virus. A participant asks, "How can you get the West Nile virus?" The nurse explains that the virus can be transmitted by which source(s)?
Select all that apply.

Quick Answer: **446**
Detailed Answer: **458**

- ○ **A.** Mosquitoes
- ○ **B.** Blood transfusions
- ○ **C.** Transplanted organs
- ○ **D.** Birds
- ○ **E.** Horses

83. The nurse is teaching a client in preparation for a colonoscopy. Which would be involved in the teaching session?
Select all that apply.

Quick Answer: **446**
Detailed Answer: **458**

- ○ **A.** Consume a liquid diet a day prior to the exam.
- ○ **B.** Sedation is usually not done for the procedure.
- ○ **C.** Laxative bowel preparation is required.
- ○ **D.** Enema is given on admission.
- ○ **E.** Remain NPO 8 hr. prior to the exam.

Quick Check

Quick Answer: **446**
Detailed Answer: **459**

84. A client with osteoarthritis has been taking ibuprofen (Motrin) 600mg four times a day. It would be essential for the nurse to make which assessment on this client?

See the following exhibit to assist in answering the question.

History	Medications
Ischemic stroke 1 year ago with partial loss of function left arm	Warfarin sodium (Coumadin) 5mg PO daily
Hypertension	Amilodipine (Norvasc) 5mg once daily
Osteoarthritis	Miralax 1 capful daily for constipation

- ○ **A.** Evidence of infection
- ○ **B.** Signs of bleeding
- ○ **C.** Respiratory function
- ○ **D.** Urinary retention

85. The nurse educator on the neurological unit is teaching a new nurse colleague regarding sensoriperceptual deficits with a stroke. The nurse would select which graphic to depict homonymous hemianopia?

Quick Answer: **446**
Detailed Answer: **459**

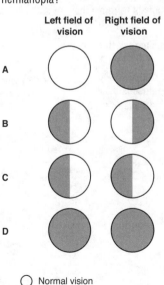

Left field of vision   Right field of vision

A

B

C

D

○ Normal vision

● Blind area

86. A client with an acute spinal cord injury is admitted to the intensive care unit. The nurse would expect to see which of the following medications ordered?
Select all that apply.

Quick Answer: **446**
Detailed Answer: **459**

- ○ **A.** Methylprednesolone (Solu-medrol)
- ○ **B.** Dopamine (Intropin)
- ○ **C.** Ondansetron (Zofran)
- ○ **D.** Diphenhydramine (Benadryl)
- ○ **E.** Amantidine (Symmetryl)

87. A client requires log rolling after back surgery. Correctly provide the sequence of steps the nurse should follow when performing the procedure.

Quick Answer: **446**
Detailed Answer: **459**

- _____ **A.** Obtain assistance; three nurses are preferable.
- _____ **B.** Maintain client's position in alignment with pillows.
- _____ **C.** Position two nurses on the side the client will be turned to and the third nurse on the opposite side of the bed.
- _____ **D.** Designate the person at the head of the bed to be in charge of coordinating the move.
- _____ **E.** Place a pillow between the client's knees.
- _____ **F.** Move the client in one coordinated movement when the nurse at the head of the bed signals to move the client.
- _____ **G.** Instruct the client to place the arms across the chest.

88. A client with a head injury has an order for dexamethasone (Decadron) 10mg IV; push every 6 hours. The dose is available Decadron 4mg/mL. How much will the nurse administer?

Quick Answer: **446**
Detailed Answer: **459**

Fill in the blank.

_____ mL(s)

Quick Answer: **446**
Detailed Answer: **459**

89. The nurse is planning for discharge teaching to a client after a total hip replacement. Which teaching points will be included? Select all that apply.

    ○ **A.** Avoid separating the legs.

    ○ **B.** Maintain fluid intake and a high fiber diet.

    ○ **C.** Seek immediate attention for shortening or internal rotation of the leg.

    ○ **D.** Prevent flexing the hips over 90 degrees.

    ○ **E.** Sleep on the affected side.

Quick Answer: **446**
Detailed Answer: **459**

90. A client with a diagnosis of Amyotrophic Lateral Sclerosis (ALS) has been prescribed riluzole (Rilutek). Which does the nurse include when teaching the client about this drug? Select all that apply.

    ○ **A.** Avoid the use of alcohol.

    ○ **B.** Take the medication with food.

    ○ **C.** Report any fever to the health care provider.

    ○ **D.** Medication should be taken at the same time each day.

    ○ **E.** Laboratory test will be monitored regularly.

Quick Answers

1. A, B, D

2. A, C

3. E, F, G

4. B, E, F

5. B

6. C, F

7. C

8. B, E

9. B, D, D

10. B, D, C, A

11. C, D

12. A, C, D

13. A, B, C

14. A, B, C, D

15. B, D

16. A, B, C, D, E, G

17. Stage I decubitus

18. A, B, E

19. C

20. C

21. A, B, C

22. 4, 3, 2, 1

23. 1170ml

24. A, B, C, F

25. 1805

26. A, B, D, E

27. A

28. A, B, D

29. B, E

30. C, E, F

31. B, D, E

32. A, B, C, D

33. G (1), D (2), C (3), F (4), E (5), B (6), A (7)

34. A (U), B (E), C (E), D (NU), E (U), F (E)

35. A, C, E

36. See figure in Answers and Rationales

37. C, E, F

38. A, B, C, I, J

39. Respiratory acidosis

40. See figure in Answers and Rationales

41. See figure in Answers and Rationales

42. A, C, D, F

43. B, C, E

44. 12,096mL

45. Airway obstruction and excessive bleeding

46. D, E

47. D. See figure in Answers and Rationale

48. 60mEq/L

49. B, D, E

50. Serotonin syndrome

51. C rice cereal (1), E vegetables (2), D fruits (3), A strained meats (4), and B whole milk (5)

52. 21 pounds

53. D. See figure in Answers and Rationales

54. 3 liters

55. B, D, E, F

56. A, D

57. A, D, E

58. A, B, D

59. A, C, E

60. B, C, E

61. A, C, F

62. A, B, F

63. B

64. A, B, C

65. A, B, C

66. B, D, E

67. A

68. B, C, D

69. C, B, D, A

70. A

71. 950

72. A, C, E

73. A, B

74. A

75. D

76. A, B, E

77. A, B, D

78. A, B, C, E

79. A, B, C

80. A, B, C

81. A, B

82. A, B, C

83. A, C, E

84. B

85. C

86. A, B, C

87. A, E, C, D, G, F, and B

88. 2.5mL

89. B, C, and D

90. A, C, D, and E

Alternative Items Answers and Rationales

1. Answers A, B, and D are correct. These actions should be carried out prior to the bath. C, E, and F are incorrect since these actions are done during or after the bath.

2. Answers A and C are correct. The nurse should not delegate to the unlicensed assistive personnel the task of giving a bath to the client with a closed head injury, since this client will have an intracranial pressure monitor. Should the line be pulled out during the bath, the nurse that did the delegation is responsible. The unlicensed assistive personnel should not be assigned to give intramuscular medication, subcutaneous medication, or intravenous medications. B, D, and E are incorrect because the unlicensed assistive personnel can be assigned to do these tasks. The unlicensed assistive personnel should be taught about the dangers of aspiration pneumonia with a nasogastric tube. The nurse should check for placement and teach the unlicensed assistive personnel how to check for placement and that the client should be in high Fowler position during the tube feeding and for 30 minutes after the feeding. The unlicensed assistive personnel is skilled in basic life-support measures. They also know the correct method of performing perineal care for the client with an indwelling urinary catheter.

3. Answers E, F, and G are correct. These actions would hamper the staff's learning. A, B, C, and D are incorrect since these actions by the educator will facilitate learning.

4. Answers B, E, and F are correct. Answers A, C, and D are incorrect since these are signs of acidosis.

5. Answer B is correct. The diagram is describing Trousseau's sign. Trousseau's sign is elicited by placing a blood pressure cuff on the arm and inflating to a pressure greater than the systolic blood pressure. In the absence of blood flow, the patient's hypocalcemia and subsequent neuromuscular irritability will induce spasm of the muscles of the hand and forearm causing the wrist and hand to flex down and contract. This is indicative of hyperreflexia. A, C, and D are incorrect since they are not indicated by Trousseau's sign.

6. Answers C and F are correct. The best sites for obtaining a pulse oximeter in the neonate (birth to 28 days) are the hand and feet. The other sites may be used for older individuals and are, therefore, incorrect.

7. Answer C is correct. When the examiner's finger depresses the skin to 6mm, the client is described as having 3+ pitting edema. A, B, and D are incorrect since 1+ edema is 2mm depression, 2+ edema is 4mm depression, and 4+ edema is a 8mm depression.

8. Answers B and E are correct. Hepatitis B is transmitted by blood and body fluids. Blood can be present on the toothbrush. Health care workers, such as the dentist, may come in contact with blood and body fluids and should, therefore, be alerted to the diagnosis. A, C, and D are incorrect since Hepatitis A is spread by oral fecal route. The nurse should instruct the client to wash fresh fruits and vegetables prior to eating if on immunosuppressant. The nurse should instruct the client with hepatitis A and E to clean the commode after each bowel movement. Answer D is incorrect since there is no need to boil water prior to drinking. Any client that is immune suppressed, such as those being treated for hepatitis, should place open containers in the refrigerator to decrease bacterial growth.

9. Answers B, C, and D are correct. Varicella requires airborne precautions; therefore, A is incorrect. E and F are incorrect since these require contact precautions.

10. The correct sequence according to the CDC is B, D, C, and A. Gloves, eyewear, gown, and mask is the correct sequence.

11. Answers C and D are correct. The normal level of sodium is 135-145 mEq/L, and the normal Calcium level is 8.5-10.5 mg/dL. A, B, and E are normal findings.

12. Answers A, C, and D are correct. All these test results will be elevated in the client with a suspected myocardial infarction. B, E, and F are incorrect because these values will be elevated in liver disease.

13. Answers A, B, and C are correct. Prior to the Cardiac Computer Tomography Angiography, the nurse should check renal function by reviewing the creatinine levels, question the client regarding allergies to shellfish and iodine, and obtain a permit for the procedure. Answer D is incorrect since a cardiac CTA does not affect hearing. Answer E is incorrect since drinking increased amounts of fluid should be done after the exam. There is no need to force fluids prior to the exam.

14. Answers A, B, C, and D are correct. When the nurse is collecting a sputum specimen, the nurse should collect the specimen in the morning prior to the meal, transport the collected specimen to the laboratory immediately after collection, and offer mouth care after collecting the specimen. The nurse should also collect a specimen for three consecutive days for the best diagnostic results. Answer E is incorrect since the client can rinse the mouth with water, but not an antiseptic solution.

15. Answers B and D are correct. Botulism can be spread by ingestion of the toxin or C-botulism can be contracted by direct contact with a contaminated wound, for example if the client cuts his/her skin with a contaminated knife. A is incorrect since botulism is not spread from person to person. West Nile virus and malaria are examples of diseases that are transmitted by a contaminated mosquito. Goat saliva and contaminated cat litter can spread toxoplasmosis, not botulism, so these answers are incorrect.

16. Answers A, B, C, D, E, and G are correct. These actions facilitate client independence. F and H are incorrect since these actions will not facilitate independence.

17. Answer is stage I decubitus. Stage I is nonblanchable erythema signaling potential ulceration. Stage II, partial thickness skin loss, involves an abrasion, shallow crater, or blister. This stage involves the epidermis and may involve the dermis. Stage III is a full thickness skin loss that involves damage and/or necrosis of subcutaneous tissue. Stage IV is a full-thickness skin loss with tissue necrosis. This stage may involve the bone, muscle, and fascia.

18. Answers A, B, and E are correct. These tasks can be performed by the licensed practical nurse. C and D are responsibilities of the RN.

19. Answer C is correct. This diagram is of a client in Trendelenburg position. This position will relieve pressure of the fetal presenting part from the umbilical cord. A, B, and D will not relieve pressure on the umbilical cord.

20. Answer C is correct. Anisocoria is unequal pupil size. A is conjunctivitis or reddening of the conjunctivitis. B is a diagram of strabismus or cross-eyes. D is ptosis or drooping eyelid. These answers are therefore incorrect.

21. Answers A, B, and C are correct. Minocycline, Tazorac, and Devonex are category X medications and should not be given during pregnancy since they are teratagenic.

22. Answer:

    4   Withdraw the NPH insulin.

    3   Withdraw the regular insulin.

    2   Inject air into the vial of regular insulin.

    1   Inject air into the vial of NPH insulin.

    To prevent cross-contamination, regular insulin should be withdrawn first.

23. Answer 1170ml is correct. A scrambled egg is not on a full liquid diet. The other foods are full liquid.

24. Answers are A, B, C, and F. These illnesses can result in a false positive test. The RPR is a screening test for Syphilis.

25. Answer: 1805 hours. If the infusion is begun at 2ml per minute, 120ml will infuse in one hour. Therefore, it will take two hours and 5 minutes to infuse.

26. A, B, D, and E can all be performed by the licensed practical nurse. Removing a peripherally inserted central line should be performed by the RN or the doctor.

27. Answer A is correct. EKG strip indicates atrial fibrillation. The irregular rhythm predisposes the patient to develop blood clots. Anticoagulants, such as aspirin, are given to prevent an ischemic stroke due to clot formation. The other NSAIDS listed are not commonly given to prevent clot formation.

28. Answers A, B, and D are correct. If the client is experiencing hypovolemic shock related to blood loss in surgery, the hemoglobin (oxygen carrying capacity) will be lowered. The central venous pressure will drop with hypovolemic shock. Pulmonary artery wedge pressure indicates left ventricular function. The hematocrit is the number of red blood cells per cubic millimeter. The troponin is elevated, but indicates cardiac muscle damage, not hypovolemia.

29. Answers B and E are correct. The diaphragm should be washed in warm water, not hot water; therefore, A is incorrect. The client should use contraceptive gel in conjunction with the diaphragm. The client should not douche after intercourse; therefore, C is incorrect. There is no need to resize the diaphragm every six months. The diaphragm should be resized if the client gains or loses 10 pounds, has a baby, or has abdominal surgery. The client should leave the diaphragm in for six hours after intercourse.

30. Answers C, E, and F are correct. A blood glucose level of 740mg/dl is extremely high. The nurse should call the physician, prepare to give regular insulin, and assess the client's level of consciousness.

31. Answers B, D, and E are correct. Droplet transmission based precautions should be used when caring for the client with influenza. Answer A is incorrect since airborne transmission based precautions are not required when caring for the client with influenza. Answer C is incorrect because contact transmission-based precautions are not required when caring for the client with influenza.

32. Answers A, B, C, and D all affect the accuracy of pulse oximetry readings. Diminished peripheral perfusion, a brightly lit environment, dark skin color, acrylic nail polish, and acrylic fingernails can lower the accuracy of pulse oximetry readings.

33. Answer: The correct sequence for performing tracheostomy suctioning is G (1), D (2), C (3), F (4), E (5), B (6), A (7). A sterile suction kit and sterile gloves are used each time tracheostomy suctioning is performed.

34. Answer: A (U), B (E), C (E), D (NU), E (U), F (E). Emergent conditions require immediate interventions because of the increased risk of death or permanent disability. Emergent conditions include major burns, chest pain, cardiac arrest, respiratory distress, blunt or penetrating trauma, and hemorrhage. Urgent conditions require care as soon as possible, usually within one hour, because of the possibility of deterioration in the patient's status. Urgent conditions include temperature greater than 101°F in an infant less than 3 months of age, abdominal pain, stable fractures, headache, lacerations with controlled bleeding, and dehydration. Non-urgent conditions require routine care, usually within two hours. Non-urgent conditions include colds, sore throat, and abrasions.

35. Answer: A, C, and E are correct. Before the procedure, the nurse should weigh the client, obtain vital signs, and check the blood pressure with the client in a standing and lying position. Protective eyewear, gown, and gloves should be worn by the nurse during the hemodialysis procedure to prevent accidental exposure to blood. The partial thromboplastin time or other standard laboratory studies are monitored according to protocol since heparin is used as an anticoagulant during the procedure. Answers B, D, and F do not apply to the care of the client receiving hemodialysis; therefore, they are incorrect.

36.

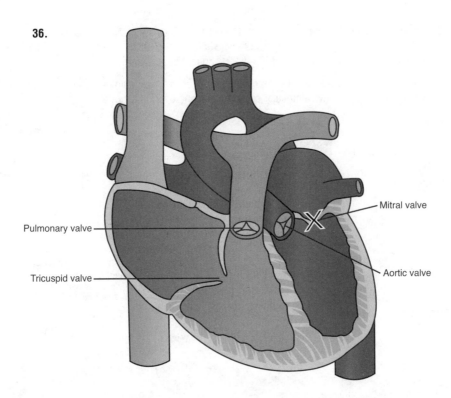

Pulmonary valve

Tricuspid valve

Mitral valve

Aortic valve

37. Answers C, E, and F are correct. Joint Commission has established the following protocols to prevent surgical errors. The operative site is to be identified using a facility designated mark after confirming the information with the patient. No ambiguous marks are to be used. Patient information is verified three times: at the time the surgery is scheduled, during admission, and when the patient is transferred to another caregiver. Observance of a pre-op time out prior to surgery allows for a final verification of the patient, the procedure being performed, and confirmation of the surgical site. Answers A, B, and D are not part of Joint Commission's protocol for preventing surgical errors; therefore, they are incorrect.

38. Answer: A, B, C, I, and J are correct. Foods high in oxylate include asparagus, beets, celery, cabbage, fruits, tomatoes, green beans, chocolate, and nuts. Beer, colas, and tea are also high in oxylate. Cheese, whole grains, cranberries, rhubarb, and eggs are not high in oxylate; therefore, answers D, E, F, G, and H are incorrect.

39. Answer: Respiratory acidosis is correct. The pH 7.2 indicates acidosis (normal pH 7.35 – 7.45). The pCO2 of 50mm Hg indicates acidosis (normal pCO2 is 35 – 45mm Hg). The HCO3 of 28 is elevated (normal HCO3 is 22 – 26mEq/L).

40. The four separate defects that comprise Tetralogy of Fallot are pulmonic stenosis, right ventricular hypertrophy, ventricular septal defect, and overriding aorta.

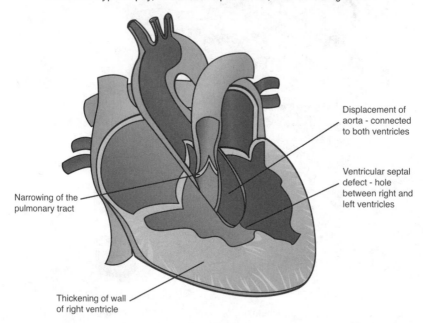

Displacement of aorta - connected to both ventricles

Ventricular septal defect - hole between right and left ventricles

Narrowing of the pulmonary tract

Thickening of wall of right ventricle

41. The first chamber of a closed chest drainage system, the suction control chamber, helps to re-establish negative intrathoracic pressure. The chamber is filled with water to a level that regulates the amount of suction, usually 20cm. The second chamber is the water seal chamber. The water seal chamber is filled to the 2cm mark with sterile water to maintain an underwater seal. This prevents air in the drainage tubing and collection chamber from flowing back into the chest cavity. Fluctuations in the water seal chamber can be seen as the client breathes. The third chamber is the drainage collection chamber. This chamber collects drainage and may be marked once per shift or more often in order to monitor the amount of chest drainage over time.

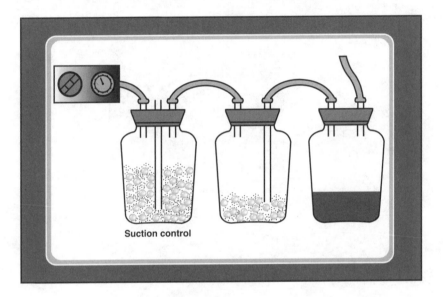

Suction control

42. Answer: A, C, D, and F are correct. Sources of lead include ceramic wares, stained glass, collectible toys, and lead-based paint. Houses constructed before 1950 are more likely to have leaded paint as well as leaded pipes. Drinking from disposable plastic bottles and non-stick cookware are not associated with increased lead exposure.

43. Answer: B, C, and E are correct. Presbyopia, a decreased elasticity of the lens, makes focusing on near objects more difficult. Discoloration and opacification of the lens reduces the perception of colors, especially green, blue, and violet. Development of enophthalmos (sinking in) of the eyes limits peripheral vision. Answers A and D are incorrect because there is decreased pupil dilation and decreased eye mobility in the elderly.

44. Answer: The client's 24-hour fluid requirement is 12,096mL.

Using the Rule of Nines, each of the client's legs represents 18% TBSA, for a total of 36%. Conversion of the client's weight from 185 pounds to kilograms (185 pounds divided by 2.2 pounds) = 84.09kg or 84kg. Using the Parkland formula, (4 X 84 X 36) = 12,096mL for the first 24-hour post-burn period.

45. Answer: Following a parathyroidectomy, the nurse should give priority to assessing the patient for **airway obstruction** and **excessive bleeding**. Signs of airway obstruction include changes in phonation, increased respiratory effort, and respiratory stridor. Bleeding that exceeds 5 mL per hour is considered excessive. The nurse should check the patient's dressing as well as behind the patient's neck for signs of bleeding. The nurse should also assess for difficulty swallowing or tracheal deviation.

46. Answer: D and E are correct. These instructions should be given to the client who has been prescribed a dry powder inhaler. Answers A, B, and C refer to the use of a metered dose inhaler; therefore, they are incorrect.

47. Answer: D is correct. If the tuberculin skin test is accurately administered, a wheal will appear at the injection site.

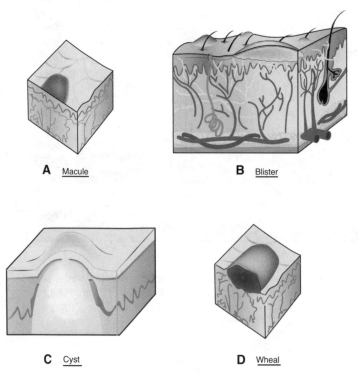

A Macule   **B** Blister

C Cyst   **D** Wheal

48. Answer: Cystic fibrosis is confirmed by a sweat chloride greater than **60mEq/L**.

49. Answer: B, D, and E are correct. Answer A is incorrect because items of clothing should be separated and placed in paper bags. Answer C is incorrect because the nurse should avoid cutting through blood stains, tears, and dirt, as this may alter physical evidence.

50. Answer: **Serotonin syndrome**, a potentially fatal condition, can occur when antidepressant medications, such as Cymbalta (duloxetine), are used with certain herbals, like St. John's wort. Symptoms of serotonin syndrome include confusion, hypomania, agitation, hyperthermia, hyperreflexia, tremors, rigidity, and gastrointestinal upset.

51. Answer: C rice cereal (1), E vegetables (2), D fruits (3), A strained meats (4), and B whole milk (5). The diet for the first six months of life should be limited to breast milk or formula. After six months, other items are introduced one at a time to detect any potential allergies. Rice cereal is offered first followed by green and yellow vegetables, fruits, and strained meat. Whole milk should not be offered until the infant is 1 year of age.

52. Answer: 21 pounds. Infants can be expected to triple their birth weight by 1 year of age.

53. Answer: D. Gower's sign or Gower's maneuver is commonly observed in patients with Duchenne muscular dystrophy. The patient maneuvers from a sitting to standing position by flexing his trunk at the hips and placing his hands on his knees. He then extends the trunk by using his hands to walk up his legs to assume an upright position. Answer A is incorrect since Allis' sign is seen in patients with hip dysplasia. Answer B is incorrect since Turner's sign is seen in patients with acute pancreatitis or abdominal trauma. Answer C is incorrect because Trendelenburg's sign is seen in patients with weak or paralyzed abductor muscles of the hips.

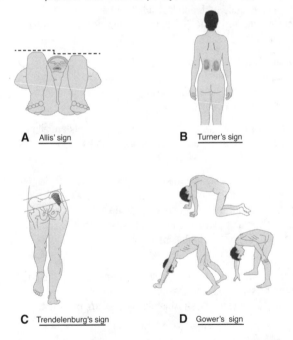

A Allis' sign

B Turner's sign

C Trendelenburg's sign

D Gower's sign

54. Answer: **3** liters. A weight loss of 2 pounds is equivalent to 1 liter; therefore, a loss of 6 pounds is equal to a loss of 3 liters of fluid.

55. Answer: B, D, E, and F are correct choices. Sources of dietary iron include organ meats, green leafy vegetables (such as collards), beans, molasses, raisins, egg yolk, and peanut butter. Milk and dairy products, carrots, and potatoes have limited amounts of dietary iron.

56. Answer: A and D are correct. Following the repair of retinal detachment in which silicone oil was instilled, the client should be placed in a prone position. When sitting upright, the client should be instructed to keep his head bowed. Answers B, C, and E do not apply to the care of the client with repair of a retinal detachment using silicone oil; therefore, they are incorrect.

57. Answer: A, D, and E are correct. Administering an oral antihistamine is indicated in the care of patients with stings, not snake bites; therefore, answer B is incorrect. Obtaining a complete history, including a history of previous snake bites, can be done after the patient is stable; therefore, answer C is incorrect.

58. Answer: A, B, and D are correct. The client should have an increased fluid intake over 1000mL/day; therefore, answer C is incorrect. The client is not restricted to bed and should be encouraged to ambulate; therefore, answer E is incorrect.

59. Answer: A, C, and E are correct. Skates and bicycles require greater motor development than that possessed by the 2–3 year old; therefore, answers B and D are incorrect.

60. Answer: B, C, and E are correct. The 18-month old can be expected to remove his/her clothes, point to at least one named body part, and kick a ball forward. Answer A is incorrect since it is an expected behavior of the 2–3 year old. Answer D is incorrect since it is an expected behavior of the 3 year old.

61. Answers A, C, and F are correct. Night cramps, anorexia, and nausea are usually caused by a deficiency in Vitamin B12. Petechiae, E, occur with aplastic anemia; cheiolosis, D, with an iron deficiency; and splenomegaly, B, is usually caused by a hemolytic anemia making them incorrect choices.

62. Answers A, B, and F are correct. Broccoli, green leafy vegetables, and milk are all good sources of folic acid. The foods in C, D, and E are not adequate sources of folic acid, so they are incorrect.

63. Answer B is correct. Therapeutic phlebotomy is a method of treatment for the diagnosis of polycythemia vera. The client's vital signs do not warrant notification of the HCP as in A. Smoking cessation is important, but is not an appropriate action on admission, nor is there any information noting that the client smokes, so choice C is incorrect. Aspirin is given once daily to prevent thrombosis, not as an analgesic in this case, so D is incorrect.

64. Answers A, B, and C are correct. Jaundice, splenomegaly, hepatomegaly, and mild to moderate anemia are symptoms associated with thalassemia. Headaches and epistaxis, options D and E, are associated with aplastic anemia, so they are incorrect.

65. Answers A, B, and C are correct. Controlling environmental smells, sucking on hard candy, and omitting food immediately before chemotherapy treatment are all measures to prevent nausea or vomiting. Hot and spicy foods as in option D and lying down after meals, option E, can cause nausea and vomiting, so they are incorrect.

66. Answers B, D, and E are correct. Best evidence and support for the standards include research articles, literature reviews, expert opinions, and practice guidelines. Client preferences, as in option A, are taken into consideration, but don't provide as much evidence or support. The care plans are not considered a source of evidence, so C is incorrect.

67. Answer A is correct. The image in A indicates the correct procedure utilized for assessment of carpel tunnel. The image in B (Bulge test) and C (Ballottement) depict the tests used to check for fluid in the knee joint, so they are incorrect. Option D is an image that illustrates the difference in clients with normal and low hemoglobin levels, so it is incorrect.

68. Answers B, C, and D are correct. Appropriate nursing interventions for clients with a halo device for a fractured neck include frequent neurovascular checks, cleansing of the pin sites to prevent infections, and reporting any signs of infection to the physician. The answer in A is not associated with a halo device, because weights are not applied, and wire cutters (answer E) should be at the bedside of clients with wired jaws who have fractures of the jaw, so it is a wrong choice.

69. Answer sequence C, B, D, and A. The client in choice C is the unstable client due to the low GCS score and immediate care needed for a ruptured aneurysm. This client should be assessed first. A client with a brain injury and recent transfer from intensive care (option B) would be seen next and has priority over the client with a motor vehicle accident and high GCS of 13 (option D). The most stable client is the client with a migraine headache (option A).

70. Answer A is correct. The client has a low hemoglobin (normal 13.5-18g/dL) and Hct (normal 40%-54%). These results warrant further assessment for signs and symptoms of volume deficit and shock-low BP, increased heart rate, etc. The assessments in choices B, C, and D are appropriate but are not a priority with the information given, so they are incorrect.

71. 950 is the correct amount calculated. IV fluid at 75mL/hr for 8 hours= 600mL; Vancomycin fluid=250mL, Protonix 50mL, given twice=100mL.

600

250

<u>100</u>

950 Total mL

72. Answers A, C, and E are correct. The unlicensed assistive personnel can perform basic nursing care tasks. These tasks include bathing, feeding, and collecting some specimens. They cannot assume the role of assessing (option D) or performing vital signs (option B) on unstable clients.

73. Answers A and B are correct. The client with diabetes insipidus has large amounts of urine output. The lab values associated with the disorder are low specific gravity (< 1.005) in the urine and increase in the sodium level (> 145mEq/L). Options C, D, and E are all within normal range and not associated with diabetes insipidus, so they are incorrect.

74. Answer A is correct. A TPA infusion is given to destroy clots. It is contraindicated to administer the infusion with any possibility of bleeding, making this the most important information to convey to the healthcare provider. The laboratory values (option C) are within the normal range, and the medication history and dosage (options B and D) are not relevant to the TPA infusion, so they are incorrect options.

75. Answer D is correct. Seizure activity increases intracranial pressure and Dilantin would be expected to prevent another seizure from occurring. In option A, Narcotic pain medication is not usually given, and there is no evidence supporting a need for pain meds. Option B, aspirin, would be contraindicated because of the possibility of bleeding. If an antifebrile medication were given, it would be acetaminophen (Tylenol). Option C, Lasix, would not be expected to be administered. A client with a head injury and increased intracranial pressure is given an osmotic diuretic, such as mannitol (Osmitrol).

76. Answers A, B, and E are correct. Adverse effects of esomeprazole (Nexium) include headache, diarrhea, and nausea. Flushing and dizziness (options C and D) are not adverse effects of Nexium, so they are incorrect.

77. Answers A, B, and D are correct. The methods of sitting upright to eat, swallowing one bite at a time, and placing the food on the unaffected side are all practices to ensure safety and avoid aspiration. The client should eat pureed foods instead of solid food, so C is incorrect. The liquids should be of honey consistency, so E is wrong.

78. Answers A, B, C, and E are correct. There are decreased problems with the administration of IV ancyclovir (Zovirax) if it is given slowly in individuals that are well hydrated. The nurse should assess for symptoms of neurotoxicity (confusion, coma, etc.). The drug can be harmful to clients with decreased kidney function and should be used cautiously in these clients. There is no need to check the heart rate with this drug, so D is incorrect.

79. Answers A, B, and C are correct. The clinical manifestations of flu-like symptoms followed by a red painful, purplish rash that can blister and shed are associated with Stevens Johnsons syndrome and the healthcare provider should be notified. Options D and E are side effects, but are not dangerous, so they are incorrect choices.

80. Answers A, B, and C are correct. The client taking Levaquin should avoid direct sunlight, report joint pain (this could indicate a ruptured tendon), and not take any antacids within 2 hours of taking the drug. The drug should be taken with food, but no dairy products, so D is incorrect. There is no need to keep the head of the bed elevated as in option E, so it is wrong.

81. Answers A and B is correct. Clients taking Epivir may have adverse effects, such as nausea, vomiting, and diarrhea. Steatorrhea (fatty stools), neutropenia (low white blood cells [WBC]), and amnesia are not adverse effects of Epivir, so they are incorrect choices.

82. Answers A, B, and C are correct. According to the CDC, West Nile Virus can be transmitted by mosquitoes, blood transfusions, and transplanted organs. The major source of transmission is via infected mosquitoes. Birds or horses do not transmit the virus, so options D and E are incorrect.

83. Answers A, C, and E are correct. The preparation for a colonoscopy includes a bowel preparation, liquid diet the day before the procedure, and nothing by mouth 8 hours before the procedure. Clients are usually sedated for the procedure and an enema is usually not done, so B and D are incorrect choices.

84. Answer B is correct. It would be essential for the nurse to assess for any signs of bleeding on this client because of the Motrin possible adverse effects and the medication history of the drug Coumadin (an anti-coagulant). It is important to perform the assessments in A, C, and D, but they are not the priority, so they are incorrect.

85. Answer C is correct. Clients with stroke may exhibit sensoriperceptual difficulties, such as homonymous hemianopia. With this deficit, the client has a loss of visual fields; when the loss is the same half missing in each eye, it is homonymous hemianopia. Option A depicts a normal field of vision in the left eye and loss of vision in the right eye, so it is incorrect. Option B shows a loss of vision in the temporal half of both fields, bitemporal hemianopia, so it is wrong. Option D is not a demonstrated partial loss of visual field, so it is an incorrect choice.

86. Answers A, B, and C are correct. Steroids, such as solu-medrol, are given to decrease spinal cord edema. A vasopressor, Dopamine, would be given to counteract the hypotension from spinal shock. Zofran may be given to prevent vomiting. Benadryl, an antihistamine, and Symmetryl (an antiviral for influenza), as in options D and E, would not be an expected order for this client, so they are incorrect choices.

87. The correct order for logrolling the client: A, E, C, D, G, F, and B.

88. Answer 2.5mL is correct. The desired dose divided by the dose on hand multiplied by the volume = the answer.

$$\frac{10}{4} \times 1mL = 2.5mL$$

89. Answers B, C, and D are correct. Clients with total hip replacements should keep their legs abducted, maintain fluid intake and a high fiber diet, prevent flexing of the hip over 90 degrees, and seek immediate attention for prosthetic problems manifested by shortening or internal rotation of the leg on the affected side. It is generally preferable to sleep on the unoperative side; therefore, A and E are incorrect choices.

90. Answers A, C, D, and E are correct. Avoiding the use of alcohol, reporting fever, taking the medication at the same time each day, and monitoring of laboratory values are all points that are important to teach the client taking riluzole (Rilutek). Rilutek should not be taken with food, so option B is incorrect.

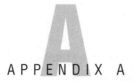

APPENDIX A

Things You Forgot

Throughout this book, we have tried to help you to simplify preparation for the NCLEX exam. This appendix includes information you have learned during nursing school but might have forgotten.

Therapeutic Drug Levels

Here are some of the therapeutic blood levels that are important for the nurse to be aware of when taking the NCLEX® exam:

- ▶ **Digoxin:** 0.5–2.0 ng/mL
- ▶ **Lithium:** 0.6–1.5 mEq/L
- ▶ **Dilantin:** 10–20 mcg/dL
- ▶ **Aminophylline:** 10–20 mcg/dL

> **NOTE**
> Lab values vary by age, and some books might have different reference values.

Vital Signs

Here are some of the normal ranges for vital signs:

- ▶ **Heart rate:** 80–100 beats per minute
- ▶ **Newborn heart rate:** 100–180 beats per minute
- ▶ **Respiratory rate:** 12–20 respirations per minute
- ▶ **Newborn respiratory rate:** 30–60 breaths per minute
- ▶ **Blood pressure:** systolic = 110–120 mm Hg; diastolic = 60–90 mm Hg

▸ **Newborn blood pressure:** 60/40 – 90/60 mm Hg

▸ **Temperature:** 98.6 F +/- 1°

Anticoagulant Therapy

These are the tests to be done for the client taking anticoagulants and their control levels. Remember that the therapeutic range is 1.5–2 times the control:

▸ **Coumadin (sodium warfarin) PT/Protime:** 11.0–13.8 seconds

▸ **International normalizing ratio (INR) is similar to the PT:** 2–3% for standard warfarin therapy and 3.0–4.5 for higher doses

▸ **Antidote for sodium warfarin:** Vitamin K

> **NOTE**
>
> Lab values vary by age, and some books might have different reference values.

▸ **Heparin and heparin derivatives actual partial thromboplastin time (aPTT):** 30-40 seconds. If the client is taking Lovenox (enoxaparin), the nurse should check the platelet count because Lovenox can cause thrombocytopenia. Therapeutic range is 1.5–2.5 times the control.

▸ **Antidote for heparin:** Protamine sulfate.

Intrapartal Normal Values

Here are some of the normal ranges to remember when caring for the client during the intrapartal period:

▸ **Fetal heart rate:** 120–160 beats per minute

▸ **Variability:** 6–10 beats per minute

▸ **Contractions:**

  ▸ **Frequency of contractions:** Every 2–5 minutes

  ▸ **Duration of contractions:** Less than 90 seconds

  ▸ **Intensity of contractions:** Less than 100 mm Hg

▸ **Amniotic fluid amount:** 500–1200 ml

Standard Precautions

Standard precautions are a set of guidelines for the nurse to take when caring for the client. These precautions protect the nurse from transmitting the disease to another client or to himself:

▶ Gloves should be worn when there is a chance of contact with blood and body fluids, when handling other potentially infected material, and when performing vascular access procedures.

▶ Gloves should be changed after each client contact and between contact procedures with the same client.

▶ Masks and protective eyewear should be worn when there is a likelihood of splashes or when body fluids might become airborne.

▶ Gloves and aprons should be worn during procedures in which there is the likelihood of splashes of blood or body fluids.

▶ Handwashing should be done immediately after contact with body fluids or other potentially infected material and as soon as gloves are removed.

▶ Needles and sharps should be disposed of in sharps containers. No recapping, bending, or breaking of needles should occur.

▶ Mouth-to-mouth resuscitation should be performed using a mouthpiece or other ventilation device.

CAUTION

Body fluids likely to transmit blood-borne disease include blood, semen, vaginal/cervical secretions, tissues, cerebral spinal fluid, amniotic fluid, synovial fluid, pleural fluid, peritoneal fluid, and breast milk. Body fluids not likely to transmit blood-borne disease unless blood is visible include feces, nasal secretions, sputum, vomitus, sweat, tears, urine, and saliva (the exception is during oral surgery or dentistry).

Airborne Precautions

Examples of infections caused by organisms suspended in the air for prolonged periods of time are tuberculosis, measles (rubella), and chickenpox. Place these clients in a private room. Healthcare workers should wear a HEPA mask or N-95 mask when dealing with such clients. These masks contain fine fibers and filter out particles, preventing them from passing through to the healthcare worker.

Droplet Precautions

Infections caused by organisms suspended in droplets that can travel 3 feet, but are not suspended in the air for long periods of time, are influenza, mumps, pertussis, rubella (German measles), diphtheria, pneumonia, scarlet fever, streptococcal pharyngitis, and meningitis. Place the client in a private room or in a room with a client who has the same illness. The clients should be no closer than 3 feet away from one another. Caregivers should wear a mask, and the door can remain open.

Contact Precautions

Infections caused by organisms spread by direct contact include RSV, scabies, colonization with MRSA, and VRE. Place the client in a private room or with a client with the same condition. Caregivers should wear gloves when entering the room and wear gowns to prevent contact with the client. Hands should be washed with an antimicrobial soap before leaving the client's room. Equipment used by the client should remain in the room and should be disinfected before being used by anyone else. The client should be transported only for essential procedures; during transport, precautions should be taken to prevent disease transmission.

Revised Life Support Guidelines (American Heart Association)

Frequently the American Heart Association releases guidelines for the care of the client experiencing dysrrhythmias. Refer to http://www.aafp.org/afp /2006050/practice.html for these guidelines.

Defense Mechanisms

Here is a quick reference to some of the defense mechanisms used by the client to help cope with stressors:

- ▶ **Compensation:** The development of attributes that take the place of more desirable ones.
- ▶ **Conversion reaction:** The development of physical symptoms in response to emotional distress.
- ▶ **Denial:** The failure to regard an event or a feeling.
- ▶ **Displacement:** The transference of emotions to another other than the intended.

▸ **Projection:** The transferring of unacceptable feelings to another person.

▸ **Rationalization:** The dismissal of one's responsibility by placing fault on another.

▸ **Reaction formation:** The expression of feelings opposite to one's true feelings.

▸ **Regression:** The returning to a previous state of development in which one felt secure.

▸ **Repression:** The unconscious forgetting of unpleasant memories.

▸ **Sublimation:** The channeling of unacceptable behaviors into behaviors that are socially acceptable.

▸ **Suppression:** The conscious forgetting of an undesirable memory.

Nutrition Notes

It is important for the nurse to be aware of different diets used in the disease processes we have discussed. Table A.1 provides a quick reference to help you remember the diets.

TABLE A.1   Dietary and Nutrition Notes to Remember

Nutritional Consideration	Foods to Include	Foods to Avoid
Bone marrow transplant	Cook or peel and wash all foods.	Avoid foods from salad bars, foods grown on or in the ground, and foods that are cultured.
Celiac/gluten-induced diarrhea	Milk, buttermilk, lean meats, eggs, cheese, fish, creamy peanut butter, cooked or canned prunes, juice, corn, bread stuffing from corn, cornstarch, rice, soybeans, potatoes, bouillon, and broth.	Malted milk, fat meats, luncheon meats, wheat, salmon, plums, rye, oats, barley, and soups thickened with gluten containing grains.
Congestive heart failure	Meats low in cholesterol and fats, breads, starches, fruits, sweets, vegetables, dairy products.	Foods high in salts, canned products, frozen meats, cheeses, eggs, organ meats, fried foods, and alcohol.

Nutritional Consideration	Foods to Include	Foods to Avoid
Inflammatory bowel disease	Meats, breads, fruits, vegetables, dairy products.	Whole grains, legumes,nuts, vegetables with skins, prune juice, and gristly meats.
Full liquid diets for clients who require a decrease in gastric motility	Milk, ice cream, soups, puddings, custards, plain yogurt, strained meats, strained fruits and vegetables, fruit and vegetable juices, cereal gruel, butter, margarine, and any component or combination of clear liquids.	All solid foods.
Lacto-vegetarian	Primary sources of protein, dairy products, peanut butter, legumes, soy analogs.	All animal products.
Peptic ulcer/hiatal hernia	Meats, breads, starches, fruits, vegetables, and dairy products.	Alcohol, coffee, chocolate, black or red pepper, chili powder, carminatives such as oil of peppermint and spearmint, garlic, onions, and cinnamon.
Renal transplant	Meats, dairy products, breads and starches, vegetables, and sweets.	Eggs, organ meats, fried or fatty food, foods containing salt, dried foods, salt substitutes, and fruits.

Immunization Schedule for Children and Adults

It is important for the nurse to be aware of the recommended immunization schedule for various age groups.

For a current list of recommended immunizations, consult the CDC website at http://www.cdc.gov/vaccines/schedules/index.html.

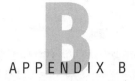

APPENDIX B

Need to Know More?

Pharmacology

http://www.druginfonet.com

http://www.fda.gov/search/databases.html

http://www.globalrph.com

http://www.mosbysdrugconsult.com

http://www.needymeds.com

http://www.nlm.nih.gov/medlineplus

http://www.nursespdr.com

Sanoski, C., and Vallerand, A. H. *Davis Drug Guide for Nurses*. 15th ed. Philadelphia: F.A. Davis, 2016.

Lehne, R. *Pharmacology for Nursing Care*. 9th ed. St. Louis: Elsevier, 2016.

Care of the Client with Respiratory Disorders

http://www.aaaai.org—The website for the American Academy of Allergy, Asthma, and Immunology

http://www.cdc.gov—The website for the Centers for Disease Control and Prevention

http://www.lungusa.org—The website for the American Lung Association

Ignatavicius, D., and Workman, M. *Medical Surgical Nursing: Patient Centered Collaborative Care*. 8th ed. St. Louis: Elsevier, 2016.

LeMone, P., and Burke, K. in *Medical Surgical Nursing: Critical Thinking in Client Care.* 5th ed. Upper Saddle River, NJ: Pearson Prentice Hall, 2012.

LeMone, P., Burke, K., Gubrud, P. and Bauldoff, G. *Medical Surgical Nursing Clinical Reasoning in Patient Care.* 6th ed. Upper Saddle River, NJ: Pearson Prentice Hall, 2014.

Lehne, R. *Pharmacology for Nursing Care.* 9th ed. St. Louis: Elsevier, 2016.

Care of the Client with Genitourinary Disorders

http://www.kidney.org—The website for the National Kidney Foundation

http://www.pkd.cure.org—The website for the Polycystic Kidney Disease Foundation

Ignatavicius, D., and Workman, M. *Medical Surgical Nursing: Patient Centered Collaborative Care.* 8th ed. St. Louis: Elsevier, 2016.

LeMone, P., and Burke, K. in *Medical Surgical Nursing: Critical Thinking in Client Care.* 5th ed. Upper Saddle River, NJ: Pearson Prentice Hall, 2012.

LeMone, P., Burke, K., Gubrud, P. and Bauldoff, G. *Medical Surgical Nursing Clinical Reasoning in Patient Care.* 6th ed. Upper Saddle River, NJ: Pearson Prentice Hall, 2014.

Lehne, R. *Pharmacology for Nursing Care.* 9th ed. St. Louis: Elsevier, 2016.

Care of the Client with Hematological Disorders

http://www.americanhs.org—The website for the American Hemochromatosis Society

http://www.aplastic.org—The website for the Aplastic Anemia and MDS International Foundation

http://www.emedicine.com/med/topic3387.htm

http://www.hemophilia.org—The website for the National Hemophilia Foundation

http://www.marrow.org

http://www.nci.nih.gov—The website for the National Cancer Institute Information Center http://www.ons.org—The website for the Oncology Nursing Society

http://www.sicklecelldisease.org—The website for the Sickle Cell Disease Association of America, Inc.

Ignatavicius, D., and Workman, M. *Medical Surgical Nursing: Patient Centered Collaborative Care.* 8th ed. St. Louis: Elsevier, 2016.

Hinkle, J. and Kerry, C. *Textbook of Medical Surgical Nursing.* 12th ed. Philadelphia: Lippincott Williams & Wilkins, 2009.

LeMone, P., Burke, K., Gubrud, P. and Bauldoff, G. *Medical Surgical Nursing Clinical Reasoning in Patient Care.* 6th ed. Upper Saddle River, NJ: Pearson Prentice Hall, 2014.

Kee, J. *Laboratory and Diagnostic Tests.* 6th ed. Upper Saddle River, NJ: Pearson, 2014.

Wilson, B., Shannon, M. and Shields, K. *Pearson Nurse's Drug Guide.* 1st ed. Upper Saddle River, NJ: Pearson Prentice Hall, 2015.

Care of the Client with Fluid and Electrolyte/Acid-Base Disorders

http://www.enursescribe.com

http://www.umed.utah.edu/ms2/renal

Ignatavicius, D., and Workman, M. *Medical Surgical Nursing: Patient Centered Collaborative Care.* 8th ed. St. Louis: Elsevier, 2016.

Hinkle, J. and Kerry, C. *Textbook of Medical-Surgical Nursing.* 13th ed. Philadelphia: Lippincott Williams & Wilkins, 2014.

Care of the Client with Integumentary Disorders

Ignatavicius, D., and Workman, M. *Medical Surgical Nursing: Patient Centered Collaborative Care.* 8th ed. St. Louis: Elsevier, 2016.

LeMone, P., and Burke, K. *Medical Surgical Nursing: Critical Thinking in Client Care.* 5th ed. Upper Saddle River, NJ: Pearson Prentice Hall, 2012.

LeMone, P., Burke, K., Gubrud, P. and Bauldoff, G. *Medical Surgical Nursing Clinical Reasoning in Patient Care*. 6th ed. Upper Saddle River, NJ: Pearson Prentice Hall, 2014.

Lehne, R. *Pharmacology for Nursing Care*, 9th ed. St. Louis: Elsevier, 2016.

Care of the Client with Sensory Disorders

Ignatavicius, D., and Workman, M. *Medical Surgical Nursing: Patient Centered Collaborative Care*. 8th ed. St. Louis, Elsevier 2016.

LeMone, P., and Burke, K. in *Medical Surgical Nursing: Critical Thinking in Client Care*. 5th ed. Upper Saddle River, NJ: Pearson Prentice Hall, 2012.

LeMone, P., Burke, K., Gubrud, P. and Bauldoff, G. *Medical Surgical Nursing Clinical Reasoning in Patient Care*. 6th ed. Upper Saddle River, NJ: Pearson Prentice Hall, 2014.

Lehne, R. *Pharmacology for Nursing Care*. 9th ed. St. Louis: Elsevier, 2016.

"Visual Impairment, Visual Disability and Legal Blindness": http://www.nlm.nih.gov/medlineplus/visionimpairmentandblindness.html

Care of the Client with Neoplastic Disorders

http://www.abta.org—The website for the American Brain Tumor Association

http://www.cancer.gov—The website for the National Cancer Institute

http://www.komen.org—The website for the Susan G. Komen Breast Cancer Foundation

http://www.leukemia.org

http://www.leukemia-research.org

http://www.ons.org—The website for the Oncology Nursing Society

http://www.skincancer.org—The website for the Skin Cancer Foundation

LeMone, P., Burke, K., Gubrud, P. and Bauldoff, G. *Medical Surgical Nursing Clinical Reasoning in Patient Care*. 6th ed. Upper Saddle River, NJ: Pearson Prentice Hall, 2014.

Kee, J. *Laboratory and Diagnostic Tests*. 6th ed. Upper Saddle River, NJ: Pearson, 2014.

Ignatavicius, D., and Workman, M. *Medical Surgical Nursing: Patient Centered Collaborative Care.* 8th ed. St. Louis: Elsevier, 2016.

Hinkle, J. and Kerry, C. *Textbook of Medical-Surgical Nursing.* 13th ed. Philadelphia: Lippincott Williams & Wilkins, 2014.

Wilson, B., Shannon, M. and Shields, K. *Pearson Nurse's Drug Guide.* 1st ed. Upper Saddle River, NJ: Pearson Prentice Hall, 2015.

Care of the Client with Gastrointestinal Disorders

http://www.asge.org—The website for the American Society for Gastrointestinal Endoscopy

http://www.ccfa.org—The website for the Crohn's and Colitis Foundation

http://www.cdc.gov—The website for the Centers for Disease Control and Prevention

http://www.uoaa.org—The website for the United Ostomy Association

LeMone, P., Burke, K., Gubrud, P. and Bauldoff, G. *Medical Surgical Nursing Clinical Reasoning in Patient Care.* 6th ed. Upper Saddle River, NJ: Pearson Prentice Hall, 2014.

Kee, J. *Laboratory and Diagnostic Tests.* 6th ed. Upper Saddle River, NJ: Pearson, 2014.

Ignatavicius, D., and Workman, M. *Medical Surgical Nursing: Patient Centered Collaborative Care.* 8th ed. St. Louis: Elsevier, 2016.

Hinkle, J. and Kerry, C. *Textbook of Medical-Surgical Nursing.* 13th ed. Philadelphia: Lippincott Williams & Wilkins, 2014.

Wilson, B., Shannon, M. and Shields, K. *Pearson Nurse's Drug Guide.* 1st ed. Upper Saddle River, NJ: Pearson Prentice Hall, 2015.

Care of the Client with Musculoskeletal and Connective Tissue Disorders

http://www.amputee-coalition.org—The website for the Amputee Coalition of America

http://www.niams.nih.gov—The website for the National Institute of Arthritis and Musculoskeletal and Skin Diseases http://www.nof.org—The website for the National Osteoporosis Foundation

http://www.orthonurse.org—The website for the National Association of Orthopaedic Nurses

LeMone, P., Burke, K., Gubrud, P. and Bauldoff, G. *Medical Surgical Nursing Clinical Reasoning in Patient Care.* 6th ed. Upper Saddle River, NJ: Pearson Prentice Hall, 2014.

Kee, J. *Laboratory and Diagnostic Tests.* 6th ed. Upper Saddle River, NJ: Pearson, 2014.

Ignatavicius, D., and Workman, M. *Medical Surgical Nursing: Patient Centered Collaborative Care.* 8th ed. St. Louis: Elsevier, 2016.

Hinkle, J. and Kerry, C. *Textbook of Medical-Surgical Nursing.* 13th ed. Philadelphia: Lippincott Williams & Wilkins, 2014.

Wilson, B., Shannon, M. and Shields, K. *Pearson Nurse's Drug Guide.* 1st ed. Upper Saddle River, NJ: Pearson Prentice Hall, 2015.

Care of the Client with Endocrine Disorders

http://www.cdc.gov/diabetes—The website for the Centers for Disease Control and Prevention

http://www.diabetes.org—The website for the American Diabetes Association

http://www.diabetesnet.com—The website for the American Association of Diabetes Educators

http://www.eatright.org—The website for the American Dietetic Association

http://www.endo-society.org—The website for the National Endocrine Society

http://www.medhelp.org/nadf—The website for the National Adrenal Disease Foundation

http://www.niddk.nih.gov—The website for the National Diabetes Clearing House

http://www.pancreasfoundation.org—The website for the National Pancreas Foundation

http://www.thyroid.org—The website for the American Thyroid Association

Ignatavicius, D., and Workman, S. *Medical Surgical Nursing: Patient Centered Collaborative Care.* 7th ed. Philadelphia: Elsevier, 2013.

Hinkle, J. and Kerry, C. *Textbook of Medical-Surgical Nursing.* 13th ed. Philadelphia: Lippincott Williams & Wilkins, 2014.

Care of the Client with Cardiovascular Disorders

http://www.americanheart.org—The website for the American Heart Association

http://www.nursebeat.com—The website for the *Nurse Beat: Cardiac Nursing Electronic Journal*

Ignatavicius, D., and Workman, S. *Medical Surgical Nursing: Patient Centered Collaborative Care.* 7th ed., Philadelphia: Elsevier, 2013.

Hinkle, J. and Kerry, C. *Textbook of Medical-Surgical Nursing.* 13th ed. Philadelphia: Lippincott Williams & Wilkins, 2014.

Care of the Client with Neurological Disorders

http://www.apdaparkinson.com—The website for the American Parkinson's Disease Association

http://www.biausa.org—The website for the Brain Injury Association

http://www.epilepsyfoundation.org—The website for the Epilepsy Foundation

http://www.gbs-cidp.org—The website for the Guillain-Barré Syndrome Foundation

http://www.nmss.org—The website for the National Multiple Sclerosis Society

http://www.parkinson.org—The website for the National Parkinson's Foundation

http://www.stroke.org—The website for the American Stroke Association

LeMone, P., Burke, K., Gubrud, P. and Bauldoff, G. *Medical Surgical Nursing Clinical Reasoning in Patient Care.* 6th ed. Upper Saddle River, NJ: Pearson Prentice Hall, 2014.

Kee, J. *Laboratory and Diagnostic Tests.* 6th ed. Upper Saddle River, NJ: Pearson, 2014.

Ignatavicius, D., and Workman, M. *Medical Surgical Nursing: Patient Centered Collaborative Care.* 8th ed. St. Louis: Elsevier, 2016.

Hinkle, J. and Kerry, C. *Textbook of Medical-Surgical Nursing.* 13th ed.

Philadelphia: Lippincott Williams & Wilkins, 2014.

Wilson, B., Shannon, M. and Shields, K. *Pearson Nurse's Drug Guide*. 1st ed. Upper Saddle River, NJ: Pearson Prentice Hall, 2015.

Care of the Client with Psychiatric Disorders

Ball, J., Bindler, R., Cowan, R. *Principles of Caring for Children*. 6th ed. Upper Saddle River, NJ: Pearson Prentice Hall, 2015.

Halter, M. Varcarolis *Foundations of Psychiatric Mental Health Nursing*. 7th ed. St. Louis, Elsevier, 2014.

Kneisl, C., and Trigoboff, E. *Contemporary Psychiatric Mental Health Nursing*. 3rd ed. Upper Saddle River, NJ: Pearson Prentice Hall, 2013.

Lehne, R. *Pharmacology for Nursing Care*. 9th ed. St. Louis: Elsevier, 2016.

Townsend, M. *Essentials of Psychiatric Mental Health Nursing: Concepts of Care in Evidenced Based Practice*. 6th ed. Philadelphia: F.A. Davis, 2014.

http://www.nami.org—The website for the National Alliance on Mental Illness

Maternal-Newborn Care

Lowdermilk, D., Perry, M. and Cashion, S. (eds.). *Maternity Nursing*. 8th ed. St. Louis: Mosby Elsevier, 2011.

Hockenberry, M., and Wilson, D. *Wong's Essentials of Pediatric Nursing*. 9th ed. St. Louis: Elsevier, 2013.

Care of the Pediatric Client

Ball, J., Bindler, R., Cowan, R. *Principles of Caring for Children*. 6th ed. Upper Saddle River, NJ: Pearson Prentice Hall, 2015.

Perry, S., Hockenberry, M., Lowdermilk, D. and Wilson, D. *Maternal Child Nursing Care*. 5th ed. St. Louis: Elsevier, 2014.

www.aaai.org—The website for the American Academy of Allergy, Asthma, and Immunology

www.aafp.org—The website for The American Academy of Family Practice

www.candlelighters.org—The website for the Candlelighters Childhood Cancer Foundation www.cdc.gov—The website for the Centers for Disease Control

www.cff.org—The website for the Cystic Fibrosis Foundation

Emergency Nursing

Ignatavicius, D., and Workman, S. *Medical Surgical Nursing: Patient Centered Collaborative Care*. 8th ed. St. Louis: Elsevier, 2016.

Lehne, R. *Pharmacology for Nursing Care*. 9th ed. St. Louis: Elsevier, 2016.

LeMone, P., Burke, K., Gubrud, P. and Bauldoff, G. *Medical Surgical Nursing Clinical Reasoning in Patient Care*. 6th ed. Upper Saddle River, NJ: Pearson Prentice Hall, 2014.

Cultural Practices Influencing Nursing Care

Hinkle, J. and Kerry, C. *Textbook of Medical-Surgical Nursing*. 13th ed. Philadelphia: Lippincott Williams & Wilkins, 2014.

Ignatavicius, D., and Workman, S. *Medical Surgical Nursing: Patient Centered Collaborative Care*. 8th ed. St. Louis: Elsevier, 2016.

Potter, P., and Perry, A. *Fundamentals of Nursing*. 8th ed. St. Louis: C.V. Mosby, 2012.

Legal Issues in Nursing Practice

Weiss, D., Whitehead, S. and Tappen, R. *Essentials of Nursing Leadership and Management: Concepts and Practice*. 6th ed. Philadelphia: F.A. Davis, 2014.

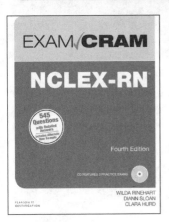

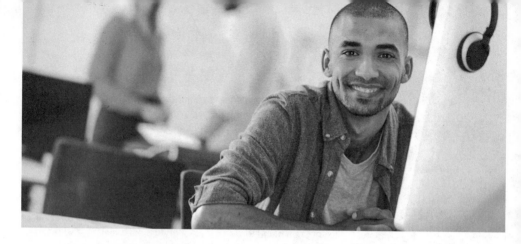

REGISTER YOUR PRODUCT at PearsonITcertification.com/register
Access Additional Benefits and SAVE 35% on Your Next Purchase

- Download available product updates.

- Access bonus material when applicable.

- Receive exclusive offers on new editions and related products.
  (Just check the box to hear from us when setting up your account.)

- Get a coupon for 35% for your next purchase, valid for 30 days. Your code will
  be available in your PITC cart. (You will also find it in the Manage Codes
  section of your account page.)

Registration benefits vary by product. Benefits will be listed on your account page
under Registered Products.

PearsonITcertification.com–Learning Solutions for Self-Paced Study, Enterprise, and the Classroom
Pearson is the official publisher of Cisco Press, IBM Press, VMware Press, Microsoft Press,
and is a Platinum CompTIA Publishing Partner–CompTIA's highest partnership accreditation.
At **PearsonITcertification.com** you can

- Shop our books, eBooks, software, and video training.
- Take advantage of our special offers and promotions (pearsonitcertifcation.com/promotions).
- Sign up for special offers and content newsletters (pearsonitcertifcation.com/newsletters).
- Read free articles, exam profiles, and blogs by information technology experts.
- Access thousands of free chapters and video lessons.

Connect with PITC – Visit PearsonITcertifcation.com/community
Learn about PITC community events and programs.

     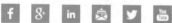

PEARSON IT CERTIFICATION

Addison-Wesley • Cisco Press • IBM Press • Microsoft Press • Pearson IT Certification • Prentice Hall • Que • Sams • VMware Press